EUTHANASIA – THE "GOOD DEATH" CONTROVERSY IN HUMANS AND ANIMALS

Edited by **Josef Kuře**

Euthanasia – The "Good Death" Controversy in Humans and Animals
Edited by Josef Kuře

Published by InTech
Janeza Trdine 9, 51000 Rijeka, Croatia

Technical Editor Mirna Cvijic

Cover Designer InTech Design Team

Additional hard copies can be obtained from orders@intechopen.com

Euthanasia – The "Good Death" Controversy in Humans and Animals,
Edited by Josef Kuře
p. cm.
ISBN 978-953-307-260-9

For EU product safety concerns:
IN TECH d.o.o., Prolaz Marije Krucifikse Kozulić 3, 51000 Rijeka, Croatia,
info@intechopen.com or visit our website at intechopen.com.

Meet the editor

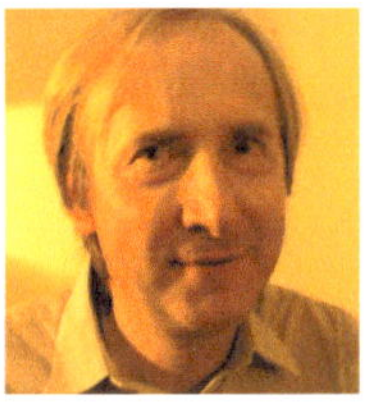

Dr. Josef Kuře, philosopher and bioethicist, is Director of the University Center for Bioethics and Head of the Department of Medical Ethics, Masaryk University, Brno, Czech Republic. After his studies at Charles University, Prague, he received his M.A. and Ph.D. (both in philosophy) from the University of Innsbruck, Austria. Dr. Kuře is Associate Professor at the Faculty of Medicine, Masaryk University, Brno. Between 2000–2003, he was Visiting Researcher at the Kennedy Institute of Ethics, Georgetown University, Washington, D.C. and Visiting Scholar at the Center for Clinical Bioethics, Georgetown University. He also serves currently as Vice-Chair of the Bioethics Committee of the Research and Development Council of the Czech Government and Chair of the Ethics Committee of the Faculty of Medicine, Masaryk University, Brno. Among his research interests are research ethics, the philosophical foundations of bioethics, prospective bioethics and the ethics of enhancement.

Contents

Preface

Few issues in contemporary health care arouse so much controversy as does the problem of euthanasia. We appear to have quite different understandings of what a "good death" is, based on diverse value judgments. Euthanasia, however, does not tolerate moral indifference. The concept of euthanasia does not allow it to be glossed over apathetically. Regardless of the way it is used, the word euthanasia always evokes strong emotions. The source of such powerful emotions and the need to draw up potent rational arguments are derived from the heart of the matter: euthanasia is about life and death. In such an arena, the fight for liberty, dignity, autonomy and individual rights does not allow for passivity and a detached view, and tends to affect both sides of the controversy to the same degree. For both proponents and opponents alike it therefore becomes a matter of principle to decriminalize euthanasia on one hand and to halt its encroachment through restrictive legislation on the other hand. The root of the dilemma is that autonomy and individual rights have to be promoted so that an individual can make the choice about his/her own life and death while the right to life has to be strongly protected. For opponents of euthanasia, there exist some similarities between the present-day debates on euthanasia as a matter of life or choice (being a compassionate choice in the case of non-voluntary euthanasia) and the debates on abortion in the 1960s and 1970s as a matter of life (pro-life) or choice (pro-choice). In both contexts "the issue" appears as a "matter of principle" and for those taking up such a stance, based on the fundamental sanctity of life, it is morally wrong to contaminate the principle itself; the principle has to be defended without any moral compromise. In contrast, as some people argue, dragging out a person's death process so that it conforms to the value system of others, which he/she believes to be a terrible contradiction of his/her life values or aspirations, is a devastating and odious form of tyranny.

While for some people euthanasia is a manifestation of the individual's autonomy at par with a responsible control of one's destiny, a compassionate responsiveness to someone's immense suffering or a clinical imperative to act in the patient's best interest, for other people euthanasia is tantamount to or merely a euphemism for killing, the violation of human life and an infringement of the human right to life, being contradictory to the sanctity of life doctrine and facilitating the abuse of vulnerable persons. Specific terms and arguments are used in euthanasia debates which have an immediate, universal appeal about them and seem to be desired, in great demand and strike a chord with our sentiments. Human dignity, humaneness and compassion belong to the first order of such terms. Nobody would doubt that people who are terminally ill, who are dying or who want to die should be treated with compassion and with respect to their (human) dignity. At a closer look, however, there are diverse semantics rooted in these terms, allowing them to be used as both arguments for and against euthanasia – depending on the individual's view. One could say that euthanasia is contrary to human dignity because the conduct of euthanasia would violate human dignity (of both persons involved), whereas one could also conclude that dying under horrible suffering would violate human dignity and therefore a request for euthanasia and its fulfilment are an expression of respect for human dignity and for a dignified death.

As a result many euthanasia discussions lack a clear semantic common ground to serve as a rational starting point. Since there is no universally agreed upon definition of "euthanasia" per se, it is essential to clarify how the word is used with regard to a particular context. Otherwise confusion dominates the debate. Both in academic literature and in public debates euthanasia is often associated with "physician assisted dying" and mixed with "(physician) assisted suicide". In some contexts euthanasia is simply assumed to refer to very general terms like "assisted death", under which assisted suicide is also subsumed. Particularly in recent years, the term "euthanasia" is used more and more in the context of that as defined by Dutch and Belgian legislation, whereby euthanasia is understood to be "administration of lethal drugs by someone other than the person concerned with the explicit intention of ending a patient's life, at the latter's explicit request". It is obvious that this definition is in need of some additional criteria specifying the conditions and situations under which euthanasia would be legal.

When euthanasia is merged with "assisted death", then under such a broader notion of "euthanasia" similar but distinct clinical situations such as medical futility, life sustaining treatment, the categorization of therapy, palliative care, and other end-of-life decisions enter into the discussion. Here one should emphasize that the decisions in palliative and intensive care medicine include a much broader spectrum of ethical dilemmas than the issue of euthanasia alone. In order for the euthanasia discussion to be meaningful, clearly accepted concepts of the terminology have to be elaborated and established before any meaningful discussion about the morality and ethics of euthanasia is initiated. Failure to keep such a sequence results in frustration. It is one of the ambitions of this book to contribute to the semantics of euthanasia. This book on euthanasia distinguishes euthanasia from other forms of killing, such as self-killing (with or without assistance) or murder. So physician assisted suicide is not covered by this book.

Euthanasia is a very old issue, with its roots in Classical thinking. Throughout the course of history, however, it has been understood differently. In recent times the concept of euthanasia has come increasingly under the spotlight due to the on-going technicization of medicine. There are several other compounding factors making the issue of euthanasia a pressing problem for contemporary society. First there has been a shift in the perception and understanding of death; death, being technicized and depersonalized, is no longer a natural event at all. Human rights have become a cornerstone of modern medicine. Particularly in Western societies, personal autonomy and autonomous choice regarding health care became a significant characteristic of the post-war period. At the same time, a focus on human dignity and an acknowledgement of people's mutual interdependency gave rise to new sensitivities in the form of an increased manifestation of solidarity and compassion for our fellow citizens. In light of these developments and the changes to civil institutions they brought with them, in certain situations, such as to prevent possible forensic consequences including law suits, physicians tend to overtreat patients, even those who are pre-terminally or terminally ill. This in turn has given rise to not only the question of distributive justice and just distribution of health care resources but also supports the idea of euthanasia as a switch from overtreatment to a "final treatment", a means of restoring the clarity and finality of death that has been protracted by modern medicine. Another common and global factor is the increasing costs of health care. In particular in countries with very limited health care resources, but not limited to these alone (health care resources are limited in all countries), the issue of euthanasia has to be addressed within the reality of limited financial resources. In economic terms, one day in an Intensive Care Unit costs hundreds or thousands of euros; while a lethal dose of morphine costs just a few euros. Another economic factor is the demographic deficit being caused by an ageing society in some areas in the world like Europe. The current and future socio-economic consequences are evident. In response, three European countries (the Netherlands, Belgium and Luxemburg) have legalized both physician assisted suicide and active euthanasia and the states of Oregon and Washington have passed legislation regulating physician assisted suicide. Drawing on the experience of these countries, it would be meaningful to examine how such proposals are affecting (and will affect) society as such and different members of society in particular, from the very young to the very old, from the healthy to the sick, handicapped and dying. It seems that the general public is more ready to embrace a compassionate approach to (physician) assisted suicide, if it is carefully managed and monitored, than to euthanasia. One can expect that the controversy surrounding the moral acceptability of euthanasia and its decriminalization will remain a challenge for our ageing societies in the twenty first century.

What distinguishes this book from other books on euthanasia is, among others, the inclusion of euthanasia in animals. This could be perceived by some people as inappropriate. Is the euthanasia of humans the same as the euthanasia of animals? If not, where do the differences lie? Why do we euthanize animals worldwide but humans legally in just a few countries (and unofficially more so)? One should be aware that there are several types of euthanasia of animals. Every day hundreds of thousands or millions of small laboratory animals (predominantly mice and rats) are euthanized after undergoing scientific experiments. Euthanasia is also used as a tool to regulate the overpopulation of animals. In veterinary medicine euthanasia is routinely used in the form of killing out of kindness severely injured and/or seriously sick animals. To not euthanatize a pet suffering from advanced cancer would be regarded as inhumane. But if this is so, why should we allow a terminally ill human cancer patient to "suffer until the end" and expect it to be regarded as humane? Why do we treat animals with compassion (euthanizing them), while not applying the same compassion to humans specifically asking for such mercy? While the book does not include a comparative and evaluative chapter which analyses the similarities and differences between the euthanasia of humans and animals outright, the material included herein will provide the reader with the sufficient grounding to make such comparisons and draw his/her own conclusions.

This edition is a collection of 12 chapters, which are organized in four parts.

The first part of the book is devoted to tackling what a confounding and intricate issue euthanasia really is, and how it can be understood. This part also provides a historical overview of euthanasia and the different meanings of the term euthanasia, with extra focus on the current debates.

The second part consists of chapters dealing with the different arguments expounded regarding euthanasia and with different approaches to the issue. The focus is on voluntary active euthanasia, as employed in the Dutch and Belgian context. Some of the arguments used in euthanasia debates are presented and critically analyzed.

The third part of the book is devoted to the aspect of public policy. The perceptions and attitudes of health care professionals to euthanasia are illustrated and the impact of the Dutch legalization regarding euthanasia as to the number of requests for euthanasia is presented.

The fourth part deals with the euthanasia of animals – euthanasia as a form of controlling the dog population, as a method of zoonosis control and the euthanasia of laboratory animals.

Hopefully, the present book will provide some insight and enlightenment into the intricate issue of euthanasia, both human and animal, inspiring readers to think critically about the medical, social, philosophical, cultural and existential aspects of "good death" in our technologized, individualized and ageing society burdened with rising health care costs.

Josef Kuře
Masaryk University, Brno
Czech Republic

Part 1

Defining the Issue

1

Good Death Within Its Historical Context and as a Contemporary Challenge: A Philosophical Clarification of the Concept of "Euthanasia"

Josef Kuře
University Centre for Bioethics & Department of Medical Ethics,
Masaryk University, Brno
Czech Republic

1. Introduction

The word euthanasia evokes emotions, regardless of the way it is used. When pronounced, instead of a rational discourse, separate camps of irreconcilable proponents and opponents are drawn up. Both fight for dignity, liberty, autonomy, rights and humaneness. Few debates in the area of health care result in such polarization of opinions as euthanasia. While for some people euthanasia is a manifestation of the individual's autonomy equal with a responsible control of one's destiny, a compassionate responsiveness to someone's immense suffering or a clinical imperative to act in the patient's best interest, for other people, euthanasia is tantamount to or merely a euphemism for killing, the violation of human life and an infringement of the human right to life, being contradictory to the sanctity of life doctrine and facilitating the abuse of vulnerable persons. The controversies surrounding the moral acceptability of euthanasia and its decriminalization are characteristic of the intellectual confrontations in medical ethics and in public debates during the last decades of the twentieth century and they remain a challenge for our ageing societies in the twenty first century. As Keown (2002, p. 9) points out, "given the absence of any universally agreed definition of 'euthanasia' it is vital to be clear about how the word is being used in any particular context. The cost of not doing so is confusion." This confusion is, among others, created by semantic substitutions in which euthanasia is not distinguished from "physician assisted dying", from "assisted suicide" or from "physician assisted suicide" (Quill & Battin, 2004; Young, 2007), or being simply replaced by very general terms like "assisted death" (Lewis, 2007; Lewy, 2011), under which not only euthanasia but also assisted suicide is usually subsumed. The general public, especially in countries other than ones such as the Netherlands or Belgium, use general terms such as "assisted death" or "assisted dying" while generally not differentiating between euthanasia and assisted suicide, not understanding euthanasia in the sense used by legislation in countries where euthanasia has been legalized. This use of a broad notion of euthanasia results in various clinical situations being discussed under the scope of "euthanasia".

Once euthanasia is merged with "assisted death", then under the term "euthanasia" similar but distinct clinical situations such as medical futility, life sustaining treatment, categorization of therapy, palliative care, and other end-of-life decisions are discussed (van der Maas, 1991; Onwuteaka-Philipsen, 2003). Decisions in palliative and intensive care medicine include a much broader spectrum of ethical dilemmas than the issue of euthanasia alone (Battin et al., 2007; Kinzbrunner & Policzer, 2010). Nevertheless it happens quite frequently that two people, discussing whether 'euthanasia' is morally good and/or right and whether it should be legalized or not understand two quite different things by the same term; they fail to connect, developing two parallel monologues. Such fruitless and frustrating occurrences are characteristic of many euthanasia debates. It was one such occasion that inspired the author to study the historical semantics of euthanasia, the results of which are presented below. [1]

Since the notion of euthanasia is loaded by strong feelings, many euthanasia discussions lack clear semantic ground as a rational starting point. So instead of semantic clarification (*status questionis* in the traditional philosophical discourse), euthanasia discussions are often limited to the justification of their arguments (regardless if *pro* or *contra*) and to the critique of the arguments of the other side as a matter of principle.

This situation is further exasperated by both opponents and proponents of euthanasia often using the same arguments but with very diverse meanings. Based on the same argument, completely contrary conclusions can be drawn. Such is the case with arguments based on human dignity. One can state that euthanasia violates human dignity and therefore it should be prohibited. However, another can argue that not allowing legal euthanasia violates human dignity since one then has to die in a way which harms dignity; therefore euthanasia is a death which fully corresponds to human dignity (the law which regulates assisted suicide in Oregon State is entitled the Death With Dignity Act).

Should the euthanasia discussion be meaningful, a conceptual clarification needs to be one of the primary conditions of such a discussion. I'm arguing that prior to any argumentation either for or against euthanasia, the semantics used in such argumentations has to be clarified. "It is important to understand what euthanasia is. No one disputes the fact that euthanasia is a form of killing; so too are murder, manslaughter, suicide, capital punishment, and war. To state that each is a form of killing warns us to

[1] This chapter was written thanks to a well-known surgeon and distinguished professor's contribution to euthanasia, a presentation at a conference called "The Philosophy of Euthanasia", which both frustrated and challenged me. This motivated me to write an article in the form of a philosophical explanation of the notion of euthanasia (Kuře, 2007). The text provided here is an extended English revision. Here is a synopsis of his presentation, which took the form of a story and a conclusion. In the mountains lived a forester who lived a happy life up to the moment when he went down to a local hospital. Having been diagnosed with cancer, he returned back to his house in the forest and shot himself to death. Conclusion: euthanasia has to be legalized. So ends the surgeon's contribution.
A typical case of suicide. One isn't able to bear a depressing and burdensome situation. Under intensive stress one sees the best way out of such a situation as one's own death, accomplishing it by one's own hand, without any external help (an unassisted death). Such a person did not ask for the termination of his life, no other person was involved. In was suicide, not euthanasia; not even assisted suicide. Besides cancer there can be many different reasons for which one might commit suicide. This story illustrates the kind of conceptual inaccuracy that can be in play. The forester was not suffering extreme pain, and he could possibly have been cured. If his story is an argument for euthanasia then any trying situation in life would qualify for euthanasia, leading euthanasia to be a first and not last resort. While most would argue that one is free to commit suicide any time he/she assesses his/her life as a burden and meaningless. But suicide has here nothing to do with euthanasia.

proceed with care, but it need not to be decisive in determining the rightness or wrongness of the act. We need, therefore, to address the question of what it is about euthanasia that distinguishes it from, or places it in a separate category to, say, self-killing or murder." (Draper, 1998, p. 176).

Even a discussion which distinguishes between euthanasia and suicide is not necessarily free of conceptual inexactitudes by using terms such as "active euthanasia", "passive euthanasia", "direct euthanasia", "indirect euthanasia", "help in dying" as synonyms for euthanasia, "mercy killing" (German "*Gnadentod*") as another synonym for euthanasia, and other terms such as "voluntary euthanasia", "involuntary euthanasia", active action causing death (*actio commissionis*), passive action (non-acting) causing death (*actio ommissionis*), "killing", "letting die" ("allowing to die"), usage of "ordinary"/"extraordinary" means, "intending death", "foreseeing death" (to foresee that an unintended death will occur). Not only is the term "euthanasia" connected with considerable semantic unclearness, but it is also used and abused in various cultural and historical contexts - so for instance, in Germany the term "euthanasia" (*Euthanasie*) is used to refer to the abuse of the Nazi regime during that period (eugenic euthanasia), while the term "*Sterbehilfe*"[2] is used in current euthanasia debates.

This use of unspecified terminology - with the term "good death" being used to subsume many very diverse situations and meanings - and including the use of single terms with diverse connotations (e.g. "assisted death" or "dignity") is quite common in these debates. So semantic clarifications are therefore a necessary prerequisite for any ethical reflection on euthanasia to take place. However one of the obstacles for a meaningful discussion of euthanasia is its semantic deficiency. The non-addressed polysemantism that is present hinders understanding, reinforcing superficiality and creating misapprehensions. For instance if one makes use of the old-fashioned "active" and "passive" euthanasia terms, which can still be found in the literature, then the use of one and the same denotation, namely "euthanasia", for ethically entirely different situations (killing by high doses of opiates and allowing to die when the terminally ill person is dying, without causing dysthanasia) is considerably problematic – not only from the semantic point of view.

The aim of this chapter is to contribute to the clarification of the concept of "good death" as it appeared throughout history; its goal is to clarify what was meant by the term "euthanasia" in various historical periods. The chapter does not seek to provide "a short history of euthanasia" but to show how differently and in which semantic, cultural and philosophical frameworks the term "euthanasia" has been used in the course of history. So instead of a comprehensive history of euthanasia, a search for diverse typologies of euthanasia through history will be conducted. It seems that it is necessary to start not with the 18th century and with the "right to die"[3] as Ian Dowbiggin does (2007) but with Classical thinking. Nevertheless, Dowbiggin clearly demonstrates euthanasia's affinity to suicide,

---

[2] The term "Sterbehilfe" is ambiguous in concept; it can be used in quite contrary meanings. In one meaning it is used as an equivalent term for active euthanasia (help to die) (Bobbert, 2003; Eibach, 1998; Eid, 1985; Müller, 1997; Ritzel, 1998). While in its other meaning "Sterbehilfe" refers to the active support of a dying person (palliative care, human accompaniment for the dying patient) (Michalsen & Reinhart, 2006; Kruse & Wagner, 1986; Pöltner, 2006; Simon, 2003; Sporken, 1988, 1990).

[3] Cf. Cavan, 2000; Downing & Smoker, 1986; Ferguson, 2007; Humphry & Wickett, 1986; Sunstein, 1997; Wilshaw, 1974.

which can be conceptualized in many ways. There were times, particularly in Christian Europe, when the fear of Hell was far greater than the fear of death. He also demonstrates that distinctions are worthwhile in a historical approach to euthanasia.[4] This chapter does not delve into the *status quo* of the current euthanasia debate, nor does it provide moral or ethical "for" or "against" arguments as used within euthanasia debates. Rather it tries to illustrate the diverse backgrounds of such debates.

The methodology used in this chapter is not a pure historical overview of the notion of euthanasia. The purpose of the historical survey conducted here is to contribute to a better "contemporary reading" of the concept called "euthanasia". This approach presumes that such a historical and semantic survey can help one to understand the contemporary challenges of the technified, highly advanced and dehumanized biomedicine of our post-industrial and postmodern society. Euthanasia today is being discussed in the context of numerous other clinical and societal issues such as medical futility, patient autonomy, physician integrity, physician assisted suicide, terminal sedation, patient's rights, social death preceding biological death, increasing health care costs and palliative care. Many of the present medical circumstances such as withholding or withdrawing treatment and other life sustaining treatments have created new therapeutic situations, questioning the traditional goals of medicine.

Methodologically this chapter combines differentiated semantics with a critical history of philosophy. Within a historical survey it shows different meanings of the term "euthanasia", from a peaceful and nonviolent death to death by request and unrequested mercy killing. The goal here is to demonstrate the broad semantic spectrum of euthanasia. The search for historical semantics will be governed by the idea of "good death" and its relation to the present problems in health care, with a specific regard to current euthanasia issues. Once the notion of "good death" has been clarified, the ethics of euthanasia can be well-founded.

As a result of the historical survey, the main semantic typologies of euthanasia will be presented, e.g. peaceful natural death (Suetonius), voluntary suicide (*autothanatos*, Stoa), medically accompanied dying without life prolongation (*euthanasia exteriori*), social euthanasia, eugenic euthanasia, "easy death" and in/voluntary euthanasia. Furthermore, the recent semantic and analytical discussions on euthanasia will be summarized and their implications for ethics discussions will be outlined. In addition, the importance of some of the philosophical background discussions for the conceptual understanding of euthanasia (e.g. human rights) will be highlighted.

2. Common desire as the common ground

In etymological terms, the word "euthanasia" in Classical Greek means "good death" (εὐ = good, θάνατος = death). With respect to the polysemantics of the adjective *εὐ*, one could, as the proper equivalent to the term "euthanasia", interpret it to mean not only "good death" but also expressions like "nice death", "beautiful death", "happy death", "lucky death", or in a tropological sense also "mild death", "easy death", "peaceful death", "nonviolent

[4] Notwithstanding the fecund contribution of Dowbiggin's historical study (2007), it overlooks two needed aspects: clear distinctions and more distance in evaluation. One would expect from a historian that he would write in the sense of the old historians' rule *sine ira et studio*.

death" or "painless death".[5] From an etymological point of view, it is obvious that "euthanasia" is not primarily about something so specific as administrating a deadly injection upon a patient's request but about the concept of a "good death".

There is a general consensus at this semantic level: as we are mortal, probably everybody, excluding those with psychopathologies, wishes to die a "good death". From this perspective, the desire for εὐ θάνατος is a panhuman one. It is difficult to imagine that someone without a pathological disorder would wish any other death than εὐ θάνατος in its original meaning. What does vary, where we differ, and remaining a lasting subject of controversy, is the context of this εὐ. All disagreements regarding euthanasia are disputes about the "good", what kind of death is a good one, what are the characteristics of a "good death". Why does the denotation "good" cause such a strong diversity of options, implacable contrapositions and ripples of emotions? There is an easy answer to this question: because such a denotation of "good" is related to the basic concepts of life, to the fundamental values, philosophical views, metaphysical and religious beliefs and *a priori* positions. Therefore the context of this "good" in its relation to death will be examined.

3. Concepts of "a good death": A historical overview

First let's look at how the concept of "a good death" has been understood over the history of philosophical thinking, which values, circumstances and actions have been assigned to this concept and how it has been conditioned by cultural, historical, social and religious factors. It is very important to note that the discussions about euthanasia in the 21st century and the good death controversy are nothing new and that these discussions have been going on within a historical context that started in the Classical era. (Brody, 1989). However, the current context of the euthanasia debate with regard to the present stage and form of medicine is new, different and peerless. (Vanderpool, 2004). The controversial concept of euthanasia has to be investigated not only with regard to what has been attributed to the adjective "good" but foremost with regard to attitudes towards death as such. The following research provides an overview of the different concepts of "good death" over the course of history, stemming from attitudes towards death in general, which, throughout our history and beyond the controversies about "good death", has been a more common source of human angst.

3.1 Antiquity

The concept of euthanasia does not start with Bacon as some people believe but with ancient Greek thinking. The term εὐ θάνατος first appears in Hellenic literature side by side with the term εὐγίρια (giras = old age). Initially looming sporadically, later a similar concept called *mors bona*[6] (good death) appears in Roman literature. The term *mors bona* denominates an honest and happy way of dying. *Felici vel honesta morte mori* (to die in a lucky and honest way) was an ancient ideal.

Already in mythological times, sleep was regarded as the brother of death. In the Odyssey, Homer lets the healthy and old citizens of the utopian island Siri die in a painless and quick

[5] In modern Greek εὐθανασία not only means "mild death" or "painless death" but also "famous death" or "glorious death".

[6] L. A. Seneca, *Epistulae* 67,9.

way: they are "saved" by the god Apollo, who kills them peacefully. In this way euthanasia was often perceived as the best gift that one could get from the gods. (Mystakidou et al., 2005). In the Classical period, in some regions, Greek citizens used to end their lives after obtaining the consent of the community. As part of *eugiria* (to grow old in a "good" way) and to prevent a life of senility and weakness, illness and fragility, they used to prefer the abandonment of life en masse by drinking hemlock within a "last festivity", being regarded in such as heroes by the community. (Mystakidou et al., 2005). In Ancient Greece there was generally a positive attitude towards suicide.

When Plato describes the death of Socrates (*Phaidon*), who prefers hemlock to exile, he notes that Socrates' act was in fact a good death. In cases where abnormality was identified, for the good of the individual citizens and for the good of the polis (society), these sick citizens were left to die. Plato justifies this in *Politeia*[7]: those who have bad (unhealthy) bodies have to be abandoned to die, those who have a bad (unhealthy) and irremediable soul have to be killed.[8]

In Antiquity, two traditions can be traced: one originating with Hippocrates and his school (*Corpus Hippocraticum*), and the other founded on Greek and Roman philosophy, in particular on the teachings of Plato, Aristotle and the Stoics. The Hippocratic tradition, whose core is the Hippocratic Oath, prohibits the killing of a human being, just as it forbids any aid in suicide (in present-day terminology in "physician assisted suicide"): "To please no one will I prescribe a deadly drug nor give advice which may cause his death." Euthanasia as a direct killing of the patient, regardless if upon his/her request or without any request, is not forbidden by the Hippocratic Oath directly. But such a prohibition can be deduced, *a fortiori*, from the prohibition of any help in suicide. So euthanasia as the killing of a patient by the physician is not in accordance with either the Hippocratic Oath or the spirit of the Hippocratic tradition. Within this tradition, health is regarded as one of the highest forms of good. So the intentional termination of a patient's life is discordant with Hippocratic medical practice, dedicated to caring for the health and life of people. Features typical of the Hippocratic tradition are a preventive and therapeutic approach to the medical art. Prevention has to protect and preserve the wellbeing of the healthy, while therapy has to return the sick to health. An integral part of this approach to the medical art is that of limitation, which has to be accepted: where no cure is available and where the patient has already been overwhelmed by disease, there no therapy should be attempted. In this case treatment should not be started, any protraction of the life of a deadly ill person was held to be inconsistent with the medical ethos.[9] The Hippocratic tradition, based on a Pythagorean sect and on ancient Greek mythological polytheism in which the gods were both protectors and proprietors of human beings, later resonated with Jewish and Christian teaching according to which God is the master who possesses dominion over life; human beings receive life as a gift. The concept of "good death" in its original version as an ancient tradition is based on a mythological sacredness of life. A modified version of this concept survived not only to the Middle Ages but to Modern Era.

The second source of the concept of euthanasia was philosophical tradition, which produced certain tension due to its contrast to the Hippocratic tradition. While the Hippocratic

---

[7] Plato, *Politeia* (III), 410a (κατα τήν ψυχήν κακοφυεις ανιατους αυτοι αποκτενουσιν).

[8] Although this passage in *Politeia* is interpretatively disputable, one can educe from this passage that euthanasia as (regardless if merciful or pragmatic) killing could be morally justifiable.

[9] Hippocrates, Of Art (VI, 3). In: Hippocrates, 1923, Vol. 2, p. 193.

tradition prohibits euthanasia as a form of killing and likewise bans physician assisted suicide, philosophers such as Plato, Aristotle and the Stoics approved of the killing of seriously and/or incurably sick patients who consume the resources of the community (polis); either the community should abandon care of them or they should be killed outright. A similar destiny, for the good the community, they held, should encounter handicapped and seriously ill children. This can be seen in the practise of the laws of Sparta: newborn children were brought to an examination which had to prove the viability of the child; any child evaluated as non-viable was killed. For Plato, a human being is the possession of the gods and suicide is a contradiction to this concept, but the gods approved of suicide in cases where the necessity to die is evident (e.g. the death of Socrates). The next sphere of exceptions which justify suicide is, according to Plato, the shame of extreme suffering, poverty, or disaster, akin to supreme deprivation and dishonour or irreversible disgrace of fate. Plato, in the Laws (Nomoi) exhorts to take flight from a society of bad people and to appreciate everything that is beautiful and fair. And if one cannot escape from heavily incorrigible maleficence or from unredeemable crimes, then it is more beautiful to choose death and to depart from life.[10] For those who find themselves in an incurable state which can be interpreted as "sickness of the soul", it is better not to live any longer. By their departure from life they would benefit others twofold: first they would become an admonitory example which warns from doing injustice; secondly the community would be free of those people.[11] The aforementioned tracts of Plato's Laws refer to both suicide and to the capital punishment.

For Aristotle death is the worst of all things. One can act towards death in a sublime and noble way, facing death courageously or spinelessly. Facing death, one also can commit injustice towards the community if one takes his/her own life. Moreover, according to Aristotle, the one who destroys him/her self suffers - as „state punishment" - a certain loss of civil rights on the ground that he/she has treated the state unjustly. The justification of this punishment is the correlation between the individual and community: if an individual treats him/her self unjustly, simultaneously he/she also treats the community unjustly.[12] In his treatise on courage Aristotle speaks about the beautiful death the courageous person faces without any fear.[13] Beautiful death can also be death in which a person gives up his own life without fear but also death which a person faces stoutly; such death is simultaneously good (αγαθόν). However suicide seems to be contrary to such courage: to die to escape from a miserable situation such as poverty or pain is not the mark of a brave person, but rather of a coward. To fly from what is troublesome is softness and frailty. To

[10] Plato, *Nomoi* (IX), 854c.

[11] Plato, *Nomoi* (IX), 862e.

[12] Aristotle, *Nicomachean Ethics,* V/15, 1138a.

Aristotle's argument about suicide as injustice towards the state (just acts are those in accordance with virtue prescribed by the law and since the law does not expressly permit suicide, and what it does not expressly permit it forbids, suicide is a violation of the law which harms others and therefore a person committing suicide is acting unjustly) was later adopted by Thomas Aquinas, who connected this argument with natural law.

[13] "Now death is the most terrible of all things; for it is the end, and nothing is thought to be any longer either good or bad for the dead. But the brave man would not seem to be concerned even with death in all circumstances, e.g. at sea or in disease. [...] He will be called brave who is fearless in face of a noble death (καλον θάνατον), and of all emergencies that involve death." Aristotle, *Nicomachean Ethics,* III/9, 1115a.

commit suicide does not mean to endure death because it is noble but because one is trying to escape from evil.[14]

While for Aristotle suicide is a sign of weakness, for Seneca suicide is a mark of sublimity. Seneca equates death to non-being: *mors est non esse*[15], holding as sublime the termination of life in the face of the cruelty of disease or of people. This is valid in particular for the elite of society: it is more appropriate to terminate one's own life than to face humiliation, fear of the future, sickness or old age.[16] The decision about *autothanatos* (suicide) is not a big decision, it is important to die in an honest, peaceful and courageous way. A substantial part of the stoical concept of a good death is serenity and equableness;[17] one leaves composedly when the inevitable hour of death comes.[18] Seneca also formulated a truth which is still valid and even more significant in our societies, where death has become taboo and something that has to be suppressed and curbed: *Non mortem timemus sed cogitationem mortis* (We do not fear death but the thinking on death).[19]

An exemplary good death in ancient times was that narrated of the death of the Roman emperor Augustus, who died at 75, and can be given as it was described by the historian Suetonius (69–122): "Then, having admitted his friends to his presence, he asked them whether they thought he had acted well his part on the stage of life [...]. After which, having dismissed them all, [...] he gave up the ghost. [...] Thus he died a very easy death, such as he himself had always wished for. For as often as he heard that any one had died quickly and without pain, he prayed that he and his might have the like *euthanasia*[20], for that was the word he made use of."[21] Here in the term "euthanasia", the whole concept of the good death as the desirable and covetable way of dying is concentrated.

In this study Diogenes Laertius (3rd century) has been selected as the last ancient author on "good death".[22] Voluntary death (*mors voluntaria*) is for him the expression of a rational concept of life. The honest reasons for a suicide lead a wise human in a good and rational way (εὔλογος) out of life, when life is loaded down by severe pain, mutilation or incurable disease.[23] Although incurable disease was at that time something different from incurable disease today (e.g. diabetes), the concept of *mors voluntaria* grounded on a good rational deliberation is in principle the same which is used in contemporary discussions on

[14] Aristotle, *Nicomachean Ethics,* III/11, 1116a.

[15] L. A. Seneca, *Epistulae* 54,4.

[16] L. A. Seneca, *Epistulae* 58,36.

[17] L. A. Seneca, *Epistulae* 67,9.

[18] "Magna res est [...] cum adventat hora illa inevitabilis, aequo animo abire." (It is a great thing to leave with a serene spirit when the inevitable hour comes). (L. A. Seneca, *Epistulae* 30,4).

[19] Seneca, *Epistulae* 30,17.

[20] In this passage, the original Latin text is interrupted and the Greek word *euthanasia* is inserted: "Nam fere quotiens audisset cito ac nullo cruciatu defunctum quempiam, sibi et suis *euthanasian* similem (hoc enim et verbo uti solebat) precabatur." (Suetonius, *De vitis ceasarum*, II/99. Available at http://www.thelatinlibrary.com/suet.html, cited 20.03.2011.)

[21] Suetonius, *Lives of the Twelve Caesars*, II, 99 (Wordsworth Editions Limited, Ware, UK, 1997, p. 122)

[22] It has to be noted that from the 4th century, the way death and euthanasia were perceived changed after Christianity became the state religion. After this point, both suicide and euthanasia as they were understood in Classical times became incompatible with Christianity and its fundamental assumptions, such as life seen as a gift from God, the decision about the moment of death belonging exclusively to God, lead to euthanasia being considered as a terrible sin.

[23] Diogenes Laertius, *Vitae philosophorum,* VII, 130.

euthanasia - with the difference that *mors voluntaria* was understood as suicide. Arguments given in these ancient discussions for voluntary euthanasia (*mors voluntaria*) could be deduced by *eulogos*, by good rational considerations.

The introduced examples demonstrate that euthanasia in Antiquity was understood in several distinctly diverse meanings. In one line, from Plato to Seneca, euthanasia is equal to a legitimate killing of unwelcome people, of those with incurable diseases or with severe handicaps who, for the good of society, have to be abandoned or directly killed. This form of "good death" can be called social euthanasia. Individuals with certain features become a burden on society and since the capacity of the society cannot bear such a load the life of these individuals will be taken, directly or indirectly. The justification of such killing is not to be found in the autonomous choice or the good of those individuals suffering, but in the best interest of the society as a whole. It is the good of the society and society's best interest that constitutes the justification for such involuntary death. To them, this could be called "a good death" (εὐ θάνατος) - despite the fact that involuntary death was not labelled as euthanasia as such in the Classical period. Therefore the term "social euthanasia" - whereby the good of the community overweighs the good of an individual - defines the good socially, not individually. Thus, such social euthanasia was perceived as a "good" death. One could argue that this is an ancient form of social utilitarianism.

The next meaning of euthanasia in Antiquity was *mors voluntaria,* voluntary death. In certain circumstances it was regarded not only as morally permissible to die a freely chosen death but even as morally right and desirable to do so in such circumstances. In this second sense, as it was an imperative to demonstrate courage, bravery and moral excellence (αρετή) in one's daily life, when faced with a situation of experiencing humiliation, inhuman suffering or inconclusiveness of a given situation (such as heavy doom, unbearable suffering, incurable disease) to choose death was an expression of human freedom, dignity and nobility. Such termination of life was even used as a preventive measure against foreseeable humiliation such as impending capture or future fate caused by the weakness of old age or by a serious disease. Voluntary death, an optional death which was chosen as a free choice from the heart and mind of the person, without any external pressure, force or violence was regarded as a *good* death. In such a way has *mors voluntaria* been understood, by the Stoics in particular. One can argue that this voluntary and rational suicide was simultaneously euthanasia.

The third meaning of euthanasia in the ancient period was a peaceful, quick, easy and painless death. The best example for this hermeneutics of euthanasia is the death of the emperor Augustus. One could argue that in this sense euthanasia is a way of dying that everybody would probably appreciate.

Finally, we find the prohibition of euthanasia (induced death or assisted death) in the Hippocratic tradition. The reasoning for such a ban is the mythological understanding of human life: the gods are in charge of life and death, life is not completely at human disposal. More philosophical support for this idea would come from Plato's metaphysics, where life is regarded as one of the important forms of good, which embodies elements from the world of ideas. The Hippocratic tradition can be regarded as the ancient version of the later doctrine of the sanctity of life.

Compared to the ancient approaches to good death introduced here, euthanasia in our time is prevalently perceived as the painless termination of life (and suffering) by a physician. Today we distinguish euthanasia from natural death (the death the emperor Augustus died) and from (physician) assisted voluntary suicide. Euthanasia in Antiquity was associated with peaceful death and with mercy killing as well, despite the fact that mercy killing was not referred to as such. Nevertheless the concept of voluntary death as it appears in ancient times and as defined by the ancient term *mors voluntaria* bears some kinship to in the contemporary discussion of euthanasia. The Platonic tradition, despite the fact that Plato also deemed life as a gift of the gods and therefore beyond human intervention, can be seen as very supportive of the contemporary idea of euthanasia, even for unrequested (non-voluntary and involuntary) euthanasia. Plato's style of argumentation and decision-making is currently used not only in discussions but also in practise, such as the euthanasia of children or of incompetent patients. The Aristotelian tradition, however, is much more reserved about the rightness of suicide, focusing on the harm to society caused by a suicide. The Stoic tradition would fully support (assisted) suicide; and one can extrapolate that the Stoic tradition would also support contemporary (physician) assisted suicide and active euthanasia.

In sum, just as most aspects of modern civilization can trace its roots to Classical times, so too can the philosophical foundations and rudiments of our contemporary discussions on euthanasia. It is not only the modern concept of autonomy but also a broader philosophical and cultural tradition which has further enriched our current discussions. And one should be aware that we are today discussing issues which are new for our advanced biomedicine and for our postmodern society. However at the same time they are very old, they are ancient, and they have already been discussed in similar forms throughout the course of history. One can hope that an awareness of such a greater historical context will improve our understanding.

3.2 The Middle Ages

In the Middle Ages a common concept of good death was shared. This concept came from Biblical literature, in particular from Decalogue and in connection with Augustine's interpretation of the commandment "You shall not kill"[24] where he equates suicide to homicide.[25] Authors of the Middle Ages, for obvious reasons, do not deal with the issue of euthanasia as we handle it today. Yet they deal intensively with the question of killing, both the killing of another person (e.g. execution) or suicide. While in the first case, to differentiate, they allow killing in certain cases such as capital punishment (death as a penalty within retributive justice), in the case of suicide, they do not allow it, holding it unequivocally as morally wrong and sinful, and as fundamentally opposed to the Christian tradition.[26]

Thomas Aquinas summarises the moral prohibition of suicide into the following three arguments:

---

[24] "Quanto magis intellegendum est non licere homini se ipsum occidere, cum in eo, quod scriptum est: Non occides, nihilo deinde addito nullus, nec ipse utique, cui praecipitur, intellegatur exceptus!" (How much greater reason have we to understand that a man may not kill himself, since in the commandment "Thou shall not kill" there is no limitation added nor any exception made in favour, and least of all in favour of him on whom the command is laid.) – Augustinus Aurelius, *De civitate Dei,* I, 20.

[25] "Non occides, nec alterum ergo nec te. Neque enim qui se occidit aliud quam hominem occidit." (Therefore you shall kill neither another nor yourself, for he who kills himself still kills nothing else than a human being.) - Augustinus Aurelius, *De civitate Dei,* I, 20.

[26] If suicide is a fundamental contradiction to the Christian tradition, then analogically such an evaluation is also valid for assisted suicide and about euthanasia as direct killing upon request.

1. Suicide is against the natural law and against love.[27]

Suicide is not in harmony with the objective order, being in discrepancy to the natural law (*lex naturalis*). Therefore suicide is unnatural and naturally immoral. Moreover it is a vitiation of one's relation to oneself; it is natural to love oneself, to take care of oneself, to keep oneself alive and to resist any loss of life. Suicide is contrary to this natural inclination of man to preserve one's life.

2. Suicide is against society.

Building on Aristotle[28], Aquinas, making use of the complexity argument, points out that suicide results in injury of the whole, i.e. society: every part, as such, belongs to the whole. As every human being is part of the community, and so, belonging to society. Therefore the one who commits suicide also injures the community (*iniuriam communitati*).[29]

3. Suicide is against God and against justice.

Because life is a gift from God, suicide means to take possession of life which is not owned and by nature cannot be owned by man. To usurp ownership of something that does not belong to one but that has been commended is an offence to justice. One can only decide about those things which belong to life but to decide about life as such is out of the scope of free human decisions. So no human can decide about departing from life.[30]

One can conclude that suicide is the worst of all terrible wrongdoings, devastation on all three levels of existence: suicide is against one's self (personal area), against society (societal area), and against the Divine order (transcendental area). So not only by Thomas Aquinas and other authors of the Middle Ages, but also by the later Christian churches, suicide was classified as one of the most grave of sins. Its gravity is based on the fact that it affects all areas, being an act "against all", enhanced by the fact that the person is now dead, without the possibility to regret and rectify. So not only medieval theologians but also many Christians in the coming centuries were horrified by the idea of suicide. Within the mentioned paradigm, one was not able to imagine anything more terrible than suicide.

Consequently a heavy penalty for suicide was inevitable. *Ipso facto* the heaviest "temporal" and "eternal" punishments were applied; the committer was to be excluded from society (in

---

[27] "...naturaliter quaelibet res seipsam amat, et ad hoc pertinet quod quaelibet res naturaliter conservat se in esse et corrumpentibus resistit quantum potest. Et ideo quod aliquis seipsum occidat est contra inclinationem naturalem, et contra caritatem, qua quilibet debet seipsum diligere. Et ideo occisio sui ipsius semper est peccatum mortale, utpote contra naturalem legem et contra caritatem existens." (Everything naturally loves itself, the result being that everything naturally keeps itself in being, and resists corruptions so far as it can. Wherefore suicide is contrary to the inclination of nature, and to charity whereby every man should love himself. Hence suicide is always a mortal sin, as being contrary to the natural law and to charity.) – Thomas Aquinas, *Summa Theologica*, II – IIae, q. 64, a. 5.

[28] Aristotle, *Nicomachean Ethics*, V/15, 1138a.

[29] "Quilibet autem homo est pars communitatis, et ita id quod est, est communitatis. Unde in hoc quod seipsum interficit, iniuriam communitati facit." - Thomas Aquinas, *Summa Theologica*, II – IIae, q. 64, a. 5.

[30] "... quia vita est quoddam donum divinitus homini attributum, et eius potestati subiectum qui occidit et vivere facit. Et ideo qui seipsum vita privat in Deum peccat, sicut qui alienum servum interficit peccat in dominum cuius est servus; et sicut peccat ille qui usurpat sibi iudicium de re sibi non commissa. Ad solum enim Deum pertinet iudicium mortis et vitae." (Life is God's gift to human beings; life is subject to God's power, only God kills and makes to live. So whoever takes his own life, sins against God, even as the one who kills another's slave, sins against that slave's master, and as the one who usurps to himself judgment of a matter not entrusted to him. For it belongs to God alone to pronounce sentence of death and life.) - Thomas Aquinas, *Summa Theologica*, II – IIae, q. 64, a. 5, ad 3.

space and time) and the church punishment of "excommunication" applied, which included burial *extra murales*, (out of the Christian cemetery), the suicide would then be punished by God with the committer excluded from heaven (out of space and time).[31] From such criminalization of suicide, moral rigorousness and intransigence follows and hence the religious and social abhorrence of suicide characteristic of a large part of historical Christianity. One should add that to some extent, this form of moral terrorism still survives, albeit a Christian burial has been allowed for several decades now. This historical context has been mentioned because there are people even today (and not as very rare exceptions) who think in a very similar way as the very late medieval theologians.

Paradoxically, within Aquinas' argumentation, contemporary involuntary euthanasia would be more justifiable than voluntary (active) euthanasia. For instance, the case of someone being sentenced to death for the good of society but who will receive a milder post-mortal punishment, contrasted to the suicide victim, who might deserve a "good death", but by virtue of his/her "sin", is condemned to the worst of all possible afterlives.[32] The death penalty, avoiding a bigger "eternal punishment", does not offend all beings, as much as voluntary euthanasia does. Then such involuntary "good death", in the form of the death penalty, would be more compatible with the norm "You shall not kill" where exceptions such as "a just war" or "capital punishment" exist, than voluntary euthanasia, which assumes that the person requesting death freely would affront each and all. Within the Thomist framework, based on Aquinas theology, mercy related to death would take the form of the "mercy killing" of a serious criminal. This version of Christian theology does not have the same mercy with a human being suffering in a devastating and possibly unbearable way.

Similar to Antiquity, with multiple viewpoints on what constituted a "good death", the Middle Ages also held another view, one which was neither rapid nor painless, namely foreseen death: death which is expected in harmony with the following wisdom: *mors certa - hora incerta* (death being certain, but with an uncertain hour of arrival). Such death finds one waiting and expectant, ready to "go". Such an expected death is peaceful because it has been accepted with equanimity. This emphasis on "good death" as a lifelong activity and continuously expected event, supported and potentiated by Christian Platonism and by the ethics of Stoa and adopted by Christianity (but "rid of" *autothanatos*) has markedly transformed the biblical message and this can be found in the Christianity of nowadays. In this approach the soul is in the body as if in a prison, all throughout life awaiting the moment of liberation, which coincides with death. There is a reciprocity of arts: the art of living well corresponds to the art of dying well (*ars vivendi – art moriendi*). Thus the art of dying (*ars moriendi*) is part of the concept of "good death".

---

[31] The theological penalization ("eternal damnation") was followed by a secular penalization which spread extensively in the period from the 16th to 18th century. The medieval argumentation against suicide gained a simplified form: As suicide is a crime against God, against society, and against natural law, it is so against the king as well. Therefore it was up to the king (monarch) to introduce punishment for the crime committed against his majesty in the case of suicide. So suicide became a crime of great castigation such as the confiscation of the suicide's property. It took a long time to revoke this crime of suicide. For instance in England, the penalty for suicide was suspended in 1823 with suicide ultimately decriminalized in 1961 (Markson, 1969).

[32] Cf. Thomas Aquinas, *Summa Theologica*, II – IIae, q. 25, a. 6, ad 2.

While suicide was treated by the medieval authors mainly in abstract theological categories (and as a morally forbidden item), in the Renaissance attention in the evaluation of suicide shifted to empirical categories and to the situation of the individual suicide. The metaphysical psychology was replaced by an empirical one. As a result, it was determined that suicide is not the worst thing under the Sun and the morality of suicide was assessed differently from the model "sin against all". Further developments in the understanding of suicide came with the Reformation[33] and the Age of Reason.

3.3 The modern era

From the era of the Renaissance one particular thinker is worthy of mention in the context of euthanasia, namely the humanist Thomas More (1478-1535). In his Utopia (1516), he proposed euthanasia as an option for hopelessly sick patients. His concept of euthanasia is different from that used in Antiquity (and later by Francis Bacon) where euthanasia means a peaceful nonviolent death. For Thomas More, euthanasia was a kind of last option for patients without any hope of cure. Euthanasia was for the Lord Chancellor, also known as Saint Thomas More, a compassionate answer to human suffering and tragedy. Besides medical hopelessness, there were two other conditions for euthanasia. First, euthanasia has to be a "voluntarily death", chosen by a person "with a torturing and lingering pain"[34]; a request for euthanasia can only be accepted in medically desperate situations where nothing has been left undone that can contribute to health ("they use all possible ways to cherish them and to make their lives as comfortable as possible"[35]). No one can be forced to ask for euthanasia, similarly no one can be killed against his/her will. It is regarded as legitimate to "choose rather to die since they cannot live in much misery"[36]. Persons in such misery are exhorted by priests and by magistrates, that, "since they are now unable to go on with the business of life, are become a burden to themselves and to all about them, and they have really out-lived themselves, they should no longer nourish such a rooted distemper"[37]. They can be persuaded to end their life but "if they cannot be persuaded to it, this does not induce them to fail in their attendance and care of them."[38] The second condition concerns approval by public authorities, both civil and religious. Then a death chosen voluntarily and "upon such an authority"[39] is deemed very honourable. Failing in this public approval means violation.[40] More's concept of euthanasia includes both (assisted) suicide[41] and intentional

---

[33] Within the Reformation tradition, since approximately the 1930s, the intellectual streams which admit euthanasia as an act of mercy (mercy killing) have won recognition; clergy of diverse confessions played an important role in establishing associations which supported euthanasia. One of the most prominent proponents of euthanasia understood as *mercy killing* was (originally Episcopalian minister) Joseph F. Fletcher (1905–1991) - see Fletcher, 1954, 1979.

[34] More, T. (2011). *Utopia.* Available at http://www.gutenberg.org/. Cited 20.03.2011.

[35] Ibidem.

[36] Ibidem.

[37] Ibidem.

[38] Ibidem.

[39] Ibidem.

[40] "If any man takes away his own life without the approbation of the priests and the senate, they give him none of the honours of a decent funeral, but throw his body into a ditch." (More, 2011).

[41] "They starve themselves of their own accord, or take opium, and by that means die without pain." - Ibidem.

killing.[42] More believed that his concept of voluntary and involuntary death is legitimate: "They think they behave not only reasonably but in a manner consistent with religion and piety; because they follow the advice given them by their priests, who are the expounders of the will of God."[43] Fortunately enough for him the concept of euthanasia was a utopian concept appropriate for the best state in the new island Utopia.[44] (How could More be canonized today as a public supporter of euthanasia?) Utopia literary means no-place, however More in the context of the English pronunciation of the word "utopia" is transforming "utopia" into "eutopia" (good place), a place of felicity.[45] This concept of euthanasia inspired praxis of euthanasia in England in the 16th century (Graziani, 1969). It is difficult to extrapolate to what extent More would apply his euthanasia (with the semantics he used) - limited to fiction solely or into the real world of current biomedicine. One can guess that his esteem for autonomy, mercy and public approval would lead him to be supportive of active voluntary euthanasia.

One of the first modern thinkers who significantly influenced later conceptions of science and scientific knowledge (*scientia est potentia*)[46] and who came out with a new concept of euthanasia was the English late Renaissance philosopher Francis Bacon (1561-1626). His new understanding of science indirectly affected medicine as well: medicine should include both science and art, which enables a physician to help the patient to die in an easy and natural way. According to Bacon, medicine should include both scientific knowledge and practical skills that enable physicians to help their patients die an easy and peaceful death. When describing this medical art, he uses the term "euthanasia exteriori"[47] (a good death coming from outside) (Bacon, 2000). Simultaneously a good death should come from inside (euthanasia interiori) in a form of a sweet and calm dying while the soul of the patient is being prepared (caring for the dying). Apparently Bacon makes use of the term "euthanasia" in the context used by Suetonius when he reported the death of the emperor Augustus.[48] By euthanasia Bacon means the quiet peaceful death of a person who is expecting it. The sense of euthanasia is for him to die non-violently and painlessly, falling asleep. Sleep is to him, similarly to the ancient understanding, a metaphor for death.[49] To aid such a peaceful death is an important task of medicine. The physician's role is to

---

42 "... being assured that if they thus deliver themselves from torture, or are willing that others should do it." - Ibidem.

43 Ibidem.

44 The full and original title of the book is "*Libellus vere aureus, nec minus salutaris quam festivus, de optimo rei publicae statu deque nova insula Utopia*".

45 In the addendum to his book, More proposed to change the semantics and to transform "utopia" to "eutopia": *"Wherfore not Utopia, but rather rightely my name is Eutopia, a place of felicity"*.

46 This aphorism can already be found in Bacon's work *Meditationes sacrae* (1597); nevertheless this aphorism is well known from his later work *Novum organum* (1620) where it established what is known today as the Baconian paradigm.

47 The original title of the work where Bacon deals with the medical art of "euthanasia exteriori" is *Of the proficience and aduancement of learning, diuine and humane* (English titled, written in Latin, published in London in 1605 by H. Tomes). Recently published under the title *The advancement of learning* (Oxford University Press, 2000).

48 *Of the Proficience and Advancement of learning, divine and humane,* Book I, X/7.

49 If Francis Bacon would have been writing his "Advancement of learning" today, he probably would include a passage about terminal sedation as a specific type of medical art that helps the patient to asleep/die peacefully.

accompany the patient in dying a painless and equable death.[50] Bacon harmonized the medical good death in its ancient meaning (peaceful death) with the medieval concept of the *ars moriendi* and with care of the dying persons that we would refer to today as palliative care. Bacon's concept of euthanasia as medical help in natural dying was the leading concept of euthanasia for medical practice until the 19th century.

The development of views about euthanasia has been strongly influenced by social progress in opinions about suicide. Since the 16th century, within the mainstream opinion which held suicide as morally unacceptable, singular voices started to appear which held suicide as morally legitimate and justifiable in cases of serious illness. This meant a breach of the erstwhile dominant moral doctrine of Christianity. To this minority opinion belong the ideas of the French Renaissance philosopher Michel de Montaigne (1533-1592). De Montaigne claimed that God allows man to take life, if man is facing conditions under which it is worse to live then to die (de Montaigne, 1946, p. 338). Within such a statement, the ancient concept of good death which was held by the Stoics in particular can be found; if someone finds oneself in a situation of enormous suffering, then it corresponds more to human dignity and nobility to abandon such a situation, even if the price of departure entails one's own life. De Montaigne, using the logic of the Stoics, provides a religious justification: in such a case, God does not oblige one to stay in such a situation at whatever the cost, instead allowing the person the possibility of choice; if one wants he/she is allowed to depart honestly, even at the price of his/her own (not another's) life. His writings were very influential, being read by Shakespeare, Rousseau, Pascal, Emerson and Nietzsche.

The Enlightenment, with its criticism, secularism and individualism, was a very powerful milestone in the development of opinions about suicide. Probably the most significant contribution of this period to the discussion of suicide comes from Hume's aptly named essay *On Suicide* (published posthumously in 1783), which remains one of the most influential philosophical treatments of suicide in modern times. In this work, David Hume (1711-1776) criticises superstition and "false religion" (Hume, 1985, p. 579) which forces humans to prolong a "miserable existence" in order not to offend God.[51] Hume turns the argument of the injustice induced to society by suicide around (Aristotle, Aquinas): the miserable existence is a burden for society, therefore an individual who chooses to exit from life in such a situation, provides benefit to society and his/her act is not condemnable but commendable.[52] "A man, who retires from life, does no harm to society. He only ceases to do good, which, if it be an injury, is of the lowest kind" (Hume, 1985, p. 586). Suicide can be in harmony with the interest of the individual and with his/her commitment to him/her

---

[50] "But the physicians contrariwise do make a kind of scruple and religion to stay with the patient after the disease is deplored; whereas in my judgment they ought both to inquire the skill, and to give the attendances, for the facilitating and assuaging of the pains and agonies of death." (Bacon, F. *Of the Proficience and Advancement of learning, divine and humane,* Book I, X/7).

[51] "...death alone can put a full period to his misery, he dares not fly to this refuge, but still prolongs a miserable existence from a vain fear left he offend his Maker, by using the power, with which that beneficent being has endowed him." (Hume, 1985, p. 583).

[52] "...suppose, that it is no longer in my power to promote the interest of the public: Suppose, that I am a burthen to it: Suppose, that my life hinders some person from being much more useful to the public. In such cases my resignation of life must not only be innocent but laudable. And most people, who lie under any temptation to abandon existence, are in some such situation. Those, who have health, or power, or authority, have commonly better reason to be in humour with the world."- Hume, D. (1985, p. 587).

self. According to Hume, it is doubtless that the hardship of old age, suffering from illness or misery of fate can be even worse than annihilation caused by suicide.[53] This argument certainly plays a role in the contemporary discussions of the morality of assisted suicide in a medical context. (Frey, 1999). For Hume, there are calamities of life, against which it is necessary to employ suicide as the fatal remedy. Hume is convinced that immense suffering and the wish to die can be understood as a challenge and invitation by which is one recalled from life. Hume, in concord with the ancient tradition, declares that suffering which does not have any positive social contribution, being in fact a burden, does not constitute any duty to prolong such life. Furthermore everybody has "*native liberty*" in which he/she arranges his/her own life. The same liberty provides the opportunity to shape a happy life ("*chance for happiness in life*").[54] Hume argues that suicide is no transgression of duty to God and everybody has the free disposal of their own life. Moreover, when pain and sorrow overcome the patience of a person and when consequently one is tired of life, it is a clear sign ("the clearest and most express terms") that the person is recalled from the station, from life (Hume, 1985). To accept a voluntary death is equal to receiving death "from the hands of the Deity as if it had proceeded from a lion, a precipice, or a fever." In line with some Classical authors, Hume thinks that there are many more things other than disease that can render life a burden. In such conditions he also considers suicide as a noble reaction to life: "If it be no crime, both prudence and courage should engage us to rid ourselves at once of existence, when it becomes a burthen." (Hume, 1985, p. 588).[55]

An antipode to Hume's approach to suicide is that of Immanuel Kant (1724-1804). Kant criticises suicide heavily. His main argument against suicide stems from the Categorical Imperative: suicide cannot become a principle of universal legislation, being contrary to the natural law. The Categorical Imperative is for Kant the basic principle that is intrinsically valid, being good in and of itself and as such it must be obeyed by all and in all situations, without exception. This general imperative as an unconditional moral duty says that one has to act in a way that the maxim of his/her will can at the same time serve as the universal natural law, anytime manifesting the universal law through the maxims of the acting person. So the fundamental obligation is to follow the maxims.[56] Then he immediately gives suicide as the first example of a duty toward oneself, concluding that by committing suicide, one would be completely inconsistent with the supreme principle of all duty.[57] Similarly in

---

[53] "That Suicide may often be consistent with interest, and with our duty to *ourselves*, no one can question who allows, that age, sickness, or misfortune may render life a burthen, and make it worse even than annihilation" (Hume, 1985, p. 588).

[54] Hume (1985, p. 588).

[55] "This is the only way, that we can then be useful to society, by setting an example, which, if imitated, would preserve to every one his chance for happiness in life, and would effectually free him from all danger of misery." (Hume, 1985, p. 588).

[56] "Handle so, als ob die Maxime deiner Handlung durch deinen Willen zum ALLGEMEINEN NATURGETZE werden sollte." Kant, I. (1996). *Grundlegung zur Metaphysik der Sitten*, p. 68.

[57] "A man reduced to despair by a series of misfortunes feels wearied of life, but is still so far in possession of his reason that he can ask himself whether it would not be contrary to his duty to himself to take his own life. Now he inquires whether the maxim of his action could become a universal law of nature. His maxim is: 'From self-love I adopt it as a principle to shorten my life when its longer duration is likely to bring more evil than satisfaction.' It is asked then simply whether this principle founded on self-love can become a universal law of nature. Now we see at once that a system of nature of which it should be a law to destroy life by means of the very feeling whose special nature it is to impel to the

the context of the Categorical Imperative formulated by ends (German *Zweck*), Kant again as a first example mentions suicide.[58] "He who contemplates suicide should ask himself whether his action can be consistent with the idea of humanity as an end in itself. If he destroys himself in order to escape from painful circumstances, he uses a person merely as a means to maintain a tolerable condition up to the end of life. But a man is not a thing, that is to say, something which can be used merely as means, but must be in all his actions always considered as an end in himself. I cannot, therefore, dispose in any way of a man in my own person so as to mutilate him, to damage or kill him."[59] So suicide is a discrepancy to the idea of humanity understood as the human being both as an individual and as the whole of mankind as an end in itself (German *Zweck an sich*). One is not allowed to dispose of one's own life in the sense of its termination. Everyone has a duty to maintain one's own life, and, according to Kant, everyone also has a direct inclination to do so (Kant, 1996, p. 80). Kant's argumentation takes the approach that suicide as a violation of the duty towards oneself in the religious sense and therefore against God.[60] So his argumentation is in line with the religiously justified prohibition of suicide.

To provide an overview on philosophical approaches to death in the modern and postmodern period is beyond this study. However it is necessary to introduce one very influential author, namely Friedrich Nietzsche (1844-1900). Concerning suicide, Nietzsche held a position very similar to that of Hume: man is an autonomous being which has the capacity and moral right to terminate his/her own life which has become unbearable and worthless. Such an act is positive both for society and for the individual, in particular if it is done as the consequence of illness, suffering or misfortune when such an individual is not useful for society, instead being a burden on society. Nietzsche formulated the new idea about free death (*frei zum Tode und frei im Tode*);[61] his leading idea being "Stirb zur rechten Zeit (die at the right moment) (Nietzsche, 1997, p. 35). He goes further than the Stoics did. For the Stoics it was an act of honesty and moral integrity to commit suicide under conditions of extreme hardship (serious illness, misfortune) or as a preventive measure in order not to be dishonoured (e.g. soldiers). For Nietzsche the "indication list" for suicide is broader; one has to determine the proper moment of death: to die in the right moment, to die when I *want*.[62] Many of Nietzsche's thoughts have inspired contemporary euthanasia: euthanasia is a *free death*. A good death is not only a desired and freely chosen one but also a quick death.[63] In Zarathustra, the desire for death (*Sehnsucht zum Tode*) appears; so one can

---

improvement of life would contradict itself and, therefore, could not exist as a system of nature; hence that maxim cannot possibly exist as a universal law of nature and, consequently, would be wholly inconsistent with the supreme principle of all duty." - Kant, I. Fundamental Principles of the Metaphysic of Morals. Available at http://www.gutenberg.org/. Cited 20.03.2011. (Kant, 1996, p. 69).

[58] "Handle so, dass du die Menschheit sowohl in deiner Person, als in der Person eines jeden anderen jederzeit zugleich als Zweck, niemals bloß als Mittel brauchst" (Kant, 1996, p. 79).

[59] Kant, I. *Fundamental Principles of the Metaphysic of Morals*. Available at http://www.gutenberg.org/. Cited 20.03.2011.

[60] Cf. Kant, I. (1990). *Die Metaphysik der Sitten*, pp. 327-334.

[61] Nietzsche, F. (1997). Also Sprach Zarathustra. In: *Werke*, Vol. II, p. 36 (Essen: Phaidon).

[62] "Meinen Tod lobe ich euch, den freien Tod, der mir kommt, weil *ich* will." (Nietzsche, 1997, p. 35)

[63] "Möchten Prediger kommen des *schnellen* Todes! Das wären mir die rechten Stürme und Schüttler an Lebensbäumen! Aber ich höre nur den langsamen Tod predigen und Geduld mit allem 'Irdischen'." (Nietzsche, 1997, p. 36)

say that with regard to Nietzsche's leading idea, a good death is the desired death. For Nietzsche, the human being is something that has to be overcome.[64] When man dies there is the possibility that the Superhuman (Übermensch) can live (Nietzsche, 1997). Thus death can be regarded as doom and as a transition.[65] The fascinating aspect of Nietzsche's thinking, concepts of extinction, doom, disappearance and "twilight", expressed by the term *Untergang* and within the context of death, has to be contemplated. Consequently, according to Nietzsche, my I has to disappear, my I has to be overcome and death is the closest, most logical and natural way how my I can be overcome in space and time.[66] Finally there is a correlation in Nietzsche's thoughts between life and heaviness: life is a weight that is borne.[67] Moreover, if one thinks of a very difficult situation in life such as disseminated carcinoma, more validity would be given to this statement. So it is not only the programmatic pessimism of Nietzsche's world (*Geist der Schwere*) but also the desperateness of various situations in life which make the heaviness and onerousness of life even that much more a burden.

Finally, in passing from the modern thinkers to the medical practice of the 20th century, Charles Darwin (1809-1892), the author of evolutionary theory needs to be mentioned. Evolutionary theory at the end of the 19th century had become a key concept for the natural and social sciences; applied to biology and sociology it gave rise to sociobiology, a very influential stream within the scientific community at the turn of the 20th century. Evolutionary theory brought new approaches to society such as concepts of development and progress, and how to deal with the problem of weak individuals, incurable patients and the handicapped accordingly. As the progress of society depends on strong individuals with appropriate features and the natural selection mechanism is the driving force of evolution, which in order to ascend further and further has to rid itself of everything that hampers this process, it was viewed that only those strong enough and properly equipped would be able to continue the evolutionary process. Contrariwise evolution frees itself of those who are weak, infirm and manifestly unfit. This evolutionary theory has been both used and abused by medicine - for instance within eugenic movements. In difference to the Kantian maxim (human being as the end in itself), within evolutionary approaches this anthropological and ethical premise has been replaced by an evolutionary maxim: evolution is the goal and the individual is a means to achieve this goal. This brings back Nietzsche's words about humans having to be overcome by the Superhuman. Both Nietzsche's philosophy and Darwinism in its reduced form contributed to the later concept of euthanasia (both as social and eugenic euthanasia) of the 19th and 20th century. Darwinians directly affected views on euthanasia, justifying euthanasia as a form of physician-induced painless death for "degenerates", "cripples" and other "unfit" persons and arguing that the doctrine of evolution justifies shortening the lives of suffering people (Vanderpool, 2004).

4. Euthanasia and medicine in the 19th and 20th century

Within a history of the meanings of euthanasia, not only philosophical concepts - which as an integral part of the Western cultural heritage have been influencing social attitudes and

---

64 "Der Mensch ist etwas, das überwunden werden soll" (Nietzsche, 1997, p. 9).

65 "Was groß ist am Menschen, das ist, daß er eine Brücke und kein Zweck ist, [...] daß er ein *Übergang* und ein *Untergang* ist" (Nietzsche, 1997, p. 10).

66 "Mein Ich ist Etwas, das überwunden werden soll" (Nietzsche, 1997, p. 20).

67 "Ja, das Leben ist schwer zu tragen!" (Nietzsche, 1997, p. 87).

medical approaches to life and to the ending of human life - have to be introduced but also the changing modes of medical practice. These modes, which have also influenced the beliefs and actions of physicians and the social perceptions of issues such as eugenics, medical advancement or "death and dying" movements have to be taken into account.

4.1 Euthanasia and the medical practice to 1870[68]

For centuries, the goal of medicine was to soften the symptoms of disease, to save and to preserve human life. From the beginning of the 17th century, euthanasia was understood as a science and art to soothe suffering, to accompany the dying patient and to help one to die easily and naturally. In this context, euthanasia was very similar to what we call palliative care today. It belonged to this realm, one of a capacity to soften pain (even at the cost of shortening life) and provide help which would change the inevitable moment of death into one of peaceful dying. In the context of Bacon's notion of euthanasia, it was a physician's duty to soothe the last moment of life, applying "that science, called euthanasia, which checks oppressing features of illness, relieves pain, and renders the [...] inescapable hour a most peaceful one"[69], as also the German physician Carl. F. H. Marx in 1826 exhorted his colleagues. It was also the physician's task to recognize when the hope for a cure had become exhausted and it had become necessary to accompany the patient towards a peaceful death. Similarly, it was the physician's duty with respect to the professional rules of nonmaleficence not to prolong life. To drag out life or to use life-maintaining treatment was held as inappropriate and wrong due to the harm and cruelty done to the patient. In contrast, the physician's presence at the bed of a dying patient was regarded as a physician's duty as a part of proper professional conduct.[70] Euthanasia only became a subject of controversy in the late nineteenth century. However, two well-known physicians, Carl Theodor Kortum (1765-1824) and Christian Ludwig Mursinna (1744-1823) had already publicly endorsed it at the beginning of the 19th century. (Stolberg, 2008).

4.2 Euthanasia and the medical practice from 1870 to the World War II

The intensive development of medicine from the late 19th century, with its increasing dependence on medical technology and institutionalization of health care, significantly affected the interpretation of good death. Since curative medicine started to exhaust more and more health care resources in terms of human resources, technical and economical means, the care for incurable and dying patients drifted out of the main focus of medical interest. Instead of the physician, it was the nurse who sat down at the bed of dying patient or this task was entrusted to clergy. Gradually physicians stopped to practise euthanasia as a way of accompanying a dying patient toward a peaceful and painless death. Furthermore, they started to apply the new possibilities of resuscitation (cardiopulmonary resuscitation in particular) to dying patients as well. A new treatment option appeared, namely the

---

[68] The periodization proposed by Vanderpool (2004) has been adopted here.

[69] Marx, C.F.H. (1952). Medical Euthanasia, *Journal of the History of Medicine and Allied Sciences*, Vol. 7, No. 4 (April 1952), pp. 401-416. First published in Latin in 1826, English translation by W. Cane in 1952; quotation from Vanderpool (2004, p. 1425).

[70] The Percival standard of medical ethics (*Code of Medical Ethics*, 1803), adopted by the American Medical Association (AMA) in 1847, assigned a professional duty to physicians to not abandon incurable patients and those who are dying because they deserve the physician's medical art in the easing of suffering and, in particular, the physician's human support. (Chauncey, 1975).

possibility to prolong life by technical means. Such prolongation of life (and suffering), being contrary to the concept of a natural death, had been previously regarded as unacceptable; however, once technically possible, it began to be practised. (Stewart, 1918). This was further compounded by the idea of evolutionary theory based on natural selection as introduced previously in the chapter, becoming increasingly influential; with individual life losing its importance. These and other factors caused a fundamental turnaround in society's understanding of good death; a new concept of good death arose, namely euthanasia as death induced by the physician for hopelessly sick patients. An important theoretical contribution to this change was the essay by Samuel D. Williams entitled "Euthanasia", published in London in 1872. According to Williams, euthanasia is a painless death for incurably and hopelessly sick persons. He goes on to state that it is even a physician's duty to recognize such a situation and if the patient wishes so, to administrate anaesthetics which would render the patient unconscious and proceed to terminate his/her suffering by a quick and painless killing.[71]

A new interpretation of good death started at the beginning of the 20th century when euthanasia became a *terminus technicus* for the killing of undesirable and "unfit" persons, usually mentally or physically handicapped people.[72] The theoretical background for euthanasia was an evolutionary approach to genetics[73] which modified genetics in its application to become eugenics. Eugenics later became a tool for racial "purification". So eugenics inspired by Darwinism was transformed into eugenic euthanasia, the elimination of those who are "unfit"[74] (Weikart, 2002).

---

[71] In his time, Williams' concept of euthanasia caused great excitement for its culturally non-traditional, legally questionable and medically unorthodox approach. For physicians, such an approach was held to be contrary to medical praxis (against *lex artis*). So until now several medical professional associations, including the World Medical Association (WMA), have repeatedly proclaimed euthanasia as contrary to medical practice. (One should add that in 1949, in the most influential International Code of Medical Ethics, the World Medical Association proclaimed that abortion is contrary to medical practice. Nevertheless, such a position is no longer held by the WMA.) - See *Policies* available at http://www.wma.net/. Cited 21.03.2011.

[72] In 1920 in Leipzig (Germany), a slim booklet (62 pages) was published by jurist Karl Binding and psychiatrist Alfred Hoche. Its original title is "*Freigabe der Vernichtung lebensunwerten Lebens: ihr Mass und ihre Form*" (Unworthy life at free disposal for its annihilation: the measure and form of this annihilation). This booklet, dealing with the possibility to destroy unworthy low quality life, became the theoretical background for the subsequent eugenic euthanasia movement; in 1933 it became a manual for mass killing during the Nazi period.

[73] Indirect resources were used, such as the works by Francis Galton (*Hereditary Genius. An Inquiry into Its Laws and Consequences,* 1869; *Inquiries into Human Faculty and Its Development*, 1883).

[74] Darwin's student Ernst Haeckel (1834-1919), looking for inspiration in Antiquity, proposed that German physicians should painlessly kill physically and mentally handicapped people. As a scientific justification, he looked to evolutionary anthropology (*Anthropogenie oder Entwickelungsgeschichte des Menschen*. Leipzig 1874).

It should be noted that in Germany, during the Nazi era from 1933, the Law for the Prevention of Hereditarily Diseased Offspring was in force (*Gesetz zur Verhütung erbkranken Nachwuchses*). Based on this law, some 300 000 people were involuntarily sterilized (6 000 of them died as a result of the surgery). The indications for this involuntary sterilization were "a serious physical of mental hereditary handicap: congenital dementia, schizophrenia, manic-depressive syndrome, congenital epilepsy, chorea Huntington, congenital blindness, congenital deafness, serious hereditary physical malformation, serious alcoholism".

On the first of September 1939, coinciding with the outbreak of the Second World War, the Reichchancellor Adolf Hitler issued a decree ordering that a "mercy death" (*Gnadentod*) be provided to those "incurably sick ones".[75] As a result, more than 100,000 psychiatric patients and thousands of seriously ill children were killed. This eugenics programme was euphemistically termed "euthanasia".[76] Related to this "euthanasia" done by German physicians on the German population, racial euthanasia ("racial hygiene") [77] focussed on the Jewish and Roma populations continued.[78]

4.3 Euthanasia and medical practice after World War II

During World War II and in the post-war period, several techniques were developed which provided new possibilities to prolong life (for instance antibiotics, pacemakers, defibrillators, dialysis) and several new fields such as transplantation or intensive care medicine arose. Advancements in cardiology made it possible to avoid a sudden death. Gradually it became common to replace the physiological functions of individual human organs with machines. With one exception (the brain), today we are able to substitute all the organs of the human body. Among many physicians, the approach requiring that everything be done that is technically possible and practically accessible to maintain the life of the patient - or more precisely, physiological functions of the human body - prevailed. Physicians became enthralled by the scientific and technological progress of medicine, even when applying it in clinically hopeless situations, unless they were stopped by multifunctional failure, by sepsis or by a clear-headed colleague. Later, depending on the concrete cultural context, this behaviour was later upheld by the courts or by the pressure of the patient's family. As the actual practice derived from the medical goal of saving life, the following guideline was being applied: If it is not possible to cure the patient and to save life then at least extend life as long as possible (as if the longest prolonged life would be the greatest success of medicine). As a result, medicine became a victim of its own success (Krämer, 1997). Medicine's task was to battle with the enemy beyond the door (death) for as long as possible. Logically the additional suffering of both patient and his/her family was produced in a non-natural way. Death ceased to be a natural event, instead a spiteful spoiler who in the end defeats a marvellous army equipped with the latest medical technology and science. This strategy of a prolongation of life also gave rise to the question of quality of life. The call for euthanasia as a mercy death was a reaction to this technologized and dehumanizing medicine (Lock, 1996). A new concept of euthanasia came into being: A good death is a merciful death (for technology does not know mercy). In this context so called "passive euthanasia" has been discussed; this "passive euthanasia" was understood as an option with or without the patient's request not to use what has been called "extraordinary means" and by an "act of omission" (Husak, 1980; Kamm, 1994) to make it possible that a person in a terminal stage will die (McMahan, 1993). According to some people death is the

[75] This one line order of Hitler's can be found in books such as that by Urban Wiesing (2004, p. 60).

[76] Therefore it is understandable that in Germany the term "euthanasia" (Euthanasie) still evokes strong associations with Nazism.

[77] A theoretical handbook for racial hygiene is the study by F. Lenz "*Menschliche Auslese und Rassenhygiene*", published 1923 in Munich (3rd edition in 1931, 593 pp.).

[78] The eugenic euthanasia as it was practised during the Nazi period is only mentioned here. For more detailed account see Michalsen & Reinhart (2006) and Vermaat (2002).

only mercy in life and it would be inhuman to deny such mercy to a person in a medically desperate situation. Moreover, to produce artificial and additional suffering by techno-medical means would be contrary to human rights: "No one shall be subjected to torture or to inhuman or degrading treatment or punishment." (Art. 4, European Charter of Fundamental Rights, 2000)

The act of mercy, avoiding any further suffering caused by advanced medical technology, has been discussed in the context of withholding and withdrawing treatment. Once a competent patient can decide if he/she will accept or refuse any medical treatment and once medical treatment is based on the legal provisions specified by international conventions such as the Convention for the Protection of Human Rights and Dignity of the Human Being with Regard to the Application of Biology and Medicine (Oviedo, 1997), it is obvious that a competent patient can refuse any life-saving treatment, regardless of whether it constitutes withholding or withdrawing, in a situation of medical futility. (Annas, 2005).There was (and still remains) a lot of haziness about the notion of euthanasia in this context. It is true that historically the term "passive euthanasia" has been used in this context. However I'm arguing that to use such a term today leads to new misapprehensions. Once the legal framework of advance directives (Cantor, 1993) and living wills have been established by the legislation of a particular country, it is meaningless to conclude that a person who has decided not to be treated by cardiopulmonary resuscitation or by other life supporting tools such as dialysis in terminal renal failure is *requesting euthanasia*!

What the post-war development of medicine has brought to the concept of good death is that of *mercy killing*, death upon the patient's request. (Behnke & Bok, 1975). Similarly there were many arguments brought forth to support *mercy death* as a refusal of dysthanasia (retention of death) or as an active voluntary termination of life.[79] As a result of these developments, a number of associations for euthanasia were born.[80]

The model of good death (mercy death) which arose in the 20th century also has another manifestation in the hospice movement, with different hermeneutics of mercy. Historically it operated on a certain modification of the model of good death as it was used in the Middle Ages and in Modern Times: mercy death meaning help and support in dying. Both the hospice model of good death and the model of good death as voluntary active euthanasia appeal to a respect of the dignity of the dying person, although the interpretation of dignity can differ considerably. The meaningless prolongation of life (and the related suffering) leads not only to a reappraisal of terms such as medical futility;[81] it also challenges the notion of euthanasia as an active termination of life when the patient is physically not able to terminate his/her own life by him/her self (suicide or

[79] Some of these arguments are discussed in the chapter "Everything under control: How and when to die. A critical analysis of the arguments for euthanasia".

[80] The Voluntary Euthanasia Legislation Society (1930), The Euthanasia Society of America (1937, later Concern for Dying), Nederlandse Vereniging voor Vrijwillige Euthanasie (The Dutch Society for Voluntary Euthanasia, 1976), Deutsche Gesellschaft für humanes Sterben (German Society for Humane Dying, 1980), The World Federation of Right To Die Societies (1980) under which can be found almost all other similar societies and associations.

[81] The former distinction "ordinary means" and "extraordinary means" used for a moral appraisal of medical futility, in particular by theologians, is thanks to the rapid scientific and technological development of (not only intensive) medicine completely futile: what was considered "extraordinary means" yesterday has become "ordinary means" today.

assisted suicide). In the meantime useful distinctions have been established and one can discriminate between the intentional shortening of life as a by-product of the pain therapy (administration of opiates such as morphine), inducing terminal sedation, terminating of life (e.g. by administration of lethal doses of morphine) and the respectful allowance of a dying patient to die (Birnbacher, 1995; Illhardt et al. 1998; Schöne-Seifert, 1997; Spaemann & Fuchs, 1997). To allow a dying patient to die with the medical support of palliative care and with the human support of interpersonal relationships - which is more difficult to provide than medical comfort - is probably the latest task and new goal of contemporary medicine.[82] Another problem is that biological death often follows the social death of the patient.

In the period between the 17th and 20th century the understanding of good death underwent fundamental changes. Initially euthanasia was understood to be the active physician's support for the dying patient within a natural death. In this model euthanasia is the good (complete) care of the dying.

From approximately the 1880s, a concept of euthanasia was implemented which meant the termination of the life of a patient in a medically hopeless situation induced by the physician. In the period leading up to the World War II, euthanasia was understood as the (involuntary) killing of "unfit" people (eugenic euthanasia) which during World War II developed into racial euthanasia (the Holocaust). In the post-war period the concept of euthanasia as mercy (assisted) death arose; its two basic forms being "letting die" (to make possible a dignified dying) and "mercy killing" (killing upon request or without request). (Bishop, 2006). In contemporary discussions the focus is not on the "mercy killing" issue but on a rational and intersubjective-communicative framework for end-of-life decision-making regarding the support of human life in its final stages in an era of very technologically advanced medicine.

5. Various historical meanings of the term 'euthanasia'

As a summary of the previous research, the main typologies of good death as they appear through history are provided below.

1. Easy, quick and serene (natural) death.

Suetonius' description of the death of Augustus serves as an example.

This concept can be found from Antiquity to the present. However this understanding of euthanasia as a peaceful, painless and swift death is not the predominant approach in the present. Furthermore a contemporary medical death is no longer perceived as a *natural* death.

Used in this sense, this euthanasia is at present perceived as an ambition and yearning which does not correspond to the present day medical reality of a prolonged and technified

---

[82] Already in 1988 the American Medical Association set the following to be a standard: "...a physician may do what is medically necessary to alleviate severe pain, or cease or omit treatment to permit a terminally ill patient whose death is imminent to die. However, he should not intentionally cause death." (AMA, 1992, p. 46). In 1987 the World Medical Association published the following: "Euthanasia, that is the act of deliberately ending the life of a patient, even at the patient's own request or at the request of close relatives, is unethical. This does not prevent the physician from respecting the desire of a patient to allow the natural process of death to follow its course in the terminal phase of sickness." Available at www.wma.net. Cited 26.03.2011.

death with additional suffering. This typology of euthanasia represents rather an escape from a medico-technical death or an alternative to this medically prolonged and technically supported dying - far from a natural death.

2. Voluntary termination of life by oneself in a situation when living holds no value or death seems to be the lesser of two evils (and the option to die seems to be the lesser evil).

The classical example is suicide (*autothanatos*) as an expression of autonomy, control over one's life, and responsibility towards oneself and towards society.

This concept has been relevant in Antiquity (voluntary death), and in Modern Times (Nietzsche: quick and free death) including the present. (Engelhardt, 1989). This form of free *autothanatos* (suicide) is often understood as euthanasia in debates on assisted suicide; euthanasia in this sense is a suicide in fact, though medically assisted. In these debates, (assisted) suicide has often been semantically incorrectly replaced by euthanasia. Once replaced by euthanasia, the (medically) assisted suicide (*A* kills *A*) cannot be distinguished from euthanasia as the death of *B* by *A* upon the explicit request of *B*. So the term "euthanasia" used as a denotation for a peaceful and painless termination of life by means of assisted suicide is euthanasia rather in a metaphorical way.

3. Medical accompaniment of a dying person (easing pain, human support, without the possibility to prolong life).

As an example the *euthanasia exteriori* as proposed by Francis Bacon can be given.

This concept can be found from Antiquity until the late 19th century, being the main concept of euthanasia in the period between the 17th and late 19th centuries.

This typology of euthanasia can be used even today as an inspiration for palliative care for seriously ill and dying patients. One of the challenges of this model of euthanasia is the re-humanization of technical medicine, well-rounded care for the dying patient and a rejection of prolonging the dying period.

4. Involuntary termination of the life of unwanted people (incurably sick, handicapped) for the good of society (secondary for the benefit of the killed person).

All cases of *social euthanasia* would come under this model.

This concept was influential in Antiquity; in Modern Times it has been used in the period between 1870 and 1939.

This form of euthanasia was in fact the elimination of persons suffering from serious incurable diseases and from physical or mental handicaps. Motivated and justified by mercy (*mercy killing, Grandentod*) this killing was a form of involuntary euthanasia, in some context even supported by law (e.g. in Germany by the Law for the Prevention of Hereditarily Diseased Offspring from the year 1933).

5. Involuntary termination of life of "unfit" people (based on genetics or race).

A specific example for this type of good death is the *eugenic euthanasia* as it was practiced under the Nazi regime during World War II.

This form of involuntary euthanasia was extended to genocide, resulting in the killing of millions of people (Jews and Roma primarily). Beside such racial eugenic euthanasia, medical eugenic euthanasia was also conducted during the Nazi regime; the previous more socially identifiable conditions, based on physical and mental handicaps were extended to medical indications such as schizophrenia, cyclothymia, blindness, deafness, homosexuality and many others. All these medical conditions qualified for mercy death (eugenic euthanasia).

6. Inducing an "easy death" by *sedatives* (including terminal sedation) - shortening of life without direct killing,[83] foreseen but nonintended death.

This model of good death has been one of the forms of euthanasia discussed in the recent past and at present.

Once the shortening of life became a de facto side-effect of pain therapy (e.g. administration of morphine), it was discussed whether and to what extent such an abbreviation of life is morally justifiable. Some authors have argued that foreseen and non intended death caused by pain therapy (administration of high doses of morphine) is acceptable while an intended death would be morally unacceptable, justifying this assessment by the double effect doctrine.[84] (Boyle, 1991; Hawryluck & Harvey, 2000; Kamm, 1999; Klein, 2004). However, the application of the double-effect doctrine is highly problematic in this context (one has to take into account not only the real shortening of life but also the probability of death being caused by the pain killers directly). To call pain therapy which also includes the acceleration of the death factor "euthanasia" is not semantically and ethically meaningful.

7. *Physician assisted suicide*

Some people classify physician assisted suicide as euthanasia, subsuming suicide under euthanasia, which is confusing and out of the semantics proposed in this chapter (the killing of another person is fundamentally different from suicide).

Historically this assisted suicide has a similarity to the ancient notion of *autothanatos* (e.g. the Stoics), however suicide as it has been known throughout history should not be intermingled with physician assisted suicide - as we understand it today as a very specific type of suicide and fundamentally different from (unassisted) suicide - for at least two reasons: first the aid to conduct suicide is solely help, not direct perpetration; therefore the modifier "assisted" is used, second the involvement of a physician, with regard to the medical profession as such and its therapeutic role, is of a specific moral relevance; this aspect is evoked by the modifier "physician". (Deigh, 1998; van der Maas, 1996; Wolf, 2008).

Should a clear semantical framework be used for euthanasia discussions, then physician assisted suicide has to be distinguished from euthanasia, and not subsumed under euthanasia. While in euthanasia the physician is the perpetrator of death, in physician assisted suicide it is the patient who causes death.

8. No application of medically futile therapy which prolongs the life (and suffering) of the terminally ill patient: *withholding* life-sustaining treatment

The typical situation is one of withholding life-sustaining treatment with or without the patient's consent because the treatment would be medically futile for that patient.

Some people consider the withholding of medically futile treatment as "passive" euthanasia while others do not call withholding of treatment "euthanasia" at all. If the withholding of

[83] The fear of an abridgment of life (even that of a dying patient) is understandable, since such a shortening of life is in contrast to the general tendency to prolong life. However, such fear should be contextualized in the situation of a terminally ill and dying patient, where pain therapy (opiates) - which alleviate suffering, and support dignity in dying but often shorten the life of the patient- is arguable necessary.

[84] The doctrine of double effect, having been developed and applied to end-of-life decision making chiefly by various Catholic theologians as an authoritative tool for assessment of moral acceptability within moral absolutism, has been intensively criticized and refuted by many authors (Donagan, 1991; Kamm, 1991; Quill, 1997). It seems to be very helpful in contemporary debates focused on the shortening of life as a side-effect of pain therapy and in the context of euthanasia.

futile treatment, thus hastening the dying process, is held as euthanasia (even as "passive" euthanasia and therefore "not so bad" as the "active" one), then the withholding of medically futile treatment is morally wrong because such an act would be equated with ("passive") euthanasia. Then two completely different notions of euthanasia have been applied in the form of a "good one" namely "passive" euthanasia (withholding, letting die) and a "bad one" namely "active" euthanasia (active killing). Thus two completely different situations have been denominated by one and the same term, then we have situations were euthanasia is "good" and "permissible" and situations where euthanasia is "evil" and "wrong". In the end we have deeply confusing semantics which causes that euthanasia discussions will be meaningless.

9. Termination of medically futile therapy which prolongs life (and suffering) of the terminally ill patient: *withdrawing* life-sustaining treatment

This type of "euthanasia" coincides with withdrawing of medically futile therapy (including life-sustaining treatment) with or without the patient's consent.

Some people hold the withdrawing of medically futile treatment as „passive" euthanasia while other people do not subsume the withdrawing of life-sustaining treatment in a situation of medical futility under euthanasia, arguing that euthanasia in the proper sense can be active (voluntary) only.

Assuming that both killing and letting die are morally wrong, then any therapy (treatment) which has been started has to continue until the death of the patient because it would be morally wrong to withdraw (any) treatment. Then the morally right approach would be "to cure until death" and to put the patient under medically conducted torture. The only prevention of such a medically generated ordeal would be the patient's timely refusal or late court decision.

In conclusion both the withholding and withdrawing of medically futile treatment shall not be called euthanasia (even if it is considered "passive").

10. Painless termination of life of an *unbearably suffering* patient by the physician upon the patient's request.

This model is called voluntary (active) euthanasia,[85] meaning that a clearly competent patient makes a voluntary and continuous request for death and the physician conducts the act of euthanasia (killing by medical means). This type of euthanasia is legally permitted in the Netherlands, Belgium and Luxemburg. Within this typology, euthanasia, being clearly defined with specifying conditions (the Rotterdam criteria), can be called the "Dutch model" of euthanasia.

It is obvious that unbearable suffering is too subjective (only the suffering person can decide if the suffering is "unbearable") and to difficult to be grasped and objectified. The criterion "unbearable suffering" does not seem to be in accordance with our objective (evidence based) medicine. Moreover this criterion could also qualify psychiatric patients (especially those suffering from depression) and somatically healthy persons suffering from "tired of life" and other states of existential suffering such as meaningless and pointlessness to request death.

11. Painless termination of life of a *terminally ill* patient (terminal stage of life) by a physician upon the patient's request.

---

[85] See the chapter "Voluntary Active Euthanasia: The Debate" by Louis-Jacques van Bogaert in this book.

This model is also called voluntary (active) euthanasia. It differs from the previous one by the primary criterion: here the primary qualifying condition is terminal illness (terminal stage), in the previous model it was unbearable suffering. It should be noted that the Dutch model does not include terminal stage as a criterion for euthanasia.

Euthanasia as the painless termination of the dying patient (with or without request) is practised in the grey zone void of regulation (beside the eventual agreement between the two actors, patient and physician or relatives and physician). If conducted without the competent patient's request, such type of euthanasia belongs to the next category.

12. Painless termination of life of a terminally ill or unbearably suffering patient by the physician without the patient's request (the patient is incompetent).[86]

This model, called *nonvolutary euthanasia*, combines two previous typologies (euthanasia in terminal stage of illness, euthanasia in unbearable suffering) with the significant difference that it is conducted without the patient's request. In this model of euthanasia one of the two criteria (terminal stage of illness or unbearable suffering) must be met and the decision to conduct euthanasia is made by the physician, without any patient's request, consent or approval (the patient is unable to give their informed consent).

13. Painless termination of life of a terminally ill or heavily suffering competent patient by the physician without patient's request or against patient's will.

This model is called *involuntary euthanasia;* euthanasia of a competent patient against their will. Involuntary euthanasia is a crime. Some people argue that crime does not refer to a "good" death and therefore it should be not called *eu*thanasia.

14. (In)voluntary painless termination of life of a person other than a terminal patient.

This type of euthanasia would for instance include quadriplegic or psychiatric patients. (Sheldon, 1994).

15. (In)voluntary painless termination of life of a terminally ill or unbearably suffering person by someone other than a physician.

This type of euthanasia differs from all other conceived forms, being that of it being conducted by any other person other than a physician, ergo euthanasia by a nurse or another health care professional or by a person who does not even belong to the health care staff, e.g. a relative.

It has been stressed that semantics is a necessary starting point for any discussion on euthanasia; it is crucial to clarify what exactly is understood by the term "euthanasia" before any argument for or against will be used. It became clear that euthanasia is not an end in itself with intrinsic value but a means to realize the end of a good death, or more precisely, a quality dying experience. (Emanuel, 1999).

Among the fifteen aforementioned typologies, one in particular should be emphasised, number eleven, which seems to be the most appropriate semantic tool for the concept of euthanasia. According to this definition, euthanasia, being different from assisted suicide (Beech, 1995; Watts & Howell, 1992) and from other scenarios of end-of-life decisions such as withholding, withdrawing or terminal sedation, is a deliberate act of termination of the life of a competent (autonomous) patient in the terminal stage of illness by a physician

[86] Specific attention should be given to the problem of the euthanasia of children, which would fall under typology 14 (newborn children with abnormalities) or older children under the legal age (typology 12 and 14) and to the issue of euthanasia in geriatric patients (with diminished cognitive capacities including conditions such as dementia).

upon an explicit and persistent request of this patient and for his/her sake. Thus under the term "euthanasia" so called active voluntary euthanasia is understood. Should these criteria not be met, a good death can be discussed within a different framework, defined by different criteria such as involuntariness, other than terminal stage of illness (e.g. psychiatric patient), another person than the physician administrating the lethal dose, and other parameters.

6. The meaning of euthanasia in current discussions

In the next section, the conceptual understanding of euthanasia in current discussions will be examined. As it follows from the previous typology of euthanasia, the current debates on euthanasia are mainly based on typologies 10 through 14; some people also include typology 8 (withholding treatment) and typology 9 (withdrawing treatment) under euthanasia, under the guise of "passive euthanasia", and thereby, in a misleading way, calling the reduction or termination of medically futile treatment "euthanasia". So attention will first be given to the distinction between "passive" and "active" euthanasia.

6.1 Euthanasia as active voluntary death

If under the term "euthanasia" are included scenarios of withholding and withdrawing treatment, medical futility and terminal sedation, then to end medical futility or even not to start medically futile treatment is euthanasia; thus to avoid such meaningless (medically futile) treatment is euthanasia. So euthanasia is omnipresent in these end-of-life decisions. If everything is considered euthanasia then we lose our ability to correctly administer (or not) treatment. Therefore what is crucial is the art of distinguishing between treatment options while maintaining an unbiased and level semantic playing field, which allows to make the dying process as humane and as dignified as possible, without applying every kind of treatment that is technically possible, but medically futile and humanely problematic (to be rather euphemistic). That's why such care cannot be called (any form of) euthanasia!

Despite the fact that so called "passive euthanasia" has appeared in the literature and in euthanasia debates for several decades and continues to appear in both the literature and in public debates - one can understand when, why, and under which circumstances this term was developed - but if euthanasia is understood as the killing of *B* by *A* upon an explicit request of *B*, then the term "passive euthanasia" remains semantic nonsense and a source of many misunderstandings, emotions and frustration. What has been called "passive euthanasia" (*A* allows *B* to die without undertaking all technically possible but medically futile steps) should rather be called "letting die" or "allowing to die" since the life of the dying person cannot be saved. This "allowing to die" is in line with the respect for human dignity and could be labelled as a "good death" but not as "euthanasia" is the sense described above. The former distinction "active" and "passive" euthanasia aimed to distinguish morally acceptable "passive euthanasia" as a form of non-obligatory passivity (omission), which did not apply so-called "extraordinary means" which had been previously regarded as morally obligatory to use, from morally unacceptable "active euthanasia" consisting of killing a person (homicide).[87]

---

[87] In the late 1960s and early 1970s both bioethicists and national medical associations started to approve, under specified conditions, "of some kinds of instances of what is called 'passive' euthanasia"

The cessation of the employment of extraordinary means to prolong life when there is irrefutable evidence that death is imminent is the decision made primarily by the patient and/or by the family and/or by physicians. But such a decision and such cessation of medical treatment is very different from what is at present considered "euthanasia". The doctrine establishing an important moral difference between "commission" and "omission", between "active" and "passive", between "ordinary means" and "extraordinary means" became useless and misleading when applied to euthanasia as it was understood in the 1970s and 1980s (Husak, 1980; Jonsen, 1998; Kamm, 1994; Walton, 1976). It follows that in one case, euthanasia is sometimes permissible, while in another case always forbidden. This doctrine, based on the distinction between act (commission) and omission, and adopted by the American Medical Association in 1973, was very soon challenged, as this would lead to decisions on life and death being made on morally irrelevant grounds (Rachels, 1975), at present not recognized by most philosophers. Moreover, active euthanasia (the "bad" one) would be in many cases more humane than passive euthanasia (the "permissible" one). So later, when medical associations issued guidelines for withholding and withdrawing treatment and for palliative and terminal sedation, they often stressed that this policy is not identical with active euthanasia, without declaring that they are authorizing "passive" euthanasia.

From the present perspective, the former distinction of "active" and "passive" euthanasia as established in the 1970s, with the aim of helping physicians adapt to the new situations they were finding themselves in and to move from a curative paradigm to a palliative paradigm (the shift from "cure" to "care") and to provide a moral rationale for the dignified treatment of terminally ill patients is a good illustration of the changes taking place and serves as an appropriate departure point to clarify terminology and then to discuss ethics. At the beginning of the 21st century, not only philosophers but physicians from palliative care units have argued that so-called "passive euthanasia" is a contradiction in terms, reasoning that palliative care which saves the dying patient from extreme pain, protects human dignity

---

because there was an acute need for some regulatory tools for the newly arisen "very pressing, widespread problems introduced by recent developments in medical technology"(Walton, 1976, p. 343). So in the case "of a terminally ill patient, who is in great pain and who is known to be about to die with overwhelming probability in a few days or a few hours, and shows symptoms of immediately imminent death" a new medical paradigm emerged, namely the option not to use all medical technology currently available to prolong life. As part of this new medical paradigm, the ideas such as "not to prolong the patient's life for a short and excruciatingly painful time" and not to use the available "active emergency methods of resuscitation" (e.g., defibrillators or heart massage) and not to "do what would constitute extreme cruelty" asserted themselves. (Walton, 1976, p. 343). Douglas Walton summarizes the debates of that time in the following way: "What is the physician to do? It has seemed to many that heroic measures should, under certain conditions, be waived. But does not such a waiver constitute 'killing' the patient? On the other side, is not a too-strenuous interference in the course of nature equally morally abhorrent, cruel, and inhumane? The latter course may not seem to serve the interests of the patient, if unthinkingly or automatically always applied." (Walton, 1976, p. 343) As a possible basis for resolving these problems the distinction "active" and "passive" euthanasia has been often cited. "The former entails active interference in the course of natural events, the taking of steps through positive action. Passive euthanasia carries with it no such requirement but only failure to institute positive action, letting nature take its course, so to speak. Thus it is sometimes felt that passive euthanasia is morally acceptable, under certain conditions, but that active euthanasia is never morally acceptable under any conditions." (Walton, 1976, p. 343).

and the patient from additional suffering and medical torture does not amount to euthanasia (Riley et at., 2009). The European Association of Palliative Care consistently refuses to call any of the following clinical procedures euthanasia: withholding futile treatment, withdrawing futile treatment or terminal sedation, emphasizing that euthanasia can be active in nature only (Materstvedt, 2003, p. 98).

In my judgement to use the term "euthanasia" within palliative care provided *lege artis* is an expression of disrespect and a violation of the efforts of palliative medicine and the health care staff who accompany the dying persons, alleviating pain, providing both human and medical comfort in dying. Naturally they cannot agree to such human support being called euthanasia, using the same word as "mercy killing" does. There is a huge difference in the "good death" of palliative care: the patient dies due to the disease, not to the physician or attending personnel who kill the dying (terminally ill) patient (Callahan, 1999).

Fortunately enough the distinction "active" and "passive" euthanasia has gradually been abandoned since the 1990s (Brock, 1992, 1993; Campbell et al. 2005; McLachlan, 2008; Warnock & Macdonald, 2008). However, not having disappeared completely, they can still be found among some authors. When for instance John Keown defines euthanasia as "the intentional termination of life by act or omission" (Keown, 2002, p.12), he bases his concept of euthanasia on the distinction "active" and "passive", holding "omission" for "passive euthanasia". Recently Gesang (2008), insisting on the distinction "active" and "passive", has proposed specified conditions to be met so as to be considered passive euthanasia, classifying many cases as such.[88] And so we are returned to "moral" and "immoral" euthanasia. Gerrard and Wilkinson (2005) examined the permissibility of so-called "passive euthanasia", emphasizing the possibility to soften the term euthanasia as a whole by including withdrawing or withholding life-prolonging treatment, as a result of their greater moral acceptance.

The important difference - not in euthanasia per se but in all acts conducted by human beings as human beings (*actus hominis*)- is the matter of intent, which is often confused with motive (Campbell, 2005). If euthanasia is defined as "intentional or foreseen life-shortening" (Keown, 2002, p.15), then the administration of morphine, which in addition to serving as pain therapy objectively shortens the patient's life, is euthanasia as well. If not only an intentional termination of life but also pain therapy falls under euthanasia, then it is really difficult to discuss euthanasia. In a similar vein Moody (2003) requires the critical attribute "*foreseen* and *intended* death", however as concurrent and simultaneous conditions. "It may be optimistic to expect the emergence of common definitions, at least in the near future, not least as the different definitions reflect different underlying moral presuppositions whose resolutions is a prerequisite to definitional consensus. Until such consensus is achieved participants should at least be open and clear about which definition they are employing and why." (Keown, 2002, p. 17). Obviously, one has to attempt to start a discussion with clarified semantics but it is also a matter of preconceptions that determines which definition is being used and why.

[88] "Passive euthanasia occurs if the general conditions for euthanasia are fulfilled and if letting it happen leads to death. If it is a case of letting it happen leads to death only those actions may be involved that withdraw a medical measure that a doctor started previously. Every other form of euthanasia is active." (Gesang, 2008, p. 179).

6.2 Euthanasia – a core definition and the specifying criteria

Within the conceptualization of euthanasia, the core notion of euthanasia as the primary definition and the set(s) of secondary criteria have to be distinguished. If for instance someone defines euthanasia as "the termination of life of an incurable patient" then any incurable diseases such as diabetes would qualify for a request for euthanasia. Obviously some additional specifying criteria should be applied. Or if euthanasia is described as "the active, intentional termination of life" (Keown, 2002, p. 10), then any suicide is at the same time euthanasia. Withal both the termination of life of an incurable patient and active termination of life apply for euthanasia, belonging to the essential conceptualization of euthanasia. If the definition proposed by Brock (1999, p. 298) - under which euthanasia is defined as "deliberate killing of an innocent person"- then some people, presuming that a late foetus is a person, could argue that there is little difference between euthanasia and abortion. The deficiency of such a definition is that not every "killing" is *ipso facto* euthanasia.

This conceptual diversity of the core definition of euthanasia has been recently shown by Quaghebeur et al. (2009). Based on this review of argument-based ethics literature, it is evident that many imprecise definitions of euthanasia can be found in the literature over the last three decades. The mentioned study demonstrates that there is a growing tendency in the preciseness and accuracy in the definition of euthanasia; while in the late 1980s and in early 1990s euthanasia was often defined as "mercy killing", "allowing to die or helping to die", "killing a patient", "bringing about of death through lethal drug dose", "taking active steps to end a patient's life", "an intentional, causally significant (either through omission or commission), foreseeable, and direct action undertaken for the purpose of ending life a person, for whatever reason", in the late 1990s and in 2000s more precise definitions such as "direct termination of a competent patient's life at the patient's request", "beneficent active voluntary euthanasia" and "deliberate action to terminate life by someone other than, and at the request of the patient" can be found (Quaghebeur et al., 2009). The said study also shows that more and more authors make use of the definition of euthanasia as it has been established by Dutch and Belgian legislation which defines euthanasia as "administration of lethal drugs by someone other than the person concerned with the explicit intention of ending a patient's life, at the latter's explicit request" (Belgian Ministry of Justice, 2002; Leenen, 1998; van der Heide et al., 2003, 2007; van der Wal & Dillmann, 1994).

Within the overview of definitions provided by Quaghebeur (2009, Table 1, 2, 3) two different types of core definitions with regard to exactness can be found. One type of these essential definitions is based on "killing the patient" ("a death brought about by someone else", "purposeful shortening of human life through active or direct assistance", "killing someone at the end stages of life", "interrupt the patient's ability to sustain life", "causing the death of an innocent person", "ending the life of another person on the grounds of unworthy living"). It has been already argued that such a definition is insufficient. Another type of these essential definitions is based on "voluntary active euthanasia" ("the direct termination of a competent patient's life at the patient's request", "the intentional bringing about of person's death at their own request in the absence of coercion"). This definition based on the concept of voluntary euthanasia (voluntary euthanasia, by definition, can never be a "passive" one) is much closer to the situations which are covered by the term euthanasia. However there are some strategies which change or manipulate the concept of euthanasia. (Campbell, 1999). So for instance if the focus is on "activeness" in euthanasia as critique or objection to so-called "passive" euthanasia then the distinction "voluntary" and "involuntary" (resp. "non-voluntary") can be cloaked and also involuntary euthanasia can be also covered by the term "euthanasia" which is obviously contradictory to the standard definition ("termination of patient's life upon their explicit request by a physician"). Only few of the definitions based on the "voluntary active euthanasia" concept include additional criteria such as physician's activity or suffering. The lack of these secondary or additional criteria demonstrates the problem we still have with the basic understanding of euthanasia in the professional literature, not to mention the perception of the general public. If we take the "better" set of essential definitions of euthanasia, understanding euthanasia to be any medical killing upon the person's own request, then any patient is eligible to request euthanasia. At the same time such a definition is of minimal help for any euthanasia discussion.

In 1988 Michael Wreen attempted to provide an analytical definition of euthanasia. It was obvious for him that "someone must kill a live creature, or let her die, if euthanasia is to occur" (Wreen, 1988, p. 637). According to Wreen (1998), person *A* committed an act of euthanasia if and only if the following conditions were fulfilled:

1. *A* killed *B* or let her die.
2. *A* intended to kill *B*.
3. The intention specified in (2) was at least partial cause of the action specified in (1).
4. The causal journey from the intention specified in (2) to the action specified in (1) is more or less in accordance with *A*'s plan of action.
5. *A*'s killing of *B* is a voluntary action.
6. The motive for the action specified in (1), the motive standing behind the intention specified in (2), is the good of the person killed.
7. The good specified in (6) is, or at least includes, the avoidance of evil.

This analytical definition of euthanasia, although staying within the former broad understanding of euthanasia which subsumes "letting die" as well, is more precise compared to other definitions. However, not specifying who decides about the good of *B*, this definition does not take into account the difference between voluntary and non-voluntary (or involuntary) euthanasia, which is of crucial importance. So if groups committed to the fundamental belief that the intentional killing of another person is wrong, despite having deep sympathy for those people who are suffering, understand euthanasia as "the intentional killing by act or omission of a dependent human being for his or her alleged benefit" [89], then a hypocrisy of "double effect" doctrine comes into play and the "life-saving" treatment in the form of medical torture have to continue which finally reinforces the argument for active euthanasia.

Another analytical definition of euthanasia was proposed by Beauchamp and Davidson (1979)[90] which is more focused on the causality and reasoning of killing then on its volition,

[89] This definition can be found at one of the leading websites dealing with euthanasia at: http://www.euthanasia.com/definitions.html. Cited 26.03.2011.

[90] "The death of a human being, A, is an instance of euthanasia if any only if (1) A's death is intended by at least one other human being, B, where B is either the cause of death or a causally relevant feature of the event resulting in death (whether by action or by omission); (2) there is either sufficient current evidence for B to believe that A is acutely suffering or irreversibly comatose, or there is sufficient current evidence related to A's present condition such that one or more known causal laws supports B's

covering rather "mercy killing" by compassion than the autonomous choice of the suffering person.

Yet in 1979 Beauchamp argued that "there are two distinctions which are commonly observed in the literature on euthanasia, and we assume that any definition which could not accommodate these distinctions is incorrect" (1979, p. 299). However in 2003 he gives a less analytical and much shorter definition of euthanasia: "Euthanasia is the act or practice of ending a person's life in order to release the person from an incurable disease, intolerable suffering, or undignified death" (Beauchamp, 2003, p. 179). Instead of the distinction between "commission" and "omission" other secondary criteria are introduced (incurable disease, intolerable suffering, or undignified death) which seems to be more important than the former distinction. The rhetoric of *killing* and *letting die* is questioned (Beauchamp, 2003). However this definition, being too general, does not discriminate between voluntary and involuntary euthanasia, though Beauchamp makes use of the terms voluntary and involuntary euthanasia (2003, p. 180).

Another definition of euthanasia has been suggested by Rosemary Firth. Her definition is more narrative then analytical. Euthanasia is (a) "the medical use of drugs to ease a painful and protracted, but inevitable death", (b) "a deliberate attempt to bring about or to hasten one's own death in sickness or suffering", (c) "actively assisting an aged, sick or handicapped person to a merciful death" (Firth, 1981). These suggested interpretations of euthanasia are rather more the phenomenology of good death. Assisted suicide comes under euthanasia (c), palliative care (a) would also come under euthanasia, the shortening of life by opiates (b) would also be considered euthanasia. Such a broad description has to be made more precise. Regarding free choice on euthanasia, Philippa Foot, already in 1977 pointed out the difficulty: Even in the case of voluntary active euthanasia, "it would be hard to devise procedures that would protect people from being persuaded into giving their consent" (Foot, 1977, p. 122).

6.3 A shift towards a more precise conceptualization of euthanasia

Recently a certain shift in the conceptualization of euthanasia can be identified in bioethics literature. While at the end of the 20th century a rather broad description of euthanasia was prevalent, in the 21st century a tendency can be observed to conceptualize euthanasia in a more precise way by applying a tighter description. This shift was reflected in the change between the first and second editions of the Encyclopedia of Ethics (Becker & Becker, 1992, 2001), which includes an article on euthanasia written by Marvin Kohl. In the first edition, Kohl (1992) tried to summarize the conceptualization of euthanasia in the following way: (a) euthanasia is "the act or method of painlessly inducing the death of a nonfetal sentient being" which distinguishes euthanasia from abortion (nonfetal sentient being), while not

belief that A will be in a condition of acute suffering or irreversibly comatoseness; (3) (a) B's primary reason for intending A's death is cessation of A's (actual or predicted) suffering or irreversible comatoseness, where B does not intend A's death for a different primary reason, though there may be other relevant reasons, and (b) there is sufficient current evidence for either A or B that causal means to A's death will not produce any more suffering than would be produced for A if B were not to intervene; (4) the causal means to the event of A's death are chosen by A or B to be as painless as possible, unless either A or B has an overridding reason for a more painful causal means, where the reasons for choosing the latter causal means does not conflict with the evidence in (3b); (5) A is a nonfetal organism." (Beauchamp & Davidson, 1979, p. 304).

distinguishing euthanasia in humans from euthanasia in animals; (b) euthanasia is "the act or method of directly causing or allowing the painless and quick death of a nonfetal being, so as to end suffering or an undesirable existence" which places "passive" euthanasia (allowing the death) under "euthanasia"; while the stated conditions (suffering, undesirable existence) remain insufficient for a suitable and applicable definition of euthanasia. Furthermore, the criterion "undesirable existence" is highly problematic since it could be interpreted to cover many diverse forms of (involuntary) euthanasia such as eugenic or social euthanasia. No distinction between euthanasia and suicide was described. Additional specific criteria would be necessary here.

It is both interesting and challenging to observe how in the second edition the same author changed his conceptualization of euthanasia: "An act of euthanasia is held to be voluntary only if there is full disclosure of relevant information to, and consent freely given by, the intended competent recipient of the act" (Kohl, 2001, p. 492).[91] First he distinguishes euthanasia from suicide, establishing a specific category of physician assisted suicide. Moreover, his concern is primarily with voluntary active euthanasia, stating that "the lines between voluntary, involuntary and non-voluntary euthanasia are crucial in a society that values both self-determination and compassion" (Kohl, 2001, p. 492). This development in Kohl's conceptualization of euthanasia demonstrates the general tendency to be more specific and not to subsume any form of killing under the term "euthanasia".

Even after such a shift to a restrictive description of euthanasia, further differentiations are necessary; the following aspects in particular have to be specified:

1. The decision-making process (competent/incompetent, patient/nonpatient, patient as decision-maker, physician/family as decision-maker…)
2. Clinical conditions (terminal stage of illness, enormous suffering, medical futility…)
3. Social context (the presence or lack of human/psychological/spiritual support…)
4. Motivation and purpose (of the persons involved).

6.4 The philosophical concepts that form the background of the euthanasia discussion

With regard to euthanasia in contemporary technologized medicine, at least three philosophical foundations can be identified that form the background of euthanasia discussions: a teleological, deontological and human rights approach. Each in turn has its respective schools of though, traditions and movements.

The teleological approach, setting out to determine what the (good) goal would be, in the context of good death often emphasizes the quality of life concept as an important purpose of human endeavour. As a part of the quality of life, health and wellbeing, good social relations and the absence of suffering can be given. Such conceptualized human life holds a high value and is therefore inviolable. However once it heads for its inevitable end, it is an important challenge and goal to aim for a dignified ending. Then autonomy in which an individual shapes his/her own life and self-determination by which one controls the circumstances are of vital significance. Therefore, the shortening of life or termination of life (and of the related suffering) are justifiable goals worthy of acting upon and realizing.

The deontological approach mainly seeks to determine our obligations towards our life and towards the lives of others. The basic obligation towards life is to care for it, to support it,

[91] In 1974, Kohl defined euthanasia as "the painless inducement of a quick death" (1974, p. 94).

and not to destroy it. Therefore suicide and euthanasia are wrong, because they violate the fundamental duty not to intentionally take life. Euthanasia thus sacrifices a person's value as a subject for the sake of his/her welfare (Luper, 2009). Since a moral obligation to terminate life cannot be positively justified, one cannot agree with the termination of life; moreover one has a duty to oppose such tendencies even against the will of the other person since the other is also bound by the duty not to take life nor to allow it to be taken. The deontological prohibition of killing is universally valid; the open question is if there are some justifiable exemptions, such as capital punishment, suicide or euthanasia.

The approach based on rights, in particular on human rights, does not identify any positive (given) or natural right to die. Therefore one cannot call for such right directly. However the right to die can be derived indirectly (e.g. from the right to life). Contrarily, the right to life belongs to human rights but one may "waive" the right to life in the case of suicide or euthanasia. Nevertheless, one is not allowed to delegate the execution of this right to another person, to allow to be legitimately killed. To take human life is morally wrong because the fundamental right to life (which is at the same time a right not to be killed) would be violated. Within liberal political philosophy, with its focus on the rights of the individual, a competent person, freely requesting the termination of his/her life which is not perceived as good and valuable anymore and having become burden to that individual, can forego his/her right to life, rendering killing as morally justifiable. In difference to the deontological approaches, within the liberal notion of rights, the duty not to be killed is limited to those who wish to live.

7. Conclusion

Euthanasia is a highly emotive and sensitive subject, causing disputes and misunderstandings. As many authors have pointed out, the term euthanasia, despite its frequent exposure in public media and in academic literature, does not reflect a clear set of concepts and definitions to be used in euthanasia debates. Thus, such debates often wind up inadequately formed and ineffectual, causing more frustration than solutions. It has become clear that any euthanasia discussion should be preceded by clarifications of the terminology to be used; semantics followed by ethics.

Nevertheless the concept of euthanasia is not a new topic; our interest in the issue has only been renewed due to the effects of contemporary medical technology. It has been demonstrated that both the concept of euthanasia and the euthanasia discourse have their roots in Antiquity. The diverse notions of euthanasia as they have appeared through history were described and their relevance to present day discussions was highlighted. Altogether 15 diverse notions (typologies) of euthanasia have been identified by this study. Many of them can be found in contemporary euthanasia debates.

Out of the many typologies of euthanasia, voluntary (active) euthanasia (typology 11) has been selected as the most relevant concept for the conceptualization of euthanasia to the current medical context. As the preferable concept of euthanasia the following definition was taken from this source: euthanasia is a deliberate act of terminating the life of a competent (autonomous) patient in the terminal stage of an illness, performed by a physician upon the explicit and lasting request of this patient and that patient's sake. So euthanasia, being different from both assisted suicide and physician assisted suicide, also differs from other instances of end-of-life decisions such as the withholding or withdrawing of life support or terminal sedation.

Consequently the conceptualization of euthanasia in recent bioethics literature was examined. As one of the results, an increasing tendency to specify the notion of euthanasia using better and more homogenized semantic precision during the last few decades was identified. This has in turn been adopted more widely, resulting in our broader understanding of euthanasia being changed towards a more precise description which distinguishes between euthanasia, suicide and (physician) assisted suicide. There has been a tendency of more and more authors understanding euthanasia as voluntary (and therefore active) euthanasia. The Dutch and Belgian legal definition of euthanasia seems to have influenced the conceptualization of euthanasia in the 21st century.
Furthermore, the most relevant philosophical approaches that form the theoretical background of stances towards euthanasia were presented (teleology, deontology, rights).
Right from the beginning, i.e. since Classical times, there has been an implicit correlation between good death and good life. Death, being not an event of life, terminates life, delimiting its boundaries as do the banks of a river. A formal determination of both good life and good death in not problematic – everybody wants a good life, including a good ending. However there is a huge discrepancy as to how to determine the content of this „good". This has led to many diverse understandings of good death existing, as the product of individual value systems and communal moralities.
One can expect that the controversy surrounding good death as an existential, emotionally sensitive and morally contentious discourse will continue to be a serious social and political challenge in this age of ever increasing medical technology, aging populations and ongoing health care debates.

8. References

American Medical Association (1992). *Code of Medical Ethics, Current Opinions: Including the Principles of Medical Ethics, Fundamental Elements of the Patient-Physician Relationship and Rules of the Council on Ethical and Judicial Affairs*, AMA Press, ISSN 15374009, Chicago, USA

Annas, G.J. (2005). The Right to Refuse Treatment. In: Beuchamp, T.L. (Ed.). *Intending Death*, pp. 109-130, Prentice Hall, ISBN 0131995553, Upper Saddle River, USA

Aristoteles (2009). *The Nicomachean Ethics*, Oxford University Press, ISBN 0199213610, Oxford, UK

Augustinus Aurelius (1909). *De civitate Dei*, University of California Libraries, ISBN 1125378921, Berkeley, USA

Bacon, F. (2000). *The Advancement of Learning*, Oxford University Press, ISBN 0198123485, Oxford, UK - New York, USA

Battin, M.P.; Leslie, F.P. & Landesman, B.M. (2007). *Death, Dying and the Ending of Life*, Ashgate Publishing, ISBN 075462174X, Burlington, USA

Beauchamp, T.L. & Childress, J.F. (2001). *Principles of Biomedical Ethics*, Oxford University Press, 5th edition, ISBN 0195143329, Cambridge, UK - New York, USA

Beauchamp, T.L. (2003). End-of-Life Decision Making. In: Beauchamp, T.L. & Walters, L. (Eds.). *Contemporary Issues in Bioethics*, 6th edition, pp. 179-185, Thomson/Wadworth, ISSN 0534584411, Belmont…, USA

Beauchamp, T.L. & Davidson, A.I. (1979). The Definition of Euthanasia, *The Journal of Medicine and Philosophy*, Vol. 4, No. 3 (September 1979), pp. 294-312, ISSN 17445019

Beech, I. (1995). Suicide and Voluntary Active Euthanasia. Why the Difference in Attitude? *Nursing Ethics*, Vol. 2, No. 2 (June 1995), pp. 161-170, ISSN 09697330

Behnke, J.A. & Bok, S. (Eds.). (1975). *The Dilemmas of Euthanasia*, Anchor Press, ISBN 0385097301, Garden City/N.Y., USA

Binding, K. & Hoche, A.E. (1920). *Freigabe der Vernichtung lebensunwerten Lebens: ihr Maß und ihre Form*, Meiner, Jena, Germany

Birnbacher, D. (1995). *Tun und Unterlassen*, Reclam, ISBN 3150093929, Stuttgart, Germany

Bishop, J.P. (2006). Euthanasia, Efficiency, and the Historical Distintion Between Killing a Patient and Allowing a Patient to Die, *Journal of Medical Ethics*, Vol. 32, No. 4 (April 2006), pp. 220-224, ISSN 14734257

Bobbert, M. (2003). Sterbehilfe als medizinisch assistierte Tötung auf Verlangen. In: Düwell, M. & Steigleder, K. (Eds.). *Bioethik. Eine Einführung*, pp. 314-322, Suhrkamp, ISBN 3518291971, Frankfurt am Main, Germany

Boyle, J. (1991). Who is Entitled to Double Effect? *The Journal of Medicine and Philosophy*, Vol. 16, No. 5 (October 1991), pp. 475-494, ISSN 03605310

Brock, D.W. (1992). Voluntary Active Euthanasia, *The Hastings Center Report*, Vol. 22, No. 2 (March-April 1992), pp. 10-22, ISSN 00930334

Brock, D.W. (1993). *Life and Death: Philosophical Essays in Biomedical Ethics*, Cambridge University Press, ISBN 0521417856, Cambridge, UK - New York, USA

Brock, D.W. (1999). Voluntary Active Euthanasia. In: Beauchamp, T.L. & Walters, L. (Eds.). *Contemporary Issues in Biomedical Ethics*, 5th edition, pp. 296-305, Thomson, ISBN 0534504760, Belmont..., USA

Brody, B.A. (Ed.). (1989). *Suicide and Euthanasia: Historical and Contemporary Themes*, Kluwer Academic Publishers, ISBN 0792301064, Dordrecht, NL - Boston, USA

Callahan, D. (1999), When Self-Determination Runs Amok, In: Curzer, H.J. (Ed.). *Ethical Theory and Moral Problems*, pp. 718-726, Wardsworth, ISBN 534529747, Belmont, USA

Campbell, A.; Gillett, G. & Jones, G. (2005). *Medical Ethics*, 4th edition, Oxford University Press, ISBN 0195584872, Oxford, UK - New York, USA

Campbell, N. (1999). A Problem for the Idea of Voluntary Euthanasia, *Journal of Medical Ethics*, Vol. 25, No. 3 (June 1999), pp. 242-244, ISSN 14734257

Cantor, N.L. (1993). *Advance Directives and the Pursuit of Death With Dignity*, Indiana University Press, ISBN 025331304X, Bloomington, USA

Cavan, S. (2000). *Euthanasia. The Debate Over the Right to Die*, Rosen Publishing Group, ISBN 082393215X, New York, USA

Deigh, J. (1998). Physician-Assisted Suicide and Voluntary Euthanasia: Some Relevant Differences, *The Journal of Criminal Law and Criminology*, Vol. 88, No. 3 (Spring, 1998), pp. 1155-1165, ISSN 00914169

Diogenes Laertius (1999). *Vitae philosophorum*, Vol. 3, Sauer Verlag, ISBN 3598713193, Munich, Germany

Donagan, A. (1991). Moral Absolutism and the Double-Effect Exception, *The Journal of Medicine and Philosophy*, Vol. 16, No. 5 (October 1991), pp. 495-509, ISSN 03605310

Dowbiggin, I. (2007). *A Concise History of Euthanasia: Life, Death, God and Medicine*, Rowman & Littlefeld Publishers, ISBN 0742531116, Lanham, USA

Downing, A.B. & Smoker, B. (Eds.). (1986). *Voluntary Euthanasia. Experts Debate the Right to Die*, P. Owen, ISBN 0391033654, London, UK

Draper, H. (1998). Euthanasia. In: Chadwick, R. (Ed.). *Encyclopedia of Applied Ethics,* Vol II., pp. 175-187, Academic Press, ISBN 012227066, San Diego…, USA

Eibach, U. (1998). *Sterbehilfe: Tötung auf Verlangen?* Brockhaus, ISBN 3417204178, Wuppertal, Germany

Eid, V. (Ed.). (1985). *Euthanasie oder Soll man auf Verlangen töten?* Grünewald, ISBN 3786711577, Mainz, Germany

Eigler, G. (Ed.). (1970). *Platon - Werke.* Griechisch und Deutsch, Wissenschaftliche Buchgesellschaft, ISBN 3534025741, Darmstadt, Germany

Emanuel, E.J. (1999). What Is the Great Benefit of Legalizing Euthanasia or Physican-Assisted Suicide? *Ethics,* Vol. 109, No. 3 (April 1999), pp. 629-642, ISSN 00141704

Engelhardt, H.T. (1989). Death by Free Choice: Modern Variations on an Antique Theme. In: Brody, B.A. (Ed.). *Suicide and Euthanasia: Historical and Contemporary Themes,* pp. 251-279, Kluwer Academic Publishers, ISBN 0792301064, Dordrecht, NL - Boston, USA

England, E.B. (Ed.). (1975). *The Laws of Plato,* Arno Press, ISBN 0405073275, New York, USA

Euthanasia Definition (2011). Available at http://www.euthanasia.com. Cited 18.03.2011

Ferguson, J.E. (2007). *The Right to Die,* Chelsea House Publishers, ISBN 0791092873, New York, USA

Firth, R. (1981). Euthanasia, *RAIN* (Royal Anthropological Institutes News), Vol . 45 (August 1981), pp. 1-4, ISSN 03076776

Fletcher, J.F. (1954). *Morals and Medicine. The Moral Problems of: the Patient's Right to Know the Truth, Contraception, Artificial Insemination, Sterilization, Euthanasia,* Princeton University Press, Princeton, USA

Fletcher, J.F. (1979). *Humanhood. Essays in Biomedical Ethics.* Prometheus Books, ISBN 0879751126, Bufallo, USA

Foot, Ph. (1977). Euthanasia, *Philosophy and Public Affairs,* Vol. 6, No. 2 (Winter 1977), pp. 85-112, ISSN 10884963

Frey, R.G. (1999). Hume on Suicide, *Journal of Medicine and Philosophy,* Vol. 24, No. 4 (June - July 1999), pp. 336-351, ISSN 17445019

Galton, F. (2006). *Hereditary Genius. An Inquiry into Its Laws and Consequences,* Prometheus Books, ISBN 1591023580, Amherst, USA (orig. London: Macmillan, 1869)

Galton, F. (1973). *Inquiries into Human Faculty and Its Development,* AMS Press, ISBN 0404081274, New York, USA (orig. London: Macmillan, 1883)

Gerrard, E. & Wilkinson, S. (2005). Passive Euthanasia, *Journal of Medical Ethics,* Vol. 31, No. 2 (February 2005), pp. 64-68, ISSN 14734257

Gesang, B. (2008). Passive and Active Euthanasia: What is the Difference? *The Hastings Center Report,* Vol. 22, No. 2 (March-April 1992), pp. 34-38, ISSN 00930334

Graziani, R. (1969). Non-Utopian Euthanasia: An Italian Report, c. 1554, *Renaissance Quarterly,* Vol. 22, No. 4 (Winter 1969), pp. 329-333, ISSN 00344338

Haeckel, E. (1910). *Anthropogenie oder Entwickelungsgeschichte des Menschen,* Edelmann, 6th edition, Leipzig, Germany (1st edition, Leipzig, 1874)

Hawryluck, L.A. & Harvey, W.R.C. (2000). Analgesia, Virtue, and the Principle of Double Effect, *Journal of Palliative Care,* Vol. 16, Supplement (October 2000), pp. S24-30, ISSN 08258597

Heide, van der, A. et al. (2003). End-of-Life Decision-Making in Six European Countries: Descriptive Study, *Lancet,* Vol. 362, No. 9381 (August 2, 2003), pp. 345–50, ISSN 01406736

Heide, van der, A. et al. (2007). End-of-Life Practices in the Netherlands under the Euthanasia Act. *New England Journal of Medicine,* Vol. 19, No. 356 (May 10, 2007), pp. 1957–1965, ISSN 00284793

Hippocrates (1923). *Works* (English and Greek, translated by W. H. S. Jones), Vol. 2, Harvard University Press, ISBN 0674995228, Cambridge, USA

Hume, D. (1985). *Essays, Moral, Political, and Literary*, Liberty Press, ISBN 0865970440, Indianapolis, USA

Humphry, D. & Wickett, A. (1986). *The Right to Die. Understanding Euthanasia,* Harper & Row, ISBN 0060155787, New York, USA

Husak, D.N. (1980). Omissions, Causation and Liability, *The Philosophical Quarterly,* Vol. 30, No. 121 (October 1980), pp. 318-326, ISSN 14679213

Chauncey, D.L. (Ed.). (1975). *Percival's Medical Ethics.* New York: R. E. Krieger Publishing, ISBN 0404133568 , New York, USA

Illhardt, F.J.; Heiss, H.W. & Dornberg, M. (Eds.). (1998). *Sterbehilfe – Handeln oder Unterlassen?* Schattauer, ISBN 379451839X, Stuttgart, Germany

Jonsen, A.R. (1998). *The Birth of Bioethics,* Oxford University Press, ISBN 0195103254, Oxford, UK

Kamm, F.M. (1991). The Doctrine of Double Effect: Reflections on Theoretical and Practical Issues, *The Journal of Medicine and Philosophy,* Vol. 16, No. 5 (October 1991), pp. 571-585, ISSN 03605310

Kamm, F.M. (1994). Action, Omission, and the Stringency of Duties, *University of Pennsylvania Law Review,* Vol. 142, No. 5 (May 1994), pp. 14931512, ISSN 19428537

Kamm, F.M. (1999). Physician-Assisted Suicide, the Doctrine of Double Effect, and the Ground of Value, *Ethics,* Vol. 109, No. 3 (April 1999), pp. 586-605, ISSN 00141704

Kant, I. (1990). *Die Metaphysik der Sitten,* Philipp Reclam, ISBN 3150045088, Stuttgart, Germany

Kant, I. (1996). *Grundlegung zur Metaphysik der Sitten,* Philipp Reclam, ISBN 315004507X, Stuttgart, Germany

Kant, I. (2011). *Fundamental Principles of the Metaphysic of Morals.* Available at http://www.gutenberg.org/. Cited 20.03.2011.

Keown, J. (2002). *Euthanasia, Ethics, and Public Policy: An Argument Against Legalisation,* Cambridge University Press, ISBN 0521804167, Cambridge, UK - New York, USA

Kinzbrunner, B.M. & Policzer, J.S. (2010). *End of Life Care. A Practical Guide,* McGraw-Hill Professional Publishing, ISBN 0071545271, New York, USA

Klein, M. (2004). Voluntary Active Euthanasia and the Doctrine of Double Effect, *Health Care Analysis,* Vol. 12, No. 3 (September 2004), pp. 225-240, ISSN 10653058

Kohl, M. (1974). *The Morality of Killing: Sanctity of Life, Abortion, and Euthanasia,* Humanities Press, ISBN 0391001957, New York, USA

Kohl, M. (1992). Euthanasia. In: Becker, L.C. & Becker, C.B. (Eds.). *Encyclopedia of Ethics,* Vol. I, pp. 335-339, Garland Publishing, ISBN 081530403X, New York, USA - London, UK

Kohl, M. (2001). Euthanasia. In: Becker, L.C. & Becker, C.B. (Eds.). *Encyclopedia of Ethics*, 2nd edition, Vol. I, pp. 492-498, Routledge, ISBN 0415936721, New York, USA - London, UK

Krämer,W. (1997). Hippokrates und Sisyphus - die moderne Medizin als Opfer ihres eigenen Erfolges. In: Kirch, W. & Kliemt H. (Eds.). *Rationierung im Gesundheitswesen*, pp. 7-19, Roderer Verlag, Regensburg, Germany

Kruse, T. & Wagner, H. (Eds.). (1986). *Sterbende brauchen Solidarität*, Beck, ISBN 3406311431, Munich, Germany

Kuře, J. (2007). Dobrá smrt. K filozofickému ujasnění pojmu eutanázie, *Filozofia*, Vol. 62, No. 3 (2007), pp. 223-234, ISSN 0046385X

Leenen, H. et al. (1998). Bill on Euthanasia and Assisting Suicide in the Netherlands, *European Journal of Health Law*, Vol. 5, No. 3 (September 1998), pp. 299-324, ISSN 15718093

Lenz, F. (1931). *Menschliche Auslese und Rassenhygiene*, Lehmanns Verlag, 3rd edition, Munich, Germany

Lewis, P. (2007). *Assisted Dying and Legal Change*, Oxford University Press, ISBN 0199212872, Oxford, UK

Lewy, G. (2011). *Assisted Death in Europa and America*, Oxford University Press, ISBN 0199746415, Oxford, UK - New York, USA

Lock, M. (1996). Death in Technological Time: Locating the End of Meaningful Life, *Medical Anthropology Quarterly*, Vol. 10, No. 4 (December 1996), pp. 575-600, ISSN 15481387

Luper, S. (2009). *The Philosophy of Death*, Cambridge University Press, ISBN 00521882491, Cambridge, UK - New York, USA

Maas, van der, P.J. et al. (1991). Euthanasia and Other Medical Decisions Concerning the End of Life, *Lancet*, Vol. 335, No. 8767, (September 1991), pp. 669-773, ISSN 01406736

Maas, van der, P.J. (1996). Euthanasia, Physician-Assisted Suicide, and Other Medical Practices Involving the End of Life in the Netherlands, 1990-1995, *The New England Journal of Medicine*, Vol. 335, No. 22 (November 28 1996), pp. 1699-1705, ISSN 00284793

Markson, D.S. (1969). The Punishment of Suicide - A Need for Change, *Villanova Law Review*, Vol. 14, No. 3 (1969), pp. 463-483, ISSN 00426229

Marx, C.F.H. (1952). Medical Euthanasia, *Journal of the History of Medicine and Allied Sciences*, Vol. 7, No. 4 (April 1952), pp. 401-416, ISSN 14684373

Materstvedt, L.J. et al. (2003). Euthanasia and Physician-Assisted Suicide: A View from An EAPC Ethics Task, *European Journal of Palliative Care*, Vol. 10, No. 2, p. 63, ISSN 1479-0793

McLachlan, H.V. (2008). The Ethics of Killing and Letting Die: Active and Passive Euthanasia, *Journal of Medical Ethics*, Vol. 34, No. 8 (August 2008), pp. 636-638, ISSN 14734257

McMahan, J. (1993). Killing, Letting Die, and Withdrawing Aid, *Ethics*, Vol. 103, No. 2 (January 1993), pp. 250-279, ISSN 00141704

Michalsen, A. & Reinhart, K. (2006). "Euthanasia": A Confusing Term, Abused Under the Nazi Regime and Misused in Present End-of-Life Debate, *Intensive Care Medicine*, Vol. 32, No. 9 (September 2006), pp. 1304-1310, ISSN 03424642

Montaigne, de M. (1946). *The Essays*, Oxford University Press, New York, USA

Moody, J. (2003). Euthanasia: A Need for Reform, *Nursing Standard,* Vol. 17, No. 25 (March 2003), pp. 40–44, ISSN 00296570

More, T. (2011). *Utopia.* Available at http://www.gutenberg.org/. Cited 20.03.2011.

Müller, A.W. (1997). *Tötung auf Verlangen: Wohltat oder Untat?* Kohlhammer, ISBN 317015110X, Stuttgart, Germany

Mystakidou, K. et al. (2005). The Evolution of Euthanasia and Its Perceptions in Greek Culture and Civilization, *Perspectives in Biology and Medicine,* Vol. 48, No. 1 (Winter 2005), pp. 95-104, ISSN 15298795

Nayernouri, T. (2011). Euthanasia, Terminall Illness and Quality of Life, *Archives of Iranian Medicine,* Vol. 14, No. 1 (January 2011), pp. 54-55, ISSN 10292977

Nietzsche, F. (1997). *Werke,* Phaidon Verlag, ISBN 3888511240, Essen, Germany

Onwuteaka-Philipsen, B.D. et al. (2003), Euthanasia and Other End-of-Life Decisions in the Netherlands in 1990, 1995, and 2001, *Lancet,* Vol. 362, No. 9381 (August 2003), pp. 395-399, ISSN 01406736

Pöltner, G. (2006). *Grundkurs Medizin-Ethik,* 2nd edition, Facultas, ISBN 3850767965, Wien, Austria

Quaghebeur, T. et al. (2009). Nursing and Euthanasia: A Review of Argument-Based Ethics Literature, *Nursing Ethics,* Vol. 16, No. 4 (July 2009), pp. 466-486, ISSN 09697330

Quill, T.E. & Battin, M.P. (2004). *Physician-Assisted Dying. The Case for Palliative Care and Patient Choice.* Johns Hopkins University Press, ISBN 0801880696, Baltimore, USA

Quill, T.E. et al. (1997). The Rule of Double Effect: A Critique of its Role in End-of-Life Decision Making, *New England Journal of Medicine,* Vol. 337, No. 24 (December 11, 1997), pp. 1768-1771, ISSN 00284793

Rachels, J. (1975). Active and Passive Euthanasia, *The New England Journal of Medicine,* Vol. 292, No. 2 (January 9, 1975), pp. 78-80, ISSN 00284793

Riley, J.; George, R. & Finlay, I. (2009). It is Our Responsiblity to Promote Care, Not Killing, *Euroepan Journal of Palliative Care,* Vol. 16, No. 3 (May 2009), p. 109, ISSN 14790793

Ritzel, G. (Ed.). (1998). *Beihilfe zum Suizid – Ein Weg im Streit um Sterbehilfe?* Roderer, ISBN 3890732445, Regensburg, Germany

Seneca, L.A. (1965). *Ad Lucilium epistulae morales,* Oxford University Press, ISBN 0198146493, Oxford, UK

Sheldon, T. (1994). Dutch Argue that Mental Torment Justifies Euthanasia. *The British Medical Journal,* Vol. 308, No. 6926 (February 12, 1994), p. 431, ISSN 09598146

Schöne-Seifert, B. (1997). Die Grenzen zwischen Töten und Sterben lassen, *Jahrbuch für Wissenschaft und Ethik,* Vol. 2, pp. 205-226, ISSN 14309017

Simon, A. (2003). *Sterbehilfe.* In: Düwell, M. & Steigleder, K. (Eds.). *Bioethik. Eine Einführung,* pp. 306-313, Suhrkamp, ISBN 3518291971, Frankfurt am Main, Germany

Spaemann, R. & Fuchs, T. (1997). *Töten oder sterben lassen?* Herder, ISBN 3451045710, Freiburg im Breisgau, Germany

Sporken, P. (1988). *Die Sorge um den kranken Menschen,* Patmos, ISBN 3491772508, Düsseldorf, Germany

Sporken, P. (Ed.). (1990). *Was Sterbende brauchen,* Herder, ISBN 3451196182, Basel, Switzerland

Stewart, H.L. (1918). Euthanasia, *International Journal of Ethics* (1890-1938), Vol. 29, No. 1 (October 1918), pp. 48-62, ISSN 1526422X

Stolberg, M. (2008). Two Pioneers of Euthanasia around 1800, *The Hastings Center Report*, Vol. 38, No. 3 (May-June 2008), pp. 19-22, ISSN 00930334

Suetonius (1997). *Lives of the Twelve Caesars*, Wodsworth Editions Limited, ISBN 185326475X, Ware, UK

Sunstein, C.R. (1997). The Right to Die, *The Yale Law Journal*, Vol. 106, No. 4 (January 1997), pp. 1123-1163, ISSN 00440094

The Belgian Ministry of Justice. (2002). *The Belgian Act on Euthanasia of 28 May 2002*. Available at http://www.ejustice.just.fgov.be. Cited 27.03.2011.

The Convention for the Protection of Human Rights and Dignity of the Human Being with Regard to the Application of Biology and Medicine (1997). Available at http://www.europarl.europa.eu/. Cited 26.03.2011.

The Charter of Fundamental Rights of the European Union (2000). Available at http://www.europarl.europa.eu/. Cited 26.03.2011.

Thomas Aquinas (1964). *Summa theologica*, McGraw-Hill, New York, USA

Van Zyl, L. (2000). *Death and Compassion: A Virtue-Based Approach to Euthanasia*, Ashgate, ISBN 0754612317, Aldershot, UK

Vanderpool, H.Y. (2004). Life-Suistaining Treatment and Euthanasia. In: Post, S.G. (Ed.), *Encylopedia of Bioethics*, Vol. III, pp. 1421-1432, Thomson & Gale, 3rd edition, ISBN 0028657748, New York, USA

Vermaat, J.A.E. (2002). 'Euthanasia' in the Third Reich: Lessons for today? *Ethics & Medicine. An International Journal of Bioethics*, Vol. 18, No. 1. (Spring 2002), pp. 21-32, ISSN 0266688X

Wal, van der, G. & Dillmann, R.J.M. (1994). Euthanasia in the Netherlands, *The British Medical Journal*, Vol. 308, No. 6940 (May 21, 1994), pp. 1346–1349, ISSN 09598146

Walton, D. (1976). Active and Passive Euthanasia, *Ethics*, Vol. 86, No. 4 (July 1976), pp. 343-349, ISSN 00141704

Warnock, M. & Macdonald, E. (2008). *Easeful Death: Is There a Case for Assisted Dying?* Oxford University Press, ISBN 0199539901, Oxford, UK - New York, USA

Watts, D.T. & Howell T. (1992). Assisted Suicide Is Not Voluntary Active Euthanasia, *The Journal of the American Geriatrics Society*, Vol. 40, No. 10 (October 1992), pp. 1043-1046, ISSN 15325415

Weikart, R. (2002). Darwinism and Death: Devaluing Human Life in Germany 1859-1920, *Journal of the History of Ideas*, Vol. 63, No. 2 (April 2002), pp. 323-344, ISSN 10863222

Wiesing, U. (Ed.). (2004). *Ethik in der Medizin*. Reclam Verlag, ISBN 3150183413, Stuttgart, Germany

Wilshaw, C. (1974). *The Right to Die. A Rational Approach to Voluntary Euthanasia*, British Humanist Association, ISBN 0901825085, London, UK

Wolf, S.M. (2008). Confronting Physician-Assisted Suicide and Euthanasia: My Father's Death, *The Hastings Center Report*, Vol. 38. No. 5 (September - October, 2008), pp. 24-26, ISSN 00930334

World Medical Association (2011). *Policies*. Available at http://www.wma.net/. Cited 21.03.2011.

Wreen, M. (1988). The Definition of Euthanasia, *Philosophy and Phenomenological Research*, Vol. 48, No. 4 (June 1988), pp. 637-653, ISSN 19331592

Young, R. (2007). *Medically Assisted Death*, Cambridge University Press, ISBN 0521880246, Cambridge, UK

2

Euthanasia: A Confounding and Intricate Issue

Isabelle Marcoux
Interdisciplinary School of Health Sciences, University of Ottawa
Canada

1. Introduction

Euthanasia is a term that often sparks heated debate, regardless of whether people are "for" or "against". It is one of the most-debated ethical issues in recent decades as revealed by the considerable number of scientific publications, media coverage of specific cases, but also proposed bills in many countries. Despite it's popularity and the fact that public opinion polls indicate increasing support, euthanasia is still illegal in most countries. Nevertheless, one of the most significant challenge in order to have an informed debate on this issue is to determine what euthanasia essentially is. In popular discourse, for example, euthanasia is often associated with expressions such as "wanting to die with dignity", "not wanting to be kept alive against one's wishes", "not wanting to suffer", and "wanting to die rather than live in a certain condition". But, logically, if in most countries euthanasia is illegal, does this mean that these wishes run counter to current practices, or even that dying with dignity be against the law? Of course not, but in the context of the debate on the legalisation of euthanasia, it is legitimate to wonder about the meaning of this loaded term. Among members of the public and even health care practitioners, the term euthanasia is apparently used to refer to situations ranging from the last injection allowing a person to pass from life to death in a context of incurable illness, through withholding treatment that would do more harm than good (futile treatment) and withdrawing life support that keeps the person alive (mechanical ventilation, feeding and hydration tubes), to relieving the pain and other symptoms of persons at the end of life whose next breath may well be their last. The use of adjectives "passive" and "active" with the term euthanasia, to describe legal and illegal practices, is undoubtedly associated with this common clustering of concepts. Given this situation, the objectives of this chapter are to delineate exactly what is meant by the term euthanasia, and to see how the variable interpretations of this term can lead to confusion and misunderstanding that often render debate pointless. Part 2 describes what euthanasia is now considered to consist in, and puts it in perspectives with other types of end-of-life decisions that characteristically arise in medical practice. Part 3 lists studies that have attempted to clarify people's understandings of euthanasia and particularly in relation to other end-of-life practices. Part 4 discusses the interpersonal, societal and political issues raised by these varied understandings of euthanasia according to various groups.

2. Meaning of euthanasia and end-of-life medical practices

Although the word euthanasia is derived from the ancient Greek *eu* (good) and *thanatos* (death), its general meaning of "good death" has changed over time. The first use of the term euthanasia in the Modern Era is attributed to early 17th-century philosopher Francis Bacon, who wrote that euthanasia referred to "a fair and easy passage from life to death without pain and dolors" (Dick, 1955). Three centuries later, however, euthanasia took on a negative connotation with the introduction of Nazi "program euthanasia", developed during World War II in order to eliminate "life unworthy of life", including persons with illnesses and disabilities. In the 1960s, in reaction to the advances in medical technology and its intensive use, serious debate took place in the Netherlands (Kater et al., 2003). At that time, the term euthanasia was placed in the highly specific context of reaction against heroic treatment. Concerns focused on the best thing to do in a life-and-death situation where the patient's wishes were central. Until the late 1970s, the term euthanasia designated a broad category of problems (for example, direct action, indirect action, refraining from action, and whether there was a request from the patient); since that time, however, it has been defined as "... the administration of drugs with the explicit intention of ending the patient's life at his/her request" (van der Mas et al., 1991). This is now the definition "officially" used in most industrialized countries. In particular, it served as a basis for regulating the practice of euthanasia in the Netherlands in the 1990s, when legislation was being amended in order to allow euthanasia in the Netherlands (2000), Belgium (2002) and Luxemburg (2009), and also for the systematic study of this practice. Thus we can see that the term euthanasia has been subjected to a variety of influences over time, and has recently been very strictly defined as a medical act that consists in intentionally bringing about the death of a patient at that person's request. Practically speaking, euthanasia is usually accomplished by giving an injection of a barbiturate, combined with a neuromuscular relaxant which bring about the patient's death (Matersvedt et al., 2003).

In order to better understand what euthanasia exactly means (or not means), we must put it in perspective with other end-of-life medical practices. In fact, there are conceptual and practical distinctions among end-of-life practices; in recent decades in a number of industrialized countries, these distinctions have made it possible to differentiate between what is considered legal and what is not. The objective here is not to pass moral judgement on whether this situation is acceptable or not, but rather to provide a factual description of the situation. First of all, **withholding treatment** means not initiating treatment that may maintain or prolong life (for example, cardiac resuscitation or blood transfusion); **treatment withdrawal** means interrupting or ceasing life-sustaining treatment (for example, a ventilator, artificial nutrition or hydration, dialysis). These decisions, made in accordance with the patient's wishes, are considered as good medical practices in most industrialized countries. Recognizing this right of refusal protects patients from possible heroic treatment and flows from physicians' duty not to harm (non maleficence). Previously, these medical decisions were sometimes labelled as "passive euthanasia" since, for some people, they considered that the result (death) was the same as in the case of active euthanasia (lethal injection with intent to induce death), even though the means to the end was different. That terminology is not only confusing but also semantically meaningless.

A physician who respects a patient's will to stop treatment that may prolong life, or that maintains life artificially, is not exonerated from the duty of providing the patient with adequate care to control pain and other symptoms. However, for some people, relieving pain with adequate doses of morphine may induce death and can therefore considered to be euthanasia. As a result, to ensure that patients receive the treatment needed for adequate pain relief, the principle of "double effect" was introduced. The "**double effect**" arises from the fact that adequate pain relief sometimes calls for significant doses that could accelerate death as a side effect. In situations of this type, the intent is to relieve pain, not to induce death. Nevertheless, as we shall see, the results of recent research strongly challenge this principle of "double effect", indicating that, on the contrary, administration of medication needed for adequate pain relief would have the effect of prolonging, not shortening, life. Furthermore, and still with the objective of controlling pain and other symptoms at the end of life, we see increasingly frequent references to **terminal sedation** since the last decade. This practice consists in inducing sleep until death in persons at the end of life who have treatment-resistant symptoms such as pain, respiratory disorders, moral suffering, or delirium.

Relief of pain and other symptoms is one specific objective of palliative care. In fact, according to the World Health Organization definition: "**Palliative care** is an approach that improves the quality of life of patients and their families facing the problem associated with life-threatening illness, through the prevention and relief of suffering by means of early identification and impeccable assessment and treatment of pain and other problems, physical, psychosocial and spiritual." (Sepùlveda et al., 2002). Dying with dignity is what palliative care professionals offer to persons at the end of life, but this is also the expression used by proponents of the legalization of euthanasia. Although the end is the same, in a number of countries euthanasia as a means to that end is considered irreconcilable with the concept of palliative care. In fact, palliative care is usually presented as antithetical to a debate on euthanasia: for example, persistent demand for euthanasia may be seen as a failure of palliative care; or palliative care may even be presented as the sole alternative to euthanasia. In endeavouring to counter the argument that better access to high-quality palliative care would eliminate the desire for euthanasia to end one's life, Belgium simultaneously passed two pieces of legislation: one on euthanasia (Sénat de Belgique, 2001a); and the other on palliative care, guaranteeing patients equal access to high-quality care (Sénat de Belgique, 2001b). In fact, access to palliative care is a major issue that must be addressed: for example, it is estimated that only between 16% and 30% of Canadians have access to palliative care, depending on their place of residence (Canadian Institute for Health Information, 2007), even though Canada ranks ninth out of 40 countries on a "Quality of Death" Index that takes into account factors including the availability of palliative care (Economist Intelligence Unit, 2010).

In general, withholding treatment, treatment withdrawal, relief of pain and terminal sedation are medically recognized as good practices and are legal in most industrialized countries, when implemented in accordance with the patient's wishes. However, except in a few European countries, euthanasia is still illegal, although its ethical justification is the subject of intense debate. Another practice usually considered to be illegal is **physician-assisted suicide**, which is distinguished from euthanasia by the concept of the person performing the act: in assisted suicide, it is the patient who takes the action that will induce that person's own death, while in euthanasia, it is the physician who assumes this responsibility. Three main concepts may be used to distinguish between these practices: intent; the act performed; and the person performing the act that results in death.

In theory, the current definition of euthanasia and the distinctions applied to other types of end-of-life practices have been accepted in legislative, research and medical circles. This consensus notwithstanding, groups each have their own justifications for acceptance. In legislative circles, the objective is to distinguish between legal and illegal practices on the basis of societal values. The medical associations, consistently following the Hippocratic oath, have a duty to determine what is acceptable in terms of medical practice and to ensure their members' adherence to the profession's code of ethics. In research circles and particularly empirical studies, the objective is to obtain sound internal validity by using a recognized definition of the concept being studied. On that basis, study results can be reproduced and compared with the results of former studies, for which studies conducted in the Netherlands have been a reference point. As presented in this part, then, distinguishing among end-of-life medical practices and making them operational is essentially utilitarian.

3. Understandings of euthanasia

Until now, there have been few specific studies on people's understandings of euthanasia, and these few studies have specific angles of analysis that can be classified under three headings. First, there are studies, often using a qualitative approach, on what people spontaneously think euthanasia is or how they identify components of a definition of euthanasia. Second, there are other studies on people's ability to distinguish between euthanasia and other end-of-life practices using vignettes. Third, there are studies on people's knowledge of whether euthanasia and other end-of-life practices are legally accepted in their respective countries. Aside from these different angles of analysis, these studies also diverge in two significant aspects of methodology: the country of the survey; and the target population of the survey (members of the general public; patients; significant others or natural caregivers; physicians or nurses). As well, the methods of data collection varied, as the way questions were formulated. Taking into account these significant challenges to the comparability of results, we will present these studies successively by angle of analysis; we will then endeavour to draw some conclusions about the current state of respondents' knowledge.

3.1 Spontaneous definitions of euthanasia

At a 1-day informative conference for Dutch medical students on the topic of "Dying on Request", participants were asked, before and after the training activity, to define euthanasia (Muller et al., 1996). Although the objective was certainly to check the acquisition of knowledge after the training day, the results provide some indications of participants' initial concepts. This study is interesting from two standpoints: theoretically, the participants should have had good knowledge of what constitutes euthanasia because their future profession would call upon them to address this issue ; as well, they lived in a country where (in the mid-1990s) euthanasia was already broadly debated, regulated in certain circumstances, but not yet legalized. In order to assess participants' knowledge, the researchers used as a benchmark the definition adopted in 1987 by the Dutch State Commission on Euthanasia: "Active voluntary euthanasia is the intentional termination of life, by someone other than the patient, at the patient's request". On that basis, the researchers were looking for three components of the definition of euthanasia: (1) intent to hasten death; (2) a person performing the act who is someone else than the patient; and (3) the existence of a request as evidence of compliance with the patient's wishes. Of the 137 student respondents, approximately two out of five initially provided the three expected components of the definition (41%; 39%; and 41% respectively, in regard to the components). Clearly the training day benefited participants, since most respondents' knowledge of what constitutes euthanasia in medical practice in the Netherlands improved significantly (90%; 89%; and 84% respectively, in regard to the component). Unfortunately, there is no indication of the number of persons who combined the three components in their definitions, either before or after the training activity. Nor is there any indication of other components spontaneously put forward by respondents, which might have made it possible to determine whether there was confusion with other end-of-life practices. Still, we may posit that, despite respondents' special status and a context conducive to discussion of euthanasia, initial knowledge appeared to be limited.

During the same decade, an Australian survey of 10 nurses was designed in particular to shed light on nurses' understanding of euthanasia (McInerney & Seibold, 1995). When asked: "What is your understanding of euthanasia?", six respondents spontaneously provided what the researchers considered to be an accurate definition, that is, involving intent to induce death. In fact, the researchers applied the distinction between "active" and "passive" to assess whether the definitions provided by the nurse respondents were accurate; when questioned, further, by far most respondents appeared to support this distinction. As well, nine out of the 10 respondents did not consider the "double effect" to be euthanasia, in particular because of the concept of intent. Interestingly, six of the 10 respondents did not refer to the voluntary aspect of euthanasia; that is, they did not mention the importance of a request by the patient, as required by the Dutch definition of euthanasia. In conclusion, this study states: "It was conceded that the term passive euthanasia, particularly in relation to treatment withdrawal, has served to confuse the real debate centring around active euthanasia"; this debate did indeed take place in Australia at that time, and the 1995 legislative amendment allowing euthanasia in the Northern Territory of that country was overturned a few months after being effective (Dickinson et al., 1998). Participants in this study endorsed the idea of confusion created by the use of various adjectives with the term euthanasia, and appeared to distinguish readily between passive and active euthanasia. Nevertheless, one may wonder about the representativity of the findings of this study, since two broader surveys of nurses (Aranda & O'Conner, 1995; Davis et al., 1993) expressed significant reservations about the validity of their own results, specifically because of differing interpretations of the subject of the study. For example, in referring to euthanasia, nurses gave as examples of treatment withdrawal taking a patient off a respirator or withdrawing artificial feeding, and even pain relief through increased doses of morphine at the risk of hastening death. In short, even among professionals working with patients at the end of life, concepts of euthanasia do not appear to be altogether clear.

A similar open-ended question about what constitutes euthanasia was asked of 236 persons with cancer in Australia (Parkinson et al., 2005). Main topics identified included: "assisted death" (44%), meaning that another person is involved in the process; "suffering" (41%), identifying the context in which euthanasia takes place; and "ending life" (39%), raising the issue of intent, but not indicating exactly what respondents meant. In fact, very few persons appear to have referred to the "methods" of ending life; under this heading, the researchers grouped all sorts of activities including not only euthanasia but also other end-of-life practices/terms (such as lethal injection, tablet, withdrawal or withholding treatment, and active or passive measures). According to the study, the fact that a personal choice is involved, and the fact that this choice has to do with one's own death, were more frequently referred to than the concept of voluntary death, which was not often made explicit.

However, the fact that a high percentage of respondents referred to personal choice (request, wish, choice, decision) suggests that euthanasia flows from compliance with "the patient's request" as set out in the Dutch definition of euthanasia. In summary, on the basis of the results presented, it is difficult to ascertain whether respondents distinguish between euthanasia and other end-of-life practices. In fact, the researchers indicate that people instinctively use euthanasia to mean a range of situations that could be described as active, passive, voluntary or even involuntary.

Lastly, respondents in a survey of 991 residents of Quebec, Canada, were asked: "In your opinion, what is euthanasia?" (Marcoux, 2003). First of all, one out of eight respondents indicated that they did not know what euthanasia is. Following an analysis of 825 codifiable definitions, nine initial themes were identified: (1) the type of subject (human or animal) to which the definition applied; (2) the intent underlying the act; (3) the act performed; (4) the person performing the act; (5) the existence of a request; (6) the existence of consent; (7) the presence of compassion; (8) the reasons underlying the act; and (9) the circumstances surrounding the act. However, in order to make people's understanding of euthanasia operational and in order to compare the definitions, certain strongly correlated themes were combined (for example: act and intent; reasons, circumstances and compassion), and only some themes were selected, on the basis of the minimal semantic components inherent in the definition of euthanasia (intent; the person performing the act; and compassion). For example, for a definition to be classified as euthanasia, it had to include at least these three components, justified as follows: the intent is to induce death; the person performing the act is someone else; and indicators of compassion are present. When justification was used to cross-reference the response components, only 414 of the 825 definitions provided could be classified, under the following composite headings: (1) euthanasia (17.4%); (2) assisted suicide (4.2%); (3) treatment withdrawal (3.0%); (4) ambiguous practices, that is, those in which intent cannot be determined (17.1%); (5) suicide (4.3%); and (6) murder (4.3%). General observations are as follows: very few people spontaneously know what euthanasia is; over half have a fragmented understanding of the subject; and the rest appear to be confused about the difference between euthanasia, other end of life practices such as treatment withdrawal, but also physician-assisted suicide and even suicide. Some respondents spontaneously indicated that euthanasia means murder, citing intent to cause death and the fact that the act is performed by someone else, but included no component of compassion in the definition. Still, care must be exercised in interpreting the scope of these results since the telephone survey method does not readily lend itself to questions of this type (attempting to identify people's understanding of euthanasia using an open-ended question) .

3.2 People's ability to distinguish between euthanasia and other end-of-life practices

The following studies used vignettes to focus on people's understanding of euthanasia as compared with other end-of-life practices. The methodological details and brief results of these studies are presented in Table 1. As part of a public education event on death and dying, participants were asked first to complete a questionnaire on their knowledge of this subject (Gallagher, 2001: see box 1). Although a high percentage of participants already worked in palliative care (61 of 144 participants, or 42%), according to the results, 47% of participants thought that: "Euthanasia involves withholding life-sustaining treatments such as life support machines," even though only 16% thought it is illegal to refuse treatment.

Although these results initially appear contradictory, they can be interpreted in two ways. First, it is possible that some persons think that the term euthanasia refers to a legal practice (which was not the case in Canada either when the study was conducted or when the book was published). Second, the lack of reference in the first vignette to a request by the patient could explain this variation between the two situations. Another interesting result of this study is the indication that 46% of participants believe in the principle of "double effect", that is, that pain relief using morphine may shorten a patient's life and even precipitate death, which is often a source of confusion with euthanasia, as we shall see.

Study	Year of realization	Country	Populations	Method	N (Response rate)	
Gallagher	1999[1]	Canada (British Columbia)	Public	Questionnaire	144/ (*not mentioned*)	Withholding or withdrawing life-sustaining treatment is euthanasia: 47.30%
Marcoux et al.	2002	Canada (Quebec)	Public	Phone interview	991 (49.8%)	Withholding treatment is euthanasia: 38.1% Withdrawing treatment is euthanasia: 66% "Double effect" is euthanasia: 48.8% PAS is euthanasia: 71.9% Euthanasia is euthanasia: 79.7%
Neil et al.	2004	Australia	Physicians	Mail	854 (47%)	Withholding or withdrawing is euthanasia: 13% "Double effect" is euthanasia: 20% Euthanasia is euthanasia: 62% Provided own definition: 4%
Vilela & Caramelli	2003[2]	Brazil	a. Physicians b. Caregivers	Interview	a. 30 (100%) b. 40 (100%)	Withholding or withdrawing is euthanasia a. 23.3% b. 15% "Double effect" is euthanasia a. 6.6% b. 20% Euthanasia is euthanasia a. 40% b. 25% PAS is euthanasia a. 3.3% b. 15% I don't know what is euthanasia (or other) a. 23.3% b. 20%

[1] Personal communication with author
[2] Personal communication with author

Study	Year of realization	Country	Populations	Method	N (Response rate)	
Lindblad et al.	2007	Sweden	a. Public b. Physician	Mail	a. 1202 (48%) b. 1200 (57%)	Withdrawal of ventilator (*no chance of improvement, but can live for many years*) is considered as a type of euthanasia a. 16% b. 26% Withdrawal of dialysis, depending of characteristics of the patients a. 16 and 17% b. 8 and 13%

Table 1. Distinction between euthanasia and other end-of-life decisions

Box 1.

- "Euthanasia involves withholding life-sustaining treatments such as life support machines"
- "It is illegal to refuse treatment if you have a life-threatening illness"
- "Morphine doses sufficient to relieve pain may shorten the life of the person or contribute to their death"

Gallagher (2001)

Confusion between treatment withdrawal and euthanasia was shown among members of the population, and this confusion was even more widespread about various end-of-life practices (Marcoux et al., 2007). Vignettes of different end-of-life practices were used; for each vignette, respondents were asked to indicate whether the situation involves euthanasia or not (see box 2). Nearly three out of four respondents identified physician-assisted suicide as being euthanasia; 66% identified treatment withdrawal at the patient's request as being euthanasia; 49% identified the “double effect” as being euthanasia; and 38% identified withholding life-sustaining treatment as being euthanasia. Although there was no specific question about knowledge of whether these acts are legal in Canada (euthanasia and assisted suicide were illegal when the study was conducted and when the book was published), one may nevertheless assume that the recurring public debate on the acceptability of legislative amendments to allow euthanasia has numerous connotations in the popular imagination. In short, how should the results of public opinion polls on euthanasia be interpreted when respondents think, for example, that taking a patient off a respirator at his or her request (treatment withdrawal) is *de facto* euthanasia?

Box 2

- "A dying person asks his doctor to give him a lethal injection because he could no longer stand suffering from his illness. The doctor agrees and this causes the patient's death" [Euthanasia vignette]
- "A doctor gives a terminally ill person medication the person can take to kill himself" [Physician-assisted suicide vignette]

- "At the request of a patient, a doctor disconnects machines which keep the person alive, for example, an artificial lung" [Treatment withdrawal vignette]
- "At the request of a patient, a doctor respects the person's decision to refuse treatment which would prolong his life" [Withholding treatment vignette]
- "A doctor gives a dying person drugs to relieve his suffering, but the drugs hasten his death" ["Double effect" vignette]

Marcoux et al. (2007)

In the next two studies, respondents were asked to choose, from among proposed definitions, the one that best reflected their individual definition of euthanasia. As a result, unlike the previous study, here the responses were mutually exclusive, which makes it impossible to determine whether there is juxtaposition of confusion. Neil et al. (2007) proposed three vignettes to a group of physicians (see box 3); 62% of respondents chose the statement emphasizing the intent of "hastening death" underlying the act performed as an inherent component of what constitutes euthanasia (an accurate definition according to the researchers), in comparison with two other statements that referred instead to the "double effect" (20%) and to withholding or treatment withdrawal (13%). Moreover, 4% of respondents wanted instead to suggest their own definitions, most of which emphasized the etymological meaning of the term euthanasia: "good death". These results show that the term euthanasia can have different meanings even among physicians, 83% of whom have already cared for patients at the end of life.

Box 3

Which of the following do you regard as euthanasia?

- Provision of medication or drug that doctor believes will hasten the patient's death
- As well as taking active steps, withdrawing or withholding
- Actions count as euthanasia only if acts with the primary intention of hastening death

Neil et al. (2007)

Unlike the study by Neil et al. (2007.), conducted in Australia where the legal status of end-of-life practices is the same as in most western countries, the study by Vilela & Caramelli (2009) was conducted in Brazil in 2003, a few years before that country's Federal Council on Medicine published standards of practice on the withholding or withdrawing life-sustaining treatment at the end of life (personal communication with the author). The comparison of responses by physicians and caregivers of persons with Alzheimer disease leads to different conclusions about what members of each of these two groups consider to be euthanasia (see box 4 for wording). Although the response choices were mutually exclusive, there was no real consistency in the responses by caregivers, since between 15% and 25% of them chose statements identifying treatment withdrawal, assisted suicide, "double effect", euthanasia, or "Don't know/Other". Responses by physicians were more limited, to statements identifying euthanasia (40%), treatment withdrawal (23%), and "Don't know/Other" (23%). In this context, the confusion between euthanasia and other end-of-life practices may be understandable since their legal status was not explicit at the time the study was conducted. Nevertheless, in comparison with the previous studies, this one still shows evidence of the conceptual mixture between withdrawal of life-sustaining treatment and euthanasia, much like the former terms active and passive euthanasia, which are a source of confusion in medical practice.

Box 4

"What do you understand by euthanasia?"

- It is to let one die without any kind of medical assistance
- It is to let one die without sophisticated medical assistance (mechanical ventilation, dialyse, feeding directly in the vein...)
- It is to induce death by giving, for instance, a medication with lethal effect
- It is the attempt to reduce patient suffering by giving medications that control pain but shorten life
- It is to give the patient a lethal medication to let him/her take by himself/herself the decision to shorten his/her life
- I do not know/free answer/more than one option

Vilela & Caramelli (2009)

Although the next study was not designed to identify specific knowledge or possible confusion about end-of-life practices, it does indicate that certain situations of treatment withdrawal are considered to be, not as "defensible acts", but rather as a type of euthanasia (Lindblad et al, 2010). This is true among approximately 16% of respondents from the general public, regardless of the vignette presented (see box 5). The same vignettes were also presented to physicians, who appeared to interpret the content of the acts differently depending on the vignette presented. For example, 8% and 13% of physicians respectively considered withdrawal of dialysis (case 1 and case 2) as a form of euthanasia, while one physician out of four (26%) considered withdrawal of a ventilator maintaining life (case 3) to be "a type of euthanasia". However, that wording may be criticized since in fact it

Box 5

- "A 77-year-old woman, who as a result of type 2 diabetes and chronic renal insufficiency is dependent on dialysis three times a week. In recent months she has repeatedly expressed a wish to terminate the dialysis treatment. The woman is tired of life, but cognitively clear and not suffering from any mental illness" (case 1).
- "A 36-year-old man, who 5 years earlier attempted to commit suicide. He was saved without brain injuries, but as a result of a persistent chronic kidney disorder he is still dialysis dependent. Initially, he also received psychiatric treatment. The patient is in line for a kidney transplant. During the past 6 months he has repeatedly expressed a wish to decline the kidney transplant and to terminate the dialysis treatment. A psychiatric examination does not reveal any mental illness" (case 2).
- "A 34-year-old competent man who is tetraplegic and ventilator dependent as the result of a car accident 5 years ago. There is no chance of improvement, but the patient may live for many years in his current state. During the past 6 months, the patient has repeatedly asked for the ventilator treatment to be discontinued. Neither the physician, who knows the patient well, nor a consultant psychiatrist regard the patient as clinically depressed" (case 3).

Lindblad et al. (2010)

gives the impression that there are a number of types of euthanasia, and thus the wording of the question alone may create confusion. In the present state of affairs (when the study was conducted and when the book was published) in Sweden, treatment may be refused, although euthanasia is prohibited. The fact that more physicians considered treatment withdrawal in the case of a young quadriplegic man to be euthanasia provides food for thought. The possibility of this patient's living for a number of years in this condition may have influenced the physicians' interpretation of the request and invite us to reflect in greater depth on the balance between respect for the patient's autonomy and the physician's duty to do good.

3.3 People's knowledge about legal status of euthanasia and other end-of-life practices

The following studies focus more specifically on whether people are aware of their rights in terms of end-of-life care under the legislation in force in their respective countries of residence. The methodology details and brief results of these studies are shown in Table 2.

Study	Year of realization	Country	Populations	Method	N (Response rate)	Knowledge about the legal options
Gallagher	1999	Canada	Public	Quest-ionnaire	144/(*not mentioned*)	Refusal of treatment: 84.5%
Silveira et al.	1999	US (Oregon)	Adult outpatients	Quest-ionnaire	728/1000	Refusal of treatment: 69% Treatment withdrawal: 46% "Double effect": 41% Assisted suicide: 23% Euthanasia (illegal): 32%
Kopp	2002	US (Arkansas)	Public	Mail	300/(*not mentioned*)	Refusal of treatment: 61.5% Treatment withdrawal: 33.7% "Double effect": 27.6% Assisted suicide (illegal): 70.8% Euthanasia (illegal): 79%

Study	Year of realization	Country	Populations	Method	N (Response rate)	Knowledge about the legal options
Morita et al.	2004	Japan	a. Public b. Bereaved family members	Mail	a. 2548/4974 b. 513/738	Withdrawal: 32 à 45% "Double effect": 50 à 63% Euthanasia (illegal): 66 à 75%
Mitchell & Owens	2000[3]	New Zealand	a. Physicians b. Students c. Greypower	Mail (a & c)[3] In class (b)	a. 120 (40%) b. 205 (80%) c. 595 (30%)	Euthanasia (illegal) a. 94% b. 65% c. 64%

Table 2. Knowledge about legal options at the end of life

One study was conducted among outpatients at university-affiliated clinics in Oregon, USA, in 1999, that is, approximately two years after the passage of legislation allowing the practice of physician-assisted suicide under specific conditions (Silveira et al., 2000). For each of a series of vignettes (see box 6), respondents were asked to indicate whether the practice was legal or illegal under legislation in force in Oregon. Of the 728 respondent, 69% appeared to be aware of their right to refuse life-sustaining treatment, and fewer than half (46%) appeared to be aware of their right to have this type of treatment withdrawn. Only 41% considered the "double effect" to be consistent with the legislation. Despite public debate in preceding years about the legislative amendments to allow physician-assisted suicide, only 23% of respondents were aware that they had the right to ask their physician for assistance in ending their life if their life expectancy was less than six months. A somewhat lower proportion (17%) however, erroneously believed that euthanasia was legally allowed in Oregon. Moreover, according to this study, nearly two out of three persons made no distinction between euthanasia and assisted suicide. Having personally experienced illness or the illness and death of a significant other, or having written an advance directive, were unrelated to greater awareness of one's rights in terms of end-of-life care. Nevertheless, having acted as a proxy in health care decisions for a significant other apparently had a positive effect on greater awareness of these rights.

Box 6

- "In Oregon, does a patient like John, who has less than 6 months to live, have the legal right to refuse treatment that might cure him or save his life"?
- "In Oregon, is it legal for a physician to turn off a ventilator when requested by a patient like John, with less than 6 months to live, even if it means the patient might die"?
- "In Oregon, is it legal for a physician to inject a medication that would cause a patient's immediate death if a patient like John, with less than 6 months to live, requests it"?

[3] Personal communication with author

- "In Oregon, is it legal for a physician to prescribe a medication and provide advice so that the patient can take the medication that will end his life if a patient like John, with less than 6 months to live, requests it"?
- "In Oregon, is it legal for a physician to give patients like John, with less than 6 months to live, pain medications with the goal of relieving pain and suffering even if death may occur sooner as a result"?

Silveira et al. (2000)

That study was replicated a few years later in 2002, in Arkansas, USA, among a sample of 300 persons (Kopp, 2008-2009). The results of this study differed somewhat from those of the previous study; possible explanations are the three-year time lag between the two studies, a difference in the type of respondents (outpatients at a medical clinic, as compared with respondents in households), sample size (728, as compared with 300), and the way the study was administered (a self-administered questionnaire, as compared with a mailed questionnaire). There was greater awareness in Arkansas whether euthanasia and assisted suicide are legal (79% and 71% respectively); both practices are illegal in that state. Nevertheless, for all practices there was a high percentage of "Don't know" responses, varying from 18% for euthanasia, through 31% for treatment withdrawal, to 35% for the "double effect". It should be noted that 21% of respondents believed they did not have the legal right to refuse treatment. A study conducted in Japan (Morita *et al.*, 2006) also shows a great deal of uncertainty about the legality of certain end-of-life practices, and indicates confusion that is proportionally similar to that shown by Silvera et al. (2000). However, it is difficult to draw any formal conclusions since at the time of the study the actual status of end-of-life practices in Japan did not appear to be very clear and had to be ascertained through consensus among experts. Still, it can be stated that there is significant confusion, regardless of type of end-of-life practice, although confusion appears to be more marked about withdrawing artificial hydration and the "double effect" (practices "supposedly" legally permitted in Japan at this time) than about euthanasia (illegal practice).

Mitchell & Owens (2004) focused on knowledge among physicians (n=120), students (n=205), and persons 55 and older (n=595) of whether acts of assistance in dying were legal in New Zealand. Four vignettes were presented, three of which showed situations of various levels of involvement in assisted suicide (supplying information; supplying drugs; assisting to take drugs) and one of which showed a situation involving euthanasia (see box below). Unfortunately, no situation involving treatment withdrawal was presented, which would have made it possible to compare knowledge of legal and illegal practices. According to this study, no physicians stated that it is legal in New Zealand to administer a lethal injection to a terminally ill person, at the patient's request, although 6% said they were not sure. This degree of uncertainty was even more marked among laypersons, who accounted for nearly one-third of respondents. Providing information on hastening death, and providing means to induce death, both at the request of a terminally ill person, were a particular source of confusion about the risk of legal action. In fact, in the first example, 18% of physicians believed that this practice is legal, while 26% were not sure. Among the two other respondent groups, not being sure about the legal status of these two acts ranged from 36% to 43%. In light of these few studies, then, we can see that awareness of legal rights in terms of end-of-life care is far from being optimal, among both physicians and persons who will eventually need to face these choices.

Box 7

- Patient B has a terminal illness (i.e. no hope of recovery), and pain is a constant problem, not alleviated by drugs. [...] The patient has difficulty swallowing and requests the doctor to administer a lethal injection to end the suffering. The doctor administers a lethal injection. In your understanding, is this action legal in New Zealand?

(Mitchell & Owens, 2004)

4. Repercussions of confusion about euthanasia

This confusion about what constitutes euthanasia and what are the distinctions among end-of-life practices necessarily has interpersonal, societal and political repercussions, depending on the roles of groups in society. As a result, our objectives are to review these studies and to discuss issues that characterize this societal debate from the standpoints of the various groups.

4.1 Laypersons

Public understanding does not appear to cover the subtleties of rights in terms of end-of-life care or the distinctions among end-of-life practices. In fact, when surveyed about these issues, people show a rather naïve approach: instead of distinguishing among end-of-life practices, often they consider all these practices to be euthanasia. In particular, many people appear to consider withholding or withdrawal of life-sustaining treatment to be an act of euthanasia (Gallagher, 2001; Marcoux et al., 2007), and appear to believe that they do not have the legal right to express that wish to a physician (Kopp, 2008-2009; Morita et al., 2006; Silveira et al., 2000). As well, in a context of public opinion polls, this confusion between treatment withdrawal and euthanasia appears to be associated with greater support for euthanasia (Marcoux et al., 2007). Similar conclusions were also shown in the study conducted by Kopp (2008-2009), which focused on the issue of physician-assisted suicide; the results of that study showed that greater awareness of the legality of certain practices, including treatment withdrawal and the "double effect", was associated with lower support for physician-assisted suicide. In summary, caution is advisable in interpreting the results of public opinion survey about euthanasia: the questions asked must be valid, and the conclusions must take into account the undeniable effect of the wide range of ideas that the term euthanasia evokes. Of course, the media have a decisive role to play in disseminating accurate information and thus fostering enlightened debate. Nevertheless, the sensitive and at times sensational nature of this subject makes it a strong magnet for headline-grabbing reporting that does not always reflect reality (Schwartz & Lutfiyya, 2009; Seale, 2010) and that, regrettably, helps perpetuate confusion.

Unfortunately, there are practically no studies on the actual ideas of what constitutes euthanasia, or on which end-of-life practices are legal, among persons directly concerned by these issues. Only the study by Parkinson et al. (2005) suggests that the expansive understanding of euthanasia, as compared with the "official" definition of this term, is found among patients suffering from cancer as well and influences their responses to questions on this subject. On the basis of this broader definition of euthanasia, encompassing both practices that are currently legal and those that are illegal in most countries, then, we can assume that opinions on the acceptability of euthanasia and support for its legalization both depend on a desire for a good death. This desire is influenced in particular by fear of suffering, fear of heroic treatment, fear of not having one's end-of-life wishes respected, and the wish to continue to be in control of one's life until its end. These concerns are legitimate and deserve to be heard, respected and addressed, not only by medical practice but also by means of a clear a political will, ensuring that persons do not receive medical treatment against their wishes and that no one is left in pain and suffering, and in anguish of death and dying. In this debate, there appears to be a message for the medical community about the limitations of the medical role in patients' lives; this message also raises questions about the changing therapeutic relationship between physicians and patients.

4.2 Health care professionals

Although most of the medical associations have adopted the "official" definition of euthanasia and proscribe this practice under their code of ethics (except in countries where euthanasia is legal), the delineation of what is or is not euthanasia is not always clear for physicians. In fact, some physicians appear to consider withdrawal of life-sustaining treatment, including withdrawal of a respirator or dialysis, to be euthanasia (Lindblad et al., 2010; Vilela & Caramelli, 2009). In the opinion of other physicians, the "double effect" also appears to constitute euthanasia (Neil et al., 2007; Vilela & Caramelli, 2009). These findings corroborate the conclusions of studies indicate that the prevalence of deaths by euthanasia as revealed by physicians may be inflated because of confusion, misclassification or misrepresentation of their actions (Emanuel et al., 1998; van der Maas et al., 1991), but also because of the wording of the questions (Seale, 2009; van der Maas et al., 1996). Thus we may question some physicians' capacity for enlightened discussion of the options available to patients and patient's rights in terms of end-of-life care, and even some physicians' comfort in providing appropriate patient care at the end of life. In fact, according to some studies, the principle of "double effect" is contested since increased doses of morphine might even prolong life (Sykes et al., 2003). Moreover, the unfounded fear of shortening life hinders good practices for appropriate relief of end-of-life symptoms (Bilsen et al., 2006). Among some physicians, then, this lack of awareness about what constitutes euthanasia and what distinguishes it from other end-of-life practices, and the resulting confusion between legal and illegal practices, leads to fear of legal action. As well, although according to some physicians their role includes providing assistance to die by euthanasia to patients who so wish, others see in that practice a risk of instrumentalization in which the patient's autonomy would take precedence over physicians' responsibility to do good. Clearly, this confusion about end-of-life practices is also found in some nurses and even among palliative care nurses (Aranda & O'Conner, 1995; Davis et al., 1993). While nurses are not directly responsible for medical decisions, they play an important role in educating patients and significant others because of their special relationship with these persons, not only in terms of informing them of their rights, but also in terms of reassuring them that they will receive appropriate care and relief (within the options legally available in their country of residence). Specific training for all physicians and nurses on the features of palliative care appears to be an objective of the utmost importance that needs to be achieved in the very near future.

5. Conclusion

In conclusion, as is shown by the results of a few studies conducted in various countries, there does not appear to be consensus on the official definition of euthanasia, with its objectives of making end-of-life practices operational and standardizing language. In fact, the meanings attached to the term euthanasia by various groups in light of their particular concerns appear to be sometimes incompatible. In this context, arguments for legislative amendments to allow euthanasia are perceived, particularly by laypersons, as reflecting a desire for a good death, something that is apparently inaccessible at present. A good death, then, is perceived to be tied to euthanasia, and legalizing euthanasia becomes the *de facto* objective. Nevertheless, it has been observed that, in the view of a number of patients, caregivers, nurses, physicians and even members of the general population, euthanasia goes well beyond the possibility of dying following a lethal injection when suffering is considered to be unbearable by the person, as defined in the Netherlands. Unlike the institutional community, many people consider euthanasia to be as defined in the 17th century by Francis Bacon. If we want to have enlightened debate on this issue, then, would it not be appropriate to revisit the source of the present confusion and to opt for a term other than euthanasia to designate "... the administration of drugs with the explicit intention of ending the patient's life at his/her request"?

6. References

Aranda, S., & O'Conner, M. (1995). Euthanasia, nursing and care of the dying: rethinking Kuhse and Singer. *Australian Nursing Journal*, Vol. 3, No. 2, pp. 18-21.

Bilsen, J., Norup, M., Deliens, L., Miccinesi, G., van der Wal, G., Löfmark, R., Faisst, K., & van der Heide, A.; EURELD Consortium (2006). Drugs used to alleviate symptoms with life shortening as a possible side effect: end-of-life care in six European countries. *Journal of Pain & Symptom Management*, Vol. 31, No. 2, pp. 111-21

Canadian Institute for Health Information (2007). *Health Care Use at the End of Life in Western Canada.* CIHI: Ottawa. Date of access April 24, 2010, Available from: <https://secure.cihi.ca/estore/productFamily.htm?pf=PFC876&locale=en&lang=EN&mediatype=0>

Davis, A.J., Davidson, B., Hirschfield, M., Lauri, S., Lin, J.Y., Norberg, A., Phillips, L., Pitman, E., Shen, C.H., & Vander Laan, R., et al. (1993). An international perspective of active euthanasia: attitudes of nurses in seven countries. *International Journal of Nursing Studies*; Aug, Vol. 30, No. 4, pp. 301-310.

Dick, H.G. (1955). *Selected Writings of Francis Bacon*. The Modern Library & Randon House: New-York.

Dickinson, G.E., Lancaster, C.J., Sumner, E.D., & Cohen, J.S. (1997-1998). Attitudes toward assisted suicide and euthanasia among physicians in South Carolina and Washington. *Omega (Westport)*; Vol. 36, No. 3, pp. 201-218.

Economist Intelligence Unit (2010). *The quality of death: Ranking end of life care across the world.* A report commissioned by Lien Foundation. Date of access April 24, 2010, Available from: <www.eiu.com/sponsor/lienfoundation/qualityofdeath>

Emanuel, E.J., Daniels, E.R., Fairclough, D.L., & Clarridge, B.R. (1998). The practice of euthanasia and physician-assisted suicide in the United States: adherence to proposed safeguards and effects on physicians. *Journal of the American Medical Association*, Aug 12; Vol. 280, No. 6, pp. 507-513.

Gallagher, R. (2001). Using a trade-show format to educate the public about death and survey public knowledge and needs about issues surrounding death and dying. *Journal of Pain & Symptom Management*, Jan; Vol. 21, No. 1, pp. 52-58.

Kater, L., Houtepen, R., De Vries, R., & Widdershoven, G. (2003). Health care ethics and health law in the Dutch discussion on end-of-life decisions: a historical analysis of the dynamics and development of both disciplines. *Studies in history and philosophy of biological and biomedical sciences*, Dec; Vol. 34, No. 4, pp. 669-684.

Kopp, S.W. (2008-2009). The influence of death attitudes and knowledge of end of life options on attitudes toward physician-assisted suicide. *Omega (Westport)*, Vol. 58, No. 4, pp. 299-311.

Lindblad, A., Juth, N., Fürst, C.J., & Lynöe, N. (2010). When enough is enough; terminating life-sustaining treatment at the patient's request: a survey of attitudes among Swedish physicians and the general public. *Journal of Medical Ethics*, May; 3 Vol. 36, No. 5, pp. 284-289.

Marcoux, I. (2003). *Vers une meilleure compréhension de l'opinion publique envers l'euthanasie: une étude du rôle des connaissances et autres facteurs d'influence*. Thèse de doctorat: Université du Québec à Montréal: Canada. [in French]

Marcoux, I., Mishara, B.L., & Durand, C. (2007). Confusion between euthanasia and other end-of-life decisions: influences on public opinion poll results. *Canadian Journal of Public Health*, Vol. 98, No. 3, pp. 235-239.

Materstvedt, L.J., Clark, D., Ellershaw, J., Forde, R., Boeck Gravgaard, A-M., Müller-Bushc, H.C., Porta I Sales, J, & Rapin, C.-H. (2003). Euthanasia and physician-assisted suicide: a view from an EAPC Ethics Task Force. *Palliative Medicine*, Vol. 17, pp. 97-101.

McInerney, F., & Seibold, C. (1995). Nurses' definitions of and attitudes towards euthanasia. *Journal of Advance Nursing*, Jul; Vol. 22, No. 1, pp. 171-182.

Mitchell, K., & Owens, G. (2004). End of life decision-making by New Zealand general practitioners: a national survey. *New Zealand Medical Journal*, Jun 18; Vol. 117, No. 1196, pp. U934, ISSN 1175 8716

Morita, T., Miyashita, M., Shibagaki, M., Hirai, K., Ashiya, T., Ishihara, T., Matsubara, T., Miyoshi, I., Nakaho, T., Nakashima, N., Onishi, H., Ozawa, T., Suenaga, K., Tajima, T., Akechi, T., & Uchitomi, Y. (2006). Knowledge and beliefs about end-of-life care and the effects of specialized palliative care: a population-based survey in Japan. *Journal of Pain & Symptom Management*, April, Vol. 31, No. 4, pp. 306-316.

Muller, M.T., Onwuteaka-Philipsen, B.D., Kriegsman, D.M., & van der Wal, G. (1996). Voluntary active euthanasia and doctor-assisted suicide: knowledge and attitudes of Dutch medical students. *Medical Education*, Vol. 30, No. 6, pp. 428-433.

Neil, D.A., Coady, C.A., Thompson, J., & Kuhse, H. (2007). End-of-life decisions in medical practice: a survey of doctors in Victoria (Australia). *Journal of Medical Ethics*, Dec; Vol. 33, No. 12, pp. 721-725.

Parkinson, L., Rainbird, K., Kerridge, I., Carter, G., Cavenagh, J., McPhee, J., & Ravenscroft, P. (2005). Cancer patients' attitudes toward euthanasia and physician-assisted suicide: the influence of question wording and patients' own definitions on responses. *Journal of Bioethical Inquiry*, Vol. 2, No. 2, pp. 82-89.

Schwartz, K.D., & Lutfiyya, Z.M. (2009). "What lay ahead...": a media portrayal of disability and assisted suicide. *Journal of Research in Special Educational Needs*, Vol. 9, No. 1, pp. 27-38.

Seale, C. (2009). End-of-life decisions in the UK involving medical practitioners. *Palliative Medicine*,Vol. 23, pp.198-204.

Seale, C. (2010). How the mass media report social statistics: a case study concerning research on end-of-life decisions. *Social Science and Medicine*, Sep; Vol. 71, No. 5, pp. 861-868.

Sénat de Belgique (2001a). Projet de loi relative à l'euthanasie. Document législatif 2-244/26. Date of access: April 24, 2011; Available from: <http://www.senate.be/www/?MIval=/index_senate&MENUID=21400&LANG= fr>

Sénat de Belgique (2001b). Projet de loi relative aux soins palliatifs. Document législatif 2-246/9. Date of access: April 24, 2011; Available from: <http://www.senate.be/www/?MIval=/index_senate&MENUID=21400&LANG= fr>

Sepùlveda, C., Marlin, A., Yoshida, T., & Ullrich, A. (2002). Palliative Care: the World Health Organization's global perspective. *Journal of Pain & Symptom Management, 24*, 91-96.

Silveira, M.J., DiPiero, A., Gerrity, M.S., & Feudtner, C. (2000). Patients' knowledge of options at the end of life: ignorance in the face of death. *Journal of the American Medical Association*, Nov 15; Vol. 284, No. 19, pp. 2483-2488.

Sykes, N., & Thorns, A. (2003) Sedative use in the last week of life and the implications for end-of-life decision making. *Archives of Internal Medicine*, Vol. 163, No. 3, pp. 341-344.

van der Maas, P.J., van Delden, J.J.M., Pijnenborg, L., & Looman, C.W.N. (1991). Euthanasia and other medical decisions concerning the end of life. *Lancet*, Vol. 338, pp. 669-674.

van der Maas, P.J., van der Wal, G., Havertake, I., de Graaf, C.L., Kester, J.G., Onwuteaka-Philipsen, B.D., van der Heide, A, Bosma, J.M., & Willems, D.L. (1996). Euthanasia, physician-assisted suicide and other medical practices involving the end of life in the Netherlands, 1990-1995. *New England Journal of Medicine*, Nov 28; Vol. 335, No. 22, pp. 1699-1705.

Vilela, L.P., & Caramelli, P. (2009). Knowledge of the definition of euthanasia: study with doctors and caregivers of Alzheimer's disease patients. *Revista da Associação Médica Brasileira*, Vol. 55, No. 3, pp. 263-267.

Part 2

Argumentation

3

Voluntary Active Euthanasia: The Debate

Louis-Jacques van Bogaert
Fellow of the Centre for Applied Ethics
University of Stellenbosch
South Africa

1. Introduction

Voluntary active euthanasia refers to a clearly competent patient making a voluntary and persistent request for aid in dying (Brock 1999; Ogubanjo & Knapp van Bogaert 2008). In this case, the individual or a person acting on that individual's behalf (physician or lay person, depending on the law of the country) takes active steps to hasten death (LaFollette, 1997). That active step can be either the provision of the means (i.e. a lethal drug) for self-administration (orally or parenterally), or the administration by a tier. The provision of the means to die is called assisted suicide, assistance in dying, or physician assisted suicide. The patient acts last. With voluntary active euthanasia the assistant acts last. Doctor Jack Kevorkian's (dubbed "doctor death") "Mercitron" is an example of assisted suicide. The contraption is hooked to the candidate who initiates the delivery of the lethal drug. With voluntary active euthanasia the lethal drug needs to be administered by an assistant because the candidate is physically unable to proceed unaided. In both circumstances, the individual expresses a competent and voluntary wish to die, and the conditions that would make it right to allow or assist a suicide are satisfied. In both cases the aim is to spare that person pain, indignity, emotional and financial burdens. Yet, suicide is seen as morally reprehensible but is not prohibited by any law. Voluntary active euthanasia, on the other hand, is illegal in most countries and the object of conflicting and polarised moral debates.

Physician assisted suicide involves an affirmative act, writing a prescription or providing the lethal drug. Voluntary active euthanasia requires the acts of providing *and* administering the lethal drug. In physician-assisted suicide, the individual who wishes to die poses the final act; in voluntary active euthanasia, because that individual is unable to pose the last act, a proxy acts on his or her behalf. The difference is about the person who acts last. The intention and motivation are the same. Therefore, one might wonder whether the distinction is not a kind of hypocritical hair splitting. It reminds us of the omission/commission debates and of the doctrine of double effect.

The doctrine of double effect states that for an action with two consequences, one good and one bad, to be morally permissible the bad consequence may be foreseeable but not intended, and the bad cannot be used to achieve the good. The Dutch debate about indirect euthanasia is a case in point. "Terminal sedation" is legally permissible; it consists of administering large oral doses of barbiturates to induce coma followed by neuromuscular blocking agent to cause death on request of patients hoping their death to be hastened

(Veldink et al., 2002). Death is foreseen (and in fact wished by the candidate) but not intended. Furthermore, the candidate takes the first step actively; the second step inevitably requires the active intervention of an assistant. So, here we have two actors with the same motives. Both foresee the result. To claim that it is not intended is sheer casuistry.

Many red tapes need to be overcome by those wishing to die. The main reason is to avoid the legendary "What if?" In spite of good evidence against it, the most commonly advanced reason is avoiding the slippery slope. For instance, in Switzerland, where assisted suicide and voluntary active euthanasia have been tolerated (though not legal it is not prosecuted if the assistant has no hidden agenda, i.e. personal interest in the death of the assisted person) since 1918, it accounts for 0.45 percent of deaths, only a little more than the 0.3 percent in the Netherlands (Veldink et al. 2002; Van der Heide et al., 2007). The candidate has to activate the "death machine" or has to swallow the lethal drug; in other cases the candidate first ingests the drug but the final blow is administered by a tier. The death is foreseen but not intended. Who is the actor? What is active (commission) and what is passive (omission)? Removing a feeding tube is an act of commission; since the intention is death it is killing. Not pouring sustenance in the tube is omission, letting die. The intention is the same; the type of action is different. Does it really matter? As pointed out by Sullivan (1999), the debate places the doctor at the centre instead of the applicant, it leaves out the *good* of the person who wishes to die, which is the purpose of end of life decisions.

2. Facing death

Etymologically, euthanasia means a good or happy death. Many might wonder if death could ever be a happy event. To be good, death should be desired and ought to be peaceful and painless. The concept of euthanasia would not apply to a person who slips away peacefully and painlessly without any intervention after a fulfilled life. Euthanasia requires an intervention by the person wishing to die or by a person acting on her behalf to hasten a wanted death.

The word euthanasia has three meanings: 1) a quiet, peaceful, and painless death; 2) the means of procuring it; and 3) the action inducing it. What is missing is that the three definitions leave out the good of the person whose death is in question and that the death is desired by that person and for its own sake. Euthanasia cannot be morally justified unless it benefits the person who dies (Foot, 1996), and if no one else is harmed by it (Hook, 1995).

Some might consider that death is welcome after a happy and fulfilled life. Others who had an unhappy life or who are burdened with sorrow and suffering view death as deliverance. It seems, though, that for many who are clinging to life death is the last thing on their wish list. In other words, death is inevitable and is either wished or feared.

LaFollette (1997) has argued that we have not decided to enter life, but that we should be granted the right to choose to exit life. Such view, of course, is highly debatable and debated. Those who believe in the principle of sanctity of life argue that life is God given; therefore, God only can take it back. This argument does not hold for non-believers though. The principle that life is sacred, says Dworkin (1995), "that's the easy part"; the crucial question is which decisions best respect it.

One must respect the wishes of those, believers or not, who wish to stay alive no matter what. On the other hand, to what extent should one respect the wish to die? One answer would be allowing them to commit suicide. Every one has the right to commit suicide; no single law prohibits suicide. However, one may not have the courage or the means to take that step. Considering suicide one may be discouraged by the impact it has on one's loved ones. However, this argument is double-edged. The person who plans committing suicide may well make this decision because his entourage failed him. In that case, should he refrain from the act to avoid guilt feelings and remorse among the survivors?

Is there a right to die? Is there a duty to die? If there is a right to die, is there a correlative duty of a tier party to assist in dying?

In an attempt to answer these though questions the topic of euthanasia is riddled with inconsistencies and twists. Thou shalt not kill, of course, but it needs qualification: thou shalt not kill the innocent (Battin, 1995). It is legally and ethically impermissible to take some one's life against her will. Mass murder in war, camps, or campuses is fittingly condemned. Even if this was labelled euthanasia by the Nazi regime, it was murder of innocent and non-consenting persons. This is not negotiable. Then we have the debate whether killing and letting die are one and the same thing or not. Should active voluntary euthanasia be accessible only for intractable *physical* pain? What is the difference, if any, between early terminal sedation and terminal sedation? What is the difference, if any, between ordinary and extraordinary means to keep some one alive? And last but not least, what are the duties of health care providers towards terminally ill patients? As pointed out by Sullivan (1999), the euthanasia debate tends to place the doctor in the centre of the debate instead of the candidate. It too often leaves out the good of the person who wishes to die (Angell, 1998).

All these queries illustrate our concerns with death, our own and the other's. Death is inevitably part of life; we cannot avoid taking a moral position, because we can now choose to interrupt and delay nature's progress (Gorsuch, 2006). Euthanasia claims Moreno (1995), "appears as the ultimate postmodern demand for personal dignity".

3. Euthanasia's historical background

Rachels (1993) has given a historical overview of euthanasia from which some of the following is borrowed. In Ancient Greece, there was nothing similar to the current view on the sanctity of life. Infanticide of deformed newborns and infants was seen as benefiting them by avoiding a miserable life. Currently, such practices would be regarded as offensive and a deep lack of respect for differently able persons. This is not to say that every one believes that non-existence might be preferable to existence with different abilities. Peter Singer (1994), notoriously, has argued in favour of the permissibility of infanticide in such circumstances. Needless to say that Singer's view did provoke public outrage.

Hippocratic physicians represented only a small minority of all self-proclaimed healers. Markel (2004) claims that it is doubtful that Hippocrates would recognise most pledges ascribed to him because many revisions of the oath were written under Christian influence during the Middle Ages. In those early times, it was not uncommon for physicians to recommend suicide to a patient with incurable disease.

Even if great thinkers as Plato, Aristotle, and Pythagoras considered that suicide was mostly an act of cowardice, they admitted to exceptions. It should also be noted that the Pythagorean School of medicine did not follow Hippocrates' teachings with regards to physicians' duty to refrain from assistance in dying. Pythagoras of Samos (582-507 BCE) shifted philosophy from Asia Minor to Southwest Italy, where he founded a school, a religious and mathematical community where his intellectual and moral authority was absolute (*autos ephê, ipse dixit,* the master has spoken). Against the Homeric world-view, he introduced features of the mystery religions. Pythagoras' community was influenced by Orphic mysticism. Pythagoras believed in the immortality of the soul ("*the body is a tomb*", just like later Plato's "body the dungeon of the soul"). Therefore, one should strive to give priority to the soul and respect all living beings because they are all ensouled. Purity of the soul was important (because of his belief in metempsychosis) and can be only achieved through philosophy - the quest for knowledge, understanding, and competence.

During the following twenty centuries, Western Europe was so much under the influence of Christianity that there was a silent condemnation of suicide and no discussion on euthanasia (Curzer, 1999). During the Enlightenment, Immanuel Kant clearly rejected the permissibility of suicide. His argument was rooted in the belief that persons have an incomparable worth. Suicide degrades humanity. Even during the Enlightenment, it would have been risky to express personal liberal view on any topic, in this case to contest the sanctity of life that would upset the Church's fundamentalism.

It was not until the twentieth century that the legal and ethical aspects of euthanasia came to the public fore. In 1918, a comment by the Swiss federal government on Article 115 of the first penal code stated (quoted in Hurst & Mauron, 2003):

> In modern penal law, suicide is not a crime …
> Aiding and abetting suicide can themselves
> be inspired by altruistic motives.

This is why the project incriminates them only if the author has been moved by selfish reasons (Hurst & Mauron 2003). The act is called "murder upon request of the victim", not euthanasia. *De facto*, a 1997 attempt to decriminalise euthanasia failed. The article does not require the involvement of a physician nor that the patient is terminally ill. Switzerland permits anyone to assist in another's death regardless whether the candidate is terminally ill or not (Ziegler & Bosshard, 2007). The Swiss Academy of Medical Sciences states that assistance in dying is "not part of a physician's activity". Nevertheless, like any other citizen, a physician is allowed to altruistically assist in dying.

The argument from palliative care (including pain palliation) is often used against assistance in dying because of excruciating pain. The promoters of the argument claim that no pain is beyond palliation. A survey in Switzerland showed that 73% of palliative care physicians opposed the legislation of euthanasia; however, 19% would practice euthanasia if it became legal (Hurst & Mauron, 2003).

In the Netherlands, voluntary active euthanasia is "tolerated" since 1973 (it is not lawful but not a criminal offence) provided strict guidelines, called "due care criteria" (also referred to as careful practice, and standards of care) are adhered to: 1) the claimant must be sound of mind; 2) the request must be voluntary, independent, persistent and fully informed; 3) the pain endured must be intolerable and unresponsive to all pain relief methods; and 3) the physician must consult with another independent colleague (Battin, 2002; Sleeboom-Faulkner, 2006). The physician is free to participate or not (conscience clause) (Sleeboom-Faulkner, 2006). Note that, since the *Brongersma* case of "life fatigue or existential suffering", the claimant needs not be terminally ill, and the pain must not be physical (Huxtable & Möller, 2007). The Netherlands since has formalised its policy in the *Termination of Life on Request and Assisted Suicide Act* 2001. The "due care criteria" including the intractable pain remain included. The *Euthanasia Act* was passed in 2003 to regulate ending of life by a physician at the request of a patient who is suffering unbearably without hope of relief. In 2005, 1.7% of deaths were the result of euthanasia and 0.1% of physician-assisted suicide; 80.2% of all cases were reported (*vs.* only 18.0% in 1990) (Van der Maas & Emanuel, 1998;

Van der Heide et al., 2007). Terminal sedation is legally permissible. It consists of the administration of a high dose of a sedative to relieve suffering without intending to hasten death, even if the patient might hope so (Quill, 2007). The Royal Dutch Association of Pharmacy technical guidelines of 1987 (revised in 1994 and 1998) recommend the oral administration of high doses of barbiturates to induce coma, followed by a neuromuscular blocking agent to cause death (Veldink et al., 2002). In the Netherlands, terminal sedation and the withdrawal of artificial feeding are regarded as "normal medical treatment" and thus different from euthanasia. Therefore, they cannot fall under the same legal regulation as euthanasia (Sheldon, 2003).

Australia's Northern Territory was the world's first jurisdiction to legalise euthanasia in 1996; four people were assisted under this legislation before the Australian federal government repealed it in 1997 (Parker, 2005). The Dutch practice is close to the requirements of the 1997 *Oregon's Death with Dignity Act,* namely: 1) two oral requests separated by at least two weeks; and 2) a written request witnessed by two persons. From the part of the physician: the prescribing and the consulting physician must inform of alternatives such as pain control and hospice care (Dieterle, 2007). Note that in Oregon, the applicant must be at least 18 years old, competent, and suffering from a terminal illness with less than six months to live. As we know, this sort of prediction is alarmingly imprecise. Moreover, it might be tricky to determine one's mental competency, but there is no obligation to get the opinion of a clinical psychologist or psychiatrist. Finally, any physician with a medical degree can assist.

In 2002, Belgium passed a Euthanasia Law. It carries most of the requirements and restrictions as those in the Dutch law (Lemiengre et al., 2007; Quill, 2007). In Germany, there is a legal "inconsistency" in the sense that voluntary active euthanasia is illegal but assisting in dying is tolerated. The preconditions are that the applicant should be competent and free. The *German Society for Humane Dying* provides the needed support provided the following conditions are met: 1) at least one-year membership; and 2) at least two years without treatment for depression or psychiatric illness. If these preconditions are met, the applicant is supplied with a list of drugs and their dosage for producing certain and painless death. It is recommended to acquire the drug through prescription from a physician and to sign a form where the decision is signed. A lay companion to assist is provided on request (Battin, 2002).

4. Definitions of euthanasia

Euthanasia is subdivided into voluntary and involuntary, active and passive. Involuntary means not under control of the will, unintentional, forced. Some add non-voluntary when a person has not expressed a choice (Beauchamp, 1996). Involuntary active euthanasia is killing an innocent person against his will. Since it does not refer to a "good" death, one should avoid calling it euthanasia.

There seems to be some confusion about the concept of active voluntary euthanasia, and its difference from physician assisted suicide. According to Dieterle (2007), in physician-assisted suicide "the patient him or herself is the instigator of death"; in active euthanasia "the physician is the instigator of death". Brock (1999) writes "with physician-assisted suicide, the physician administers a lethal dose often because the patient is unable to do so"; but he goes on with the example of Janet Adkins (see below) who acted last. Brock (1999) opposes this to (voluntary active) euthanasia, where "the physician acts last". Rachels (1975) writes:

> The important difference between active and passive euthanasia is that, in passive euthanasia, the doctor does not do anything to bring about the patient's death. The doctor does nothing, and the patient dies of whatever ills already afflict him. In active euthanasia, however, the doctor does something to bring about the patient's death: he kills him. The doctor who gives the patient with cancer a lethal injection has himself caused his patient's death; whereas if he merely ceases the treatment, the cancer is the cause of death.

This, again, is unhelpful. To die from any terminal illness is a natural death. Whether it is accompanied by intractable and untreatable physical pain or psychological suffering is a different matter altogether. Notice the vocabulary: the doctor is the "killer". In the euthanasia debate, the use of the verb killing should be avoided because it refers conventionally to taking a person's life against his will. The position of the American Medical Association, which Rachels tries to debunk, is "At stake is the intentional termination of life of one human being by another" (viz. of a person who did not express a consistent and free request of dying) (quoted in Rachels, 1975).

It seems that the debate has been confused by the fact that in the Netherlands, it has become common parlance to talk of active and passive while omitting the fundamental qualification voluntary and involuntary. Active voluntary euthanasia refers to a person who makes the free decision to end her life and takes the necessary steps to achieve death. The typical example is that of Janet Adkins. She was diagnosed as in the initial stage of Alzheimer's disease. She was devastated and wanted to die with dignity before the disease would take its full toll. At that time, she was a member of the Hemlock Society, and was living in Oregon where physician-assisted suicide and active voluntary euthanasia were then illegal. She flew to Michigan, where assistance in dying was not illegal. She went to Dr Jack Kevorkian who connected her to the "Mercitron", a device composed of a pump containing a lethal substance connected to an intravenous line. The physician did install the IV-line but the candidate had to press the button to initiate the injection. In other words, Janet took the free decision to be connected to the contraption, and decided to initiate the procedure all by herself (Pence, 1995). The assistance provided by Dr Kevorkian was to make the device available. Although he was a physician and assisted by making the means available, this was not physician-assisted suicide but rather active voluntary euthanasia. It was voluntary and Janet executed the final act.

Kevorkian was prosecuted for murder by the local district attorney. A local judge dismissed the case but ordered Kevorkian to desist from using the contraption. It is unclear on what grounds the judge's ruling was based since assisting in dying was not against the law. In 1992, the governor of Michigan signed a law making assisted suicide illegal. In 1994, the Michigan Court of Appeals overruled the state's ban on assisted suicide on grounds of technicalities (Pence, 1995).

The striking down of a Washington state law banning assisted suicide followed this. The federal judge Barbara Rothstein held that the Fourteenth Amendment to the Constitution that protects individual liberties was broad enough to cover women's right to abortion *and* the right of the terminally ill to be assisted in dying. In *Quill v. Vacco*, 80 F.3d 716 (2d. Cir. 1996), the Second Circuit Court of Appeals declared unconstitutional New York's law against physician-assisted-suicide because it is a violation of the constitutional right of equal protection under the law, since it denies help in dying to those without life-sustaining treatment, while permitting it for those receiving such treatment (Angell, 1998; Gorsuch, 2006).

In 1992, a referendum campaign aimed at toppling the California's law banning assisted suicide failed. In 1993, a similar campaign was successful in Oregon; legal challenges delayed the implementation of *Oregon's Death with Dignity Act* until 1997. Currently, in the vast majority of states' statutes have been retained or enacted expressly banning assisted suicides. In *Washington v. Glucksberg* (1997), the justices made it clear that there is no constitutionally protected right to physician-assisted suicide. However, they expressed concern about the inadequacies of access to and delivery of palliative care (Quill, 2004). Terri Schiavo was in the same condition as Quinlan and Cruzan. In 1990, at the age of 27 she went into permanent vegetative state. In 1998, her husband petitioned the court to withdraw the feeding tube. Florida's Supreme Court refused to hear appeals. A trial court judge ordered the removal. *Terri's Law* (2003) gave Governor Jab Bush authority to order the feeding tube to be reinserted. The US Supreme Court refused to hear an appeal brought by Governor Bush. Despite the adoption by the senate of a bill *For the Relief of the Parents of Theresa Marie Schiavo* (2005), the tube was removed and Terri died (Annas, 2005).

Passive voluntary euthanasia refers to a person who makes a fully voluntary and persistent request to put an end to life but demands assistance from a tier person, either because she does not have the courage to do the needful to achieve her goal, or because she does not have the physical ability to do it. This is the same as assistance in dying. However, here again, Brock (1999) has a different definition; for him passive euthanasia (he omits the qualification of voluntary *vs.* involuntary) consists of withholding or withdrawing life-sustaining procedures.

The first assisted death on public record was the *Postma* case in the Netherlands in 1971. She suffered a severe brain haemorrhage that left her partially paralysed, deaf, and with gross speech deficits. She repeatedly begged for death. Her physician daughter Geertruda injected morphine to induce unconsciousness and curare (an agent that paralyses all muscles including the respiratory ones) to kill her. She informed the authorities. She was found guilty of murder but was given a suspended sentence. In the aftermath, the Royal Dutch Medical association set down guidelines, the so-called "due care criteria", that were accepted by the Dutch prosecutors. Eventually, passive voluntary euthanasia or assistance in dying became rechristened as "terminal sedation", where deep sedation is induced to "an imminently dying patient". It is deemed permissible if it does not hasten death significantly (Varelius, 2007). Cellarius (2011) has argued that terminal sedation differs from early terminal sedation. He defines early terminal sedation as "palliative sedation in which deep, continuous sedation is combined with cessation of nutrition and hydration, orally or parenterally". Because it hastens death, he claims, it is "contentious but not unethical". What is contentious is debatable, disputed. This is unhelpful in the debate. Cellarius (2011) contends that deep and continuous sedation is acceptable to treat "intolerable and intractable pain", unless it hastens death. Sullivan (1999), on the other hand, states that a decision may hasten death, but that it does not follow from the fact that the intention is to bring about death that is intended. Death is only foreseeable.

This debate illustrates the contentious old doctrine of double effect, now rechristened "principle of proportionality". The doctrine states that if an action results in a foreseeable bad consequence (i.e. death), but that this end is not intended, it is morally permissible. It is quite clear that terminal sedation and early terminal sedation both aim at a single end, death. To argue that the aim is the relief of pain or suffering is hypocritical. It seems that the same sophistry is used to permit withholding of treatment, i.e. letting die.

Passive involuntary euthanasia refers to a condition where the candidate is diagnosed irreversibly comatose. She either has a living will or not. If there is a living will that stipulates clearly the conditions in which she declines life-sustaining treatment, the decision should be respected. In the absence of a living will the decision has to be made by proxy. The proxy can be close relatives or friends who know what she would have chosen in the circumstances. In their absence, the decision is incumbent to the healthcare team and should be in the best interest of the patient. Now, this is more complex than it might appear. It raises the debate between killing and letting die. It raises the issue of the person's best interest and the possible hidden agenda of the proxy decision maker(s). We will come back to these issues.

Pickering (1993) has argued that an advance directive for "voluntary euthanasia" is a volatile combination. In brief, the argument stresses that the person who made advance directives was not psychologically the same at the time of the writing and at the time of the condition leading to coma. Perhaps, if she would regain momentary or permanent consciousness she would change her mind. One cannot foresee what type of condition one might be in and how one would judge it if one was conscious. It follows, so the argument goes, that advance directives should be respected only when the candidate is in a position to reiterate the decision made by advance directive.

The argument is often presented that one has to be suffering from depression to consider suicide or assistance in dying. One cannot fully exercise one's autonomy under the influence of depression. Therefore, one should never honour the request for assistance in dying. Along these lines, Brock (1999) discusses the "expressed-wishes euthanasia" based on what the patient would say if competent and rational. He contends that it is impossible to know what incompetent patients would choose if they were competent, even if they have previously expressed their preferences.

All these arguments have some truth, but they boil down to the infamous slippery slope: what if? Granted, all life and death decisions are controversial and may be abused. None the less, one cannot negate the fact that life and its quality may degrade so badly that death is deemed a better choice.

5. Killing and letting die

The ethical dilemma is about the difference, if any, between killing and letting die. The legal conundrum shows that, mainly in the US, the legality of letting die is variously interpreted. Similar cases, such as Karen Quinlan (1975) and Nancy Cruzan (1990), were treated differently. Karen was in permanent vegetative state and on a respirator; she was fed through a naso-gastric feeding tube. The New Jersey Supreme Court ruled in favour of Karen's parents' request to disconnect the ventilator to let her die. The importance physicians placed on the distinction between withholding and withdrawing life support surprised the Court. The Court applied the right to privacy to allow proxy decision of letting die. The Roman Catholic nursing staff, unbeknownst to Karen's relatives, implemented the weaning. Unexpectedly, Karen survived after having been weaned from the respirator. It is likely that without weaning she would have died when the respirator was disconnected. She ultimately died after 10 years in permanent vegetative state (Pence, 1995).

Nancy Cruzan was also in permanent vegetative state and fed through a naso-gastric tube. The Missouri Supreme Court overturned the probate court's decision to allow the withdrawal of the feeding tube. This was because, in the eyes of the judiciary, there was no clear and convincing evidence about Nancy's wishes not to be resuscitated if she were to be in permanent vegetative state. In reviewing the Missouri Supreme Court decision, the United States Supreme Court began to recognise a right of a competent patient to informed refusal. The tube was finally removed legally and Nancy died (Pence, 1995).

The importance of the Quinlan and the Cruzan cases was that they brought about the legal permissibility of informed refusal and the right to proxy decision-making about withholding and withdrawing life-sustaining procedures. In both cases the issue was the artificial feeding. Since food and water are basic human needs, the controversy arose whether artificial feeding is an ordinary or an extraordinary means. In addition, it ignited the debate whether removing the tube would be an act of omission (letting die) or commission (killing).

The legality of assistance in dying is mostly not recognised. The US state of Oregon, however, enacted the Oregon Death with Dignity Act. Oregon's Department of Human Services has the task of auditing a sample of the records regarding each act of assisted suicide on a yearly basis. At variance with the Dutch medical guidelines, in Oregon the right to assistance in dying does not require the existence of any pain, treatable or not. The distinction between killing and letting die has connection with the elusive distinction between omission and commission, as well as with the hair splitting and hypocritical doctrine of double effect.

In *Active and Passive Euthanasia*, Rachels (1975) has argued that there is no moral difference between killing (commission) and letting die (omission), but rather that it is "a grotesque perversion of moral reasoning". He opposes the American Medical Association's denial that the withdrawal of life-sustaining interventions equals the intentional termination of life. He contends that it is "patently cruel" to withhold a treatment (letting die) because it results in a prolonged agony; therefore, it is more humane to inject a lethal drug (killing). The American Medical Association's position is that in certain circumstances it is permissible to withhold treatment (letting die), but that in no circumstances a positive step can be taken to end a patient's life (mercy killing). Note that what the American Medical Association talks about is the withdrawal (i.e. "cessation", not withholding) of "extraordinary means" when it is clear that death is imminent. To withdraw is to discontinue something that was given; to withhold is to refuse to give. Rachels appears to be mixing both withholding and withdrawing treatment.

Thought experiments are often used as a fictional situation to underpin a moral argument. In his paper, Rachels (1975) argues that there is no difference if a person who has a personal interest in the death of a child, either witnesses it drowning in the bath tub (letting die) or actively drowns it (killing). In both cases the motive and the end in view were identical. Therefore, killing and letting die are the same. Now, as Rachels (1975) acknowledges, this is irrelevant to the issue under discussion, namely withholding and withdrawing life-sustaining procedures in medicine. If it is irrelevant to the issue under discussion, it should be omitted. He also points out that what matters in the moral judgement are the motives: personal gain or a humanitarian motive (which applies to the thought experiment he offers). The twist is that, as far as Rachels' case study is concerned, the problem is about the social and parental acceptance of Down's babies, rather than killing *vs.* letting die.

Now consider the following scenarios. Bill and his wife Nancy are clear about their mutual desire not to be resuscitated in case of irreversible coma. This is written down in their living will. Both drive weekly to their respective work place in two different and far away locations. Bill is involved in a car accident. He has a life threatening head injury and is treated by paramedics at the scene of the accident. He is put on emergency life-support and transported to the nearest hospital. On arrival, the casualty medical officer judges that Bill needs to be ventilated artificially to give him any chance of survival. Bill is intubated and connected to the ventilator. Nancy is informed about the situation and rushes to the hospital. She is told that the brain damage is most likely to be irreversible. She explains that Bill has a living will that is clear about "do not resuscitate" (DNR). The doctor acted according to his professional duty to preserve life. Nancy wants to respect Bill's wishes, but the life-support procedures were initiated. There was no way the doctor could have known about Bill's DNR wish. Now what would the decision to pull the plug be, killing or letting die? Bill had expressed the will to die if such foreseeable circumstances would occur. The life-sustaining procedure should not have been commenced if his DNR will have been known, but would it? Even if the doctor had known, would he have let Bill die? Let us now change the scenario. Bill and Nancy are driving on the highway to their log cabin at the lake. A drunk driver hits their car on the passenger side. Nancy suffers a life-threatening injury, but Bill is unscathed. The paramedics arrive on the scene. Bill tells them to desist from assistance. Bill lets Nancy die. This sounds similar to Rachel's scenario where the person watches the child drowning in the bathtub. But is it? Nancy has no interest at all in Bill's death. She only wants to respect his living will. However, it is doubtful whether she will be allowed. It is very likely that she would be charged of non-assistance to a person in danger.

6. The right to die: The limits of autonomy?

In 1973, an exploding gas line burned 67 percent of Donald ("Dax") Cowart's body. At the time, he was a healthy young jet pilot and amateur rodeo performer. At the scene of the accident, he begged for a gun to shoot himself when the emergency paramedics arrived. Dax's prognosis for survival was approximately 20 percent, but his potential quality of life was deeply compromised. His request was denied. Against his will he underwent 232 days of treatment in Parkland Memorial Hospital in Dallas. Despite the fact that he was deemed competent, his repeated refusal of treatment and requests to die where consistently declined. Instead, the physicians honoured the wishes of his mother. The accident left him blind and gravely disfigured, with only partial use of his fingers. He later became a millionaire from an out of court settlement with the gas company. He graduated from law school in 1986 and got married. He also became a regular speaker for the Society for the Right to Die. His main argument has always been that his physicians had been morally wrong to treat him against his wishes (Andersen et al., 1996; Knapp van Bogaert & Ogubanjo, 2010).

The question is: Would it be an act of commission, sanctioned legally and morally, to provide someone the means to commit suicide? Recall Kevorkian's Mercitron. Janet Adkins did operate the device herself knowingly and willingly. At the time, assisted suicide was legal in Michigan. And still, Kevorkian was requested to desist from repeating assistance. Dax, however, was unable to get hold of a gun without assistance. Isn't there an inconsistency? One tends to admit that a terminally ill person has the right to assistance in dying, especially if she is in excruciating pain. When burns cover 67 percent of the body the pain is excruciating and there is generally little hope to survive. Dax was in excruciating pain (and remained in that condition for the 32 following weeks). And yet, assistance was denied.

As we have seen, the US Supreme Court recognised the legal right to informed refusal of treatment or life-sustaining interventions. Unfortunately for Dax that was in 1993, twenty years after his ordeal began.

The right to die from one's personal perception of quality of life, as it was in Dax's case, was brought to the fore with Larry McAffee in 1985. Twenty-nine years old McAffee became almost totally paralysed in a motorcycle accident. In 1989, he decided to file suit in court for the right to die because the institutions he was placed did not provide what he judged an acceptable quality of life. He designed a switch to be connected to his IV-line that would allow him to self-inject a lethal drug by blowing in certain ways into the ventilator. The County Superior Court ruled in his favour. McAffee did not commit suicide as he was eventually placed in an institution where his quality of life was improved (Knapp van Bogaert & Ogubanjo, 2010).

As commented by Pence (1995), such cases suggest that society often gives severely disabled people only three limited, grim choices: to become a burden on their families or friends, to live miserably in a public institution, or to kill themselves. Even the last option is often denied. Is there any difference between a terminally ill patient requesting assistance in dying, given the hurdles of prognostication, and an almost totally paralysed person whose lack of quality of life is unbearable? Why would one oblige to the former's wish and not to the latter?

Like many others, Beauchamp and Childress (2001) remark that if autonomy is the corner stone of medical decision-making one has to admit that double standards regulate the granting and declining of patients' autonomy. On the one hand, a patient's informed refusal to life-sustaining interventions is viewed as an affirmation of and respect for his autonomy. That is the moral (and legal) permissibility of letting die. On the other hand, the right to assistance in dying by mutual agreement between the patient and her assistant is, with some exceptions mentioned above, unlawful and regarded morally impermissible. One does not always have the ability to commit suicide; for instance, if one is paralysed one cannot exercise one's autonomy. So, killing is not the same as letting die. Rachels (1993) has argued that it is the same. If he is right, the mentioned inconsistency must be redressed.

In the clinical context, autonomy and respect for patients are linked to the notion of informed consent or refusal. It is often regarded as a *loose* expression of patient's right to choose; the health care provider has to comply with whatever the patient decides as long as she is deemed competent and properly informed about the alternatives, the risks and benefits. This view places the concept of autonomy and respect for autonomy in a narrow or minimal perspective. This, writes O'Neill (1988), is a minimal conception of autonomy that identifies autonomy with the requirements of informed consent and that regards respect for autonomy as a sufficient rather than necessary ethical justification. Instead, she argues, autonomy should be understood as a capacity for independent decisions and actions. Autonomy is not exercised in vacuo. One is autonomous from something and from someone (the health care team, the entourage). Autonomy is exercised in a *relational* (after consultation, exchange) rather than in an adversarial context. And, finally, there are degrees of independent decisions. The mere fact of being ill places us in a vulnerable situation that may affect our level of independence and degree of willingness to accept the health care professional's plan of action. On the other hand, a stronger perception of one's autonomy may easily conflict with the reasonable choices offered by the health care team.

7. Euthanasia and the slippery slope

One stands on the slippery slope when arguments against one position appear to equally apply to the counter position, leading to an undesired or undesirable situation. With euthanasia, it would mean that if assistance in dying becomes legally authorised the door is wide open to abuse. Corners will be bent so that euthanasia will be practised for other motives and outside of the requirements set by the law, let alone that people will be forced to die under false pretences. Granted that the risk cannot be denied, one should look whether the risk is real or of minimal magnitude.

Pence (1997) distinguishes three different types of slippery slope: 1) generalising to other kinds of cases; 2) unleashing the dark side of human nature; and 3) consistency. According to the first one, you first withdraw, say, the respirator, then you stop parenteral nutrition, and finally you kill. The slope slips from terminally ill patients, to formerly competent ones (e.g. senile dementia), to never competent adults (e.g. brain damaged at birth), and to infanticide. It does only if competence is disregarded or misconstrued. The second slope slips when proxy decisions are made that are not in the best interest of dying or terminally ill patient be it for material sake (e.g. the cost of terminal care, or greed) or out of convenience (e.g. the financial and emotional burden of terminal care). In this case, the person may be competent or not but coerced into accepting that she has the duty to die. In other words, the slope becomes slippery only if one calls voluntary active euthanasia what is not a willing and knowing request for help in dying.

The third slope slips if one uses criteria applicable in one case that are not applicable to another. This slippery argument, says Pence, is the weakest sometimes time and introspection will tell that criteria may have to change.

It is unfortunate that the country with the longest "experience", Switzerland, has no validated statistics. Estimates, however, suggest that only 0.45% deaths are assisted suicides and that two thirds of the requests are rejected. In Oregon 0.09% of deaths represent assisted death, and in the Netherlands they amount to 0.3% (Hurst & Mauron, 2003). These data do not mean that "assistance" is not given without the patients' explicit request. In 1990, a confidential enquiry run in the Netherlands showed that 0.8% of deaths were initiated without the patient's request. A similar enquiry was run in 1995 and resulted in a value of 0.7% showing that toleration did not result in a ripple effect. The same questionnaire used in Australia estimated the occurrence of involuntary euthanasia at 3.5%. The difference suggests that different cultures may have different potential for misuse (van der Maas & Emanuel, 1998). As pointed out by Battin (1995), "It is unlikely that Americans can fully understand why the Dutch support their practice of euthanasia, and conversely it is unlikely that the Dutch will understand why the Americans are so ambivalent about its legalisation or why they are so likely to distort the Dutch practice, until these differences are incorporated into both sides of the debate".

One of the slippery slope arguments claims that legalising euthanasia will result in pressurising the weak and the elderly to accept dying. In Oregon, however, data show that those who choose euthanasia are younger, highly educated, and used to be in control of their lives (Branthwaite, 2005).

As Rachels (1993.) comments, there is no denying that there are abuses of virtually all social practices. The question is whether the abuses would be so numerous as to justify the banning of that specific practice. Furthermore, slippery slope arguments provide no moral basis for the conclusion that some acts are morally wrong (Beauchamp 1996). With regards to assistance in dying, Pence (1997) remarks that claiming that it is immoral "only begs the question, it isn't an argument".

8. Conclusive remarks

It appears that more is written and argued against than in favour of voluntary euthanasia. This is understandable since most people wish rather to live than to die. None the less, there are people who wish to die. Their voice must also be heard. The nagging question is why, when, and how? As emphasised by Tristram Engelhardt (1995), "to establish the wrongness of voluntary euthanasia would require a hierarchy of values that subordinates the value of individual liberty to other special values".

In this case, we encounter two potentially conflicting liberties: the autonomy of the person whishing to die, and the autonomy of the individual who is asked assistance in dying. Although Switzerland has, in my opinion, resolved that conflict by permitting legally any one who has no personal profit in assisting in dying, other countries like the Netherlands reserve this right strictly to physicians. The right to autonomy is equally applicable to physicians. Ann Davis (1996) contends that one cannot be autonomous if decisions can be overruled by people who do not share our values. Beauchamp (1997) asserts that to refuse assistance in dying is harmful because it denies a person's autonomous wish. Self-determination, as long as it does not harm the other(s), is one of the main cornerstones of ethics. If the exercise of autonomy relieves us from an unacceptable lack of quality of life, it should not be morally wrong.

The legal and ethical permissibility of a patient's right to withhold (not to allow) life-sustaining interventions is widely accepted. In this case, that person knows and willingly accepts that this will result in dead. This has been dubbed "coming to peace with death" (Gorschung, 2006). It is the disease that kills (Callahan, 1999).

In the case of withdrawing life-sustaining procedures that have been initiated (killing), the intention, malevolent or not, is death. The irony is that this fuels a sophistical debate on omission and commission. For instance, the removal of a feeding tube is an act, commission. To keep the tube but not supplying fluids and nutrients is omission. In both cases, the patient will die. In both cases this was the motivation.

On the other hand, it is deemed legally and ethically impermissible to request assistance in dying (if one is unable to, say, press the button). It is killing if one is unable to press the button or suicide with some one's assistance (otherwise called "mercy killing") if one is the last person to act.

The so-called "joint view" that justifies voluntary euthanasia is based on two ethical principles: respect for autonomy, and beneficence (Huxtable & Möller 2007,). Varelius (2007) argues that respect for autonomy trumps the principle of beneficence, because the latter results in harm even if requested. However, the twist is that the defenders of terminal sedation deem it acceptable if the harm is needed to reach the intended goal, pain relief. On the other hand, by limiting the right of assistance in dying to physicians, one creates a potential conflict between the physician's duties to preserve life, and to alleviate pain and suffering. In the case of euthanasia, one of both duties must be prioritised.

By placing the doctor at the centre of the ethical dilemma, the patient's request is often disregarded, minimised, or even put in jeopardy. Furthermore, the debate is all too often around generic patients, in ideal circumstances, where the arguments appeal to abstract principles (Donchin, 2000). In line with Beauchamp & Childress (1994), one should strive to reform ethics and the law to deal with an "apparent inconsistency" between affirmation and denial of autonomy. Autonomy is given to those who consciously and willingly refuse life-sustaining interventions; but autonomy is denied to those who consciously, willingly, and repeatedly ask for assistance in dying.

9. References

Andersen, D., Cavalier, R. & Covey, P.K. (1996). *A Right to Die? The Dax Cowart case*. Routledge, ISBN 0-415-15274-7, London.

Annas, G.J. (2005). "Culture of life" politics at the bedside - The case of Terri Schiavo. *New England Journal of Medicine*, Vol. 352, No. 16 (April 2005), pp.1710-1715, ISSN 27499832.

Ann Davis, N. (1996). The right to refuse treatment. In: *Intending Death*. T.L. Beauchamp (Ed.), pp. 109-130, Prentice Hall, ISBN 0-13-199555-3, Upper Saddle River, NJ.

Angell, M. (1998). Helping desperately ill people to die. In: *Regulating How We Die*, L.L. Emmanuel (Ed.), pp. 3-20, Harvard University Press, ISBN 0-674-66654-2 Cambridge, MA.

Battin, M. P. (1995). A dozen caveats concerning the discussion of euthanasia in the Netherlands. In: *Arguing Euthanasia*, J.D. Moreno (Ed.), pp. 88-109, Simon & Schuster, ISBN 0-684-80760-2, New York.

Battin, M. P. (2002). Euthanasia: the way we do it, the way they do it. In *Applied Ethics – A Multicultural Approach. 3rd ed.* L. May, S. Collins-Chobanian & K. Wong (Eds.), pp. 579-591, Prentice Hall, ISBN 0-13-092384-2, Upper Saddle River, NJ.

Beauchamp TL. (1996). Introduction. In: *Intending Death*. T.L. Beauchamp (Ed.), pp. 1-22, Prentice Hall, ISBN 0-13-199555-3 Upper Saddle River, NJ.

Beauchamp, T.L. & Childress, J. (2001). *Principles of Biomedical Ethics*.5th ed. Oxford University Press, ISBN 0-19-508537-x, New York.

Branthwaite, M.A. (2005). Taking the final step: changing the law on euthanasia and physician assisted suicide. *British Medical Journal*, Vol. 331, No. 7518 (September 2005), pp. 681-683, ISSN 27500139.

Brock, D. (1999). Voluntary active euthanasia, In: *Ethical Theory and Moral Problems*. H.J. Curzer (Ed.), pp. 718-726, Wadsworth, ISBN 0-534-52974-7 Belmont, CA.

Callahan, D. (1999). When self-determination runs amok. In: *Ethical Theory and Moral Problems*. H.J. Curzer (Ed.), pp. 727-732, Wadsworth, ISBN 0-534-52974-7 Belmont, CA.

Cellarius, V. (2011). 'Early terminal sedation' is a distinct entity, *Bioethics* Vol. 25, No. 1 (January 2011), pp. 46-54, ISSN 0269-9702.

Cilliers, P. (1998). Complexity & Postmodernism. Routledge, ISBN 9 780415 152877, London.

Curzer, H.J. (1999). Euthanasia, suicide, and futility. In: *Ethical Theory and Moral Problems*. H.J. Curzer (Ed.), pp. 695-705, Wadsworth, ISBN 0-534-52974-7, Belmont, CA.

Derrida, J. (1995). *The Gift of Death*. University of Chicago Press, ISBN 0-226-14306-6, Chicago.

Dieterlee, J.M. (2007). Physician assisted suicide: a new look at the arguments. *Bioethics,* Vol.21, No. 3, (March 2007), pp. 127-139, ISSN 0269 9702.

Donchin, A. (2000). Autonomy, interdependence, and assisted suicide: respecting boundaries/crossing lines. *Bioethics,* Vol. 14, No. 3 (July 2000), pp. 187-204, ISSN 0269 9702.

Dworkin, R. (1995). Life is sacred: that's the easy part. In: *Arguing Euthanasia.* J.D. Moreno (Ed.), pp. 246-251, Simon & Schuster, ISBN 0-684-80760-2, New York.

Foot, P. (1996). Euthanasia. In: *Applying Ethics.* J. Olen & V. Barry (Eds.), pp. 218-230, Wadsworth, ISBN 0-534-26316-X, Belmont, CA.

Gorsuch, N.M. (2006). *The future of assisted suicide and euthanasia.* Princeton University Press, ISBN 0-691-12458-2, Princeton, NJ.

Hardwig, J. (1997). Dying at the right time: reflections on (un) assisted suicide In: *Ethics in Practice. An Anthology.* H. LaFollette (Ed.), pp. 53-65 Blackwell Publishers, ISBN 1-55786-640-6, New York.

Hook, S. (1995). In defense of voluntary euthanasia. In: *Arguing Euthanasia.* J.D. Moreno (Ed.), pp. 237-240, Simon & Schuster, ISBN 0-684-80760-2, New York.

Hurst, S.A. & Mauron, A. (2003). Assisted suicide and euthanasia in Switzerland: allowing a role for non-physicians. *British Medical Journal;* Vol.326, No. 7383 (February 2003), pp. 271-273, ISSN 27500139.

Huxtable, R. & Möller, M. (2007). Setting a principled boundary? Euthanasia as a response to "Life Fatigue". *Bioethics,* Vol. 21, No. 3 (March 2007), pp. 117-126, ISSN 0269 9702.

Kant, I. (2000). *Metaphysics of Morals.* M. Gregor (Ed.). Cambridge University Press,, ISBN 0-521-56673-8, Cambridge.

Knapp van Bogaert, D. & Ogubanjo, G.A. (2010). Assistance in dying: Dax's case and other reflections on the issue. *South African Family Practice,* Vol. 52, No 6, (December 20110), Supplement 1, ISSN 1726-426X.

LaFollette, H. (1997). Euthanasia. In: *Ethics in Practice. An Anthology.* H. LaFollette (Ed.), pp. 19-21, Blackwell Publishers, ISBN 1-55786-640-6, Cambridge, MA.

Lemiengre, J., Dierckx de Casterlé, M., Van Craen, K., Schotsman, P. & Gastmans, C. (2007). Institutional ethics policies on medical end-of life decisions: A literature review. *Health Policy.* Doi: 10.1016/j.healthpol.2007.02.013.

Markel, H. (2004). "I swear by Apollo"- on taking the Hippocratic Oath. *New England Journal of Medicine,* Vol. 350, No. 20 (May 2004), pp. 2026-2029, ISSN 27499832.

Moreno, J.D. (1995). Introduction. In: *Arguing Euthanasia.* J.D. Moreno (Ed.), pp. 11-25, Simon & Schuster, ISBN 0-684-80760-2, New York.

Ogubanjo, G.A. & Knapp van Bogaert, D. (2008). Voluntary active euthanasia: is there a place for it in modern day medicine? *South African Family Practice,* Vol. 50, No. 3, pp. 38 -39, ISSN 1726-426X.

O'Neill, O. (2002). *Autonomy and Trust in Bioethics.* Cambridge University Press, ISBN 0-521-89453-0, Cambridge.

Parker, M. (2005). End games: euthanasia under interminable scrutiny. *Bioethics* Vo. 19. No. 5-6 (October 2005), pp. 523-536, ISSN 0269 9702.

Pence, G. (1995). *Classic Cases in Medical Ethics.* 2nd ed. McGraw-Hill ISBN 0-07-038115-1, New York:

Pence, G. (1997). Why physicians should aid the dying. In: *Ethics in Practice. An Anthology.* H. LaFollette (Ed.), pp.22-32, Blackwell ISBN 1-55786-640-6, Cambridge, MA.

Pickering Francis, L. (1993). Advance directives for voluntary euthanasia: a volatile combination? *Journal of medicine and philosophy*, Vol. 18, No. 3 (June 1993), pp. 297-322, ISSN 0360-5310.

Quill, T.E. (2004). Dying and decision making. Evolution of end-of-life options. *New England Journal of Medicine*, Vol. 350, No. (2004), pp. 2029-2032, ISSN 27499832.

Quill, T.E. (2007). Legal regulation of physician-assisted death. The latest report cards. *New England Journal of Medicine,* Vol. 356, No. 19 (May 2007), pp. 1911-1914, ISSN 27499832.

Rachels, J. (1975). Active and passive euthanasia. *New England Journal of Medicine,* Vol. 292, No. 19 (May 1975), pp. 78-80, ISSN 27499832.

Rachels, J. (1993). Euthanasia. In: *Matters of Life and Death.* 3rd ed. T, Regan (Ed.), pp.30-66, McGraw-Hill, ISBN 0-07-051330-9, New York.

Sheldon, T. (2003). "Terminal sedation" different from euthanasia, Dutch ministers agree. *British Medical Journal* Vol. 327, No. (2003), p. 465, ISSN 27500139.

Singer, P. (1994). *Rethinking Life and Death. The Collapse of our Traditional Ethics.* Oxford University Press, Oxford

Sleeboom-Faulkner, M. (2006). Chinese concepts of euthanasia and health care. Bioethics Vol. 20, No. 4 (August 2006) pp. 203-212, ISSN 0206 9702.

Sullivan, T. (1999). Active and passive euthanasia: an impertinent distinction? In: *Ethical Theory and Moral Problems.* H.J. Curzer (Ed.), pp. 709-613, Wadsworth, ISBN 0-534-52974-7, Belmont, CA.

Tristram Engelhardt, H. (1995). Fashioning an ethic for life and death in a post-modern society. In: *Arguing euthanasia.* J.D. Moreno (Ed.), pp. 42-50, Simon & Schuster, ISBN 0-684-80760-2, New York.

Van der Heide, A., Onwuteaka-Philipsen, B.D., Rurup, B. (2007). End-of-life practices in the Netherlands under the euthanasia act. *New England Journal of Medicine,* Vol. 356, No. 19 (May 2007), pp. 1957-1965, ISSN 27499832.

Van der Maas, P. & Emanuel, L.L. Factual findings. In: *Regulating how we die.* LL Emmanuel, (Ed.), pp. 151-174, Harvard University Press, ISBN 0-674-66654-2, Cambridge, MA.

Varelius, J. (2007). Execution by lethal injection, euthanasia, organ-donation and the proper goals of medicine. *Bioethics,* Vol. 21, No. 3 (March 2007), pp. 140-149, ISSN 0269 9702.

Veldink, J.H., Wokke, H.J., van der Wal, G., Vianney de Jong, J.M.B., van den Berg, L.H. (2002). Euthanasia and physician-assisted suicide among patients with ALS in the Netherlands. *New England Journal of Medicine,* Vol. 346, No. 21 (May 2002), pp. 1638-1644, ISSN 27499832.

Ziegler, S. & Bosshard, G. (2007). Role of non-governmental organisations in physician assisted suicide. *British Medical Journal,* Vol.334, No. 17588 (February 2007), pp. 295-298, ISSN 27500139.

4

Euthanasia: Between Personal Moral and Civic Ethics

Begoña Román
University of Barcelona
Spain

1. Introduction

In this article we will focus primarily on the ethical debate on euthanasia and will not approach the subject from the legal field. We also do ethical reflection from civic ethics, from a secular ethics and from civic minimums that human rights are. Civic ethic is the framework of a transnational bioethics; it is the best framework to ensure the peaceful coexistence of plural morals in public sphere. In public sphere there are morals for euthanasia and morals against euthanasia. So, if the ethics of public sphere, not of personal privacy, should be fair and respect the right to choose, both options are respectable and therefore a legal level should decriminalize euthanasia. We discuss that euthanasia is a matter of personal moral and that both options, for and against euthanasia, are ethical.
From civic ethics we merely talk about respect for the final decision of an autonomous person, because autonomy is the ethical basis that every moral has to respect.
"Euthanasia" is Greek word composed by two parts: *eu*, good, and *thanatos*, death. Thus, the word simply means peaceful death. In technological societies, due to the success of medicine, it is possible to live a long time with a disease but without quality of life; in these societies it is possible to keep *alive* the biological life of a person *while* his biographical life has finished. In these circumstances some people demand to die with dignity, because they do not want to live without quality of life. In such a context, doctors don't only have to cure, heal suffering but also help to die.

2. On the right to die

2.1 What is and what is not euthanasia? About words, things and laws

There is a big confusion related to the end of live, so it is important to clarify what and what is not euthanasia. We must distinguish among five notions (Lorda et al; 2008):

a. Euthanasia
b. Assisted suicide
c. Patient's rejection of a treatment
d. Physicians' team withdrawal or withholding of a treatment
e. Terminal sedation

a. Euthanasia

We speak about euthanasia when the following four conditions take place:

1. The patient clearly demands to die once the diagnostic and prognosis are known.
2. The patient is under great suffering due to an incurable disease that deprives from living with the quality of life he wants.
3. An action carried out by medical professionals that know the patient, respect his autonomy and accept his decision of dying.
4. This medical action is the direct and immediate cause of death.

So euthanasia is an action that directly affects two people, both professional and patient, but the patient is who has the last word. He is who, in total pain conditions with no hope of recovery, asks the doctor to help him to die. Nevertheless the patient's decision must be autonomous, i.e., with knowledge of his reality and his expectations, in coherence with his concept of quality of life, and his decision must be continuous and consistent. Certainly, to make a decision on euthanasia, the patient needs a good diagnosis and prognosis. The patient has to know the reality of his illness, because without good and understandable information, the patient can not be autonomous.

The patient has to keep his decision in a consistent, persistent manner during a reasonable time, to avoid both the precipitation (as result of a moment of disorientation), as also to be influenced (result of pressure from other heteronymous factors). In fact the decision to end one's life must be really one's decision and not caused by other pressures or influences. The Patient will need the physician to take this decision.

The physician's role is necessary before, during and after the patient's decision to die:

- *Before* the patient's decision, to know his physical conditions, to have true information about his diagnosis and prognosis:

In the case of certain diseases which causes a progressive lack of health and autonomy, the doctor has to assume a special intimate relationship with the patient, for the control of symptoms, to let the patient know all the available possibilities, from the paradigm of autonomy and informed consent, but also to inform that it will be the patient, who will set the pace and make decisions. At this moment it is very important that the doctor knows how to accompany the patient to accept reality.

- *During* the patient's decision, to be giving to the patient the dose of required information:

At this point it is crucial that the doctor asks before reporting, because there is a right to know and there is also a right to not to know. It is important the doctor respects the patient's silence, his doubts; it is important that the doctor and his team have not only good technical skills, pain management, but also communication skills and skills with the biopsychosocial model (Engel, 1980), because the "total pain" is everywhere, and not only in the body.

This means a deliberative process of the patient himself; it is an inner dialogue, very intimate and deep one: he must make probably the hardest decision of his life, his final decision.

Once the decision is taken, when the patient asks his doctor for euthanasia, is when a process of dialogue begins between them, in order that both following conditions are satisfied:

It is an autonomous decision that persists in the patient for a certain period of time

It is a decision consistent with the concept of quality of life of patient.

Once verified these conditions, the patient decides when and under what circumstances he wants to die.

- *After* the patient's decision, to carry out the euthanasia in coherence with the wishes of the patient:

Documents of advanced directives and informed consent should be signed; these documents are fundamental from an ethical point of view. These documents are the key to ensure, on one hand, that the process of dialogue between patient and doctor has taken place; on the other hand, that the patient's autonomous last decision has been observed.
It is not euthanasia if the person is not competent and others decide for him. However, how important it is to have an advance directives document for ascertaining the wishes and the decisions that the patient would have made if he knew his circumstances in which he is due to illness.

b. Assisted suicide

The difference between euthanasia and assisted suicide is that the patient is who causes his death and the professional merely offers the lethal dose and other necessary means when the patient is physically incapacitated.
There is no right to die without a duty of the doctor to help to die. But in this case it is a matter of dignity of life and dignity of death. Because only the doctor has the relevant expertise to ensure a good death; and this expertise is knowledge but it also implies attitudes and values.
Doctors should have the following competences to help to die:

a. Knowledge of diagnosis and prognosis.
b. Knowledge of appropriate doses to ensure that the patient has no pain or suffering.
c. Knowledge about the patient's competence in order to ensure that patient's decision is autonomous
d. Knowledge of consistency of the arguments that patient gives with regard to his scale of values and his notion of quality of life.
e. Attitude of respect and empathy to accompany the patients in their last moments, because the doctor can do many ethically things, when nothing technically can be done. In this aspect it is very important to look carefully what the patient can need, for example, religious needs, spiritual care, or care for the patient's family. It is also essential that the doctor and his team are friendly; they must make the patient feel that he has always dignity, and no a charge for anybody nobody.

To clarify names we avoid adjectives such as voluntary, involuntary, passive or active euthanasia etc. Euthanasia is always voluntary, because the patient wants it; and euthanasia is always active because doctor's act causes the patient's death in a direct manner. Euthanasia is not only a matter of private moral; to respect these personal moral we should focus the question of euthanasia on civic ethics that defends its legalization.

c. Patient's rejection of a treatment

Patient's rejection of a treatment is not euthanasia: in euthanasia is the doctor who causes the death in a direct manner, but in the refuse of treatment, because the patient does not want to continue with the recommended therapeutic measures by the doctor, it is the disease that runs its course, to finally cause death.

d. Physicians' withdrawal or withholding of treatment

Euthanasia is not either withdrawal or withholding of treatment. In this case we are talking of a medical decision, when doctors check the futility of the treatment and the great harm it can cause, to the patient violating the principle of non maleficence (*primum non nocere*).

e. Terminal sedation

Terminal sedation is not euthanasia either. Terminal sedation is consistent with the Hippocratic principle of non maleficence. When death is imminent, in order to avoid the pain and suffering, doctors give pharmacological doses (normally morphine), and the side effect of these high doses drugs is lethal. Doctors are not looking for to cause the death but to relieve pain.

Sooner or later the result is the same, the death of the person, but not the way. To cause death trough euthanasia is different to allow deterioration. The patient has the last decision, and only he has it.

In many countries where euthanasia and assisted suicide are illegal, the rejection of treatment is legal, because to respect the refusal of treatment, even effective treatment, is the consequence of taking seriously the principle of patient autonomy. It is interesting to note that the result is always the same, the patient's death, but euthanasia and assisted suicide are looking directly to cause death, and in the rest of circumstances, the rejection of the treatment, withdrawal or withholding of treatment and terminal sedation, death is not searched, but a result of not acting. But in all these cases the ethical principles are the same, i.e., the principle to patient autonomy and the principle of non maleficence, of not harming or imposing life to the patient.

2.2 In the name of autonomy: Live and die in a plural society

Human rights are primary goods, in Kantian words, "transcendental" goods, i.e., the condition of possibility to choose other goods. Rights are the minimum goods that any person should be guaranteed in order to enjoy a decent life from which quality of life can be chosen.

We are defending a right to die from the principle of respect to patient's autonomy, because from autonomy the patient chooses his notion of quality of life.

We make the difference between quality and dignity of life: dignity is essential for choosing quality; it is the minimum choice from autonomy. Thereby dignity is the *conditio sine qua non* in order to be able to take decisions, while quality depends on subjective, personal preferences. Good life is a purpose, a personal and subjective goal, but human rights are the conditions to look for it. A fair life must make the search for good life possible.

People have the right to take decisions, among these, when to die, and this is a matter of dignity. Some people are for euthanasia and others are against euthanasia, this will depend on the meaning of their quality of life. Both options need the right to decide, and both options exist in a morally plural society. But a law against euthanasia doesn't respect the right to take decisions; because a law against euthanasia doesn't respect one of these options, it isn't respectful regarding the dignity and quality of life of a part of this plural society.

We can distinguish two concepts of autonomy:

On the one hand, the Kantian concept as stated in the formulations of Categorical Imperative, e.g, act only according to that maxim whereby you can, at the same time, will that it should become a universal law (Kant, 2002). Kant grounded dignity on the autonomy of person and autonomy is *the ratio essendi* of morality: our duty is to become autonomous.

On the other hand, the Anglo-Saxon notion of autonomy, as right to self determination of a moral agent who is an independent and rational human being. This is the notion of autonomy of J. Bentham or J.S. Mill (Mill, 1989): "The only freedom which deserves the name is that of pursuing our own good in our own way, so long as we do not attempt to deprive others of theirs, or impede their efforts to obtain it". This notion prevails in Bioethics. So the condition for being autonomous is having the ability to grasp reality and to have information in order to be able to take decisions, without obstacles or pressures (internal or external) and in coherence with the own scale of values (Beauchamps & Childress, 1989).

Nevertheless autonomy is always a degree on a continuum, a process during which we can become more or less autonomous. People tend to lose autonomy at the end of their lives; most of them will become dependent as they grow older. However vulnerability and fragility are not shameful conditions but human conditions. Therefore we can talk about the right to be cared for until the end, even includes euthanasia.

Bioethics has put too much stress on fostering and respecting autonomy, but it has not always outlined the kind of dignity that should be recognized for a person who is progressively losing autonomy (the elder, people with degenerative illness, etc.).

We are all educated to become autonomous, but not to accept our dependence, not even to treat a dependent person. Furthermore, the traditional ways of dealing with dying people can become obsolete and ethically reproachable because they are based on charity, beneficence, goodwill or paternalism.

Autonomy is hindered in elder persons. Precisely the people deserving care, like frail old people, have dignity but they are not autonomy, maybe they will be not it any more. Elder people with dementia, Alzheimer illness or people with serious intellectual disabilities are not autonomous but not due to that should they lack dignity and human rights.

We are suggesting that, further than Kant, Mill and Beauchamps & Childresss, the concepts of dignity and human rights should be reconsidered in order to make a foundation of respect for people who are not autonomous in a great degree and who don't want to live longer. We should complete the concepts of autonomy and dignity with the concept of vulnerability.

Independently of if sick people are more or less autonomous; we are talking about dignity and rights: they are persons and they always have dignity. Most of them have finished their autonomous life project, most of them are at the end of their life; all of them are progressively losing degrees of autonomy; and some of them want to die because they consider that they do not have quality of life. But they want to die with dignity and they want quality of death.

Thus, we suggest distinguishing between dignity in *lax sense and dignity in strict sense.*

Dignity in *lax sense* is the dignity which everyone has *as a person*, someone that is an End in itself, an absolute value, the source of all other values. In Kantian words (Kant, 2000): "Act in such a way that you treat humanity, whether in your own person or in the person of another, always at the same time as an end and never simply as a means". There is a great consensus in this meaning of dignity

Dignity in *strict sense* is the dignity that *only a moral agent* can have. Dignity in strict sense would be the kind of dignity that is object of personal achievement, the purpose of the human life searching a personal identity, an *ethos*. This is the meaning of true autonomy for Kant, and it is a duty: become autonomous to be worthy.

Thus, everybody all the people have dignity, also the most perverse murderer and the anencephalic child, but neither of them have dignity in the strict sense: the former because he abused his autonomy; the latter because he is unable to exercise his autonomy. But we, the ones who interact with them, gamble with our strict dignity if we, when treating them, forget they are always people, despite the immorality of the former and the disability of the latter.

We should fight against *diagnostitis* and determinisms that dictate that if one cannot live a normal life (what is a normal life?) and make a useful function in society, life is no longer worth it. As long as there is someone who makes them feel, in their own way, they are worthy, they will find their quality of life.

Who has reasons to live, finds the way. V. Frankl said it better: whoever finds a 'why' can stand any 'how' (Frankl, 2000). A society that treats frail and dependent people as worthy, is giving them a 'why' so all of us (we all are inter/dependent people) can discover how to live in a better way.

Nevertheless the question of euthanasia is not antagonistic to that of palliative care. Euthanasia is not to kill people because it is cheaper than ensuring their care!. People who want more palliative care must be respected . But we must also respect the decision of competent, autonomous people who do not want more care and want to die with medical help. We must ensure that euthanasia is also included among palliative cares.

Kant always thinks in a rational and transcendental *human being* and this is not an embodied subject, mortal and vulnerable, as is the real subject. Autonomy is inseparable from vulnerability. Euthanasia is the unavoidable consequence of a society that has based its concept of dignity on autonomy of the individual, beyond the biological life or a religious sense of life. Beyond Kant and his concept of dignity based in autonomy, we try to maintain a normative level in making decisions. From Anglo-Saxon Notion of autonomy, everything is reduced to personal options, and all private options are respectful. However, we think, according with Kant and beyond Anglo-Saxon notion of autonomy that life is more than a preference; live is a duty as transcendental condition of searching of meaning.

How to respect the autonomy of a person who is aware he will lose it due to the disease; how to respect the autonomy of a person who knows that his fate is to gradually lose autonomy but certainly not lose his life. Correcting Kant and his rejection of suicide (because such act can not become universal law), we are arguing that we should respect the final decision, the decision of a person to die, who knows he will never more be autonomous.

On the other hand, two people should be taken into consideration concerning euthanasia, patient and doctor, one with a right to die, the other with a duty to help him to die. But the doctor also has his own autonomy, his own conception of quality of life; and there are doctors who do not agree with euthanasia. Two autonomies (self-determination) are at stake.

The right to conscientious objection means that the doctor thinks it is wrong to help to die. So, for this doctor, to respect patient autonomy is something maleficent from his personal conscience.

Society must respect all these decisions: the patient's right to die, the physician's duty to help, and the right to conscientious objection by doctor.

Two conditions are needed in order to exercise the right not to act against the conscience: Ensure the patient's right to die, that means that another doctor will do what a conscientious objector does not want to do.

Do not make any pressure on the patient (underestimating his autonomy) and do not make moral judgments about his decision.

This means that in morally plural societies, we must guarantee the rights of all, but the medicine is at the service of the autonomy of patients, and not at the service of the physicians; so, the right to conscientious objection has limits.

2.3 Personal moral, professional ethics and civic ethics: Happiness, assistance quality and justice

Civic ethics is world ethics, ethics of justice, because it has to promote respect to human rights (including future generations). The criterion for making decisions in this ambit is justice, which talks about the primary goods that everyone must have guaranteed, they are universal moral demands. This is a minimal ethics because it doesn't talk about full life, how or why we should live. This Ethics is neutral regarding the way or style of life. *Civic ethics* is world ethics; it has to promote respect for human rights. We need an ethics for global society, for a shared world with morally plural societies that don't share the concept of good and the meaning of quality of life.

We need minimal ethics for the global world that propose duties and rights for every person, including responsibilities for the other living beings or for planet Earth. In certain sense it is possible to defend not only a right to live and a right to die, but also a duty to die: because the Earth has limits and it can not support too many people. And this world ethics is civic ethics, ethics for every citizen in the world. It is also previous and a *sine qua non* condition for private Ethics. Personal Ethics has to cause happiness, not in any way, but in a legitimate and fair way.

So we are defending that human rights are the content of justice; they cannot be only conventions out of random or cultural, economical or political interests. They should be defended as universal exigencies that enable us to talk about justice and to take rights seriously.

The way a society treats its elder members says a lot of about the level of justice and solidarity in this society. J. Rawls in his work *A Theory of Justice* (1971) exposed the hypothesis of the veil of ignorance: if people are unaware of their biological-social lottery, they would choose to live in a fair society rather than a random society. In the former, each member is born equal in liberty, and the most fortunate ones in that lottery have to help minimize the disadvantages of the less fortunate ones. In contrast, the law of the jungle, an animal law, prevails in a random society. In that society natural selection is the only criterion, a survival instinct that doesn't depend on our liberty. In that society it is stupid to speak about ethics, human rights or dignity, because in ethics we talk about what depends on us, about what we owe to each other; and justice depends on our management.

Thus, we can conclude that the incidence of luck in a person is inversely proportional to the level of justice in the human society in which one lives. It is *bad luck* to become ill or disabled, but it is a good luck to live in a fair society that doesn't leave one at his luck. For instance, aging is an unavoidable fact, but it is a good luck to become old person living with dignity and quality of life until the end; living in a society that respects the last personal decision about when and how to live and die.

Civic ethics talks about two categories: truth and justice.

a. We understand Truth as the validity of knowledge, a validity based on empirical proofs, on the evidence that we have at the moment.
b. We speak about Justice considered as impartiality and as the consent of the affected parties by the decisions that must be taken.

We cannot take fair decisions without true knowledge, so we need science. From the same dignity for all, civic ethics is the frame in which dialogue takes place, with information, participation and deliberation of involved persons. Therefore we talk about the right to be informed, and that's the reason for implementing the informed consent in health organizations. Civic ethics doesn't talk about quality of life. We must be able to care with justice, the same for everybody (that is dignity), but from different approaches (that is quality). Physicians and caregivers should prioritize the civic values over their personal ones, because the patient has the last word (he has private, personal values) in decision making regarding his life. So we must ensure that in hospital or at home ill people eat, drink, bathe and take their medication, but depersonalization or homogenization must be avoided: every person has a private unique life and a personal ethics with his particular values. Thus, if a person has decided that his life is meaningless because of his loss of autonomy; if this person wants to die, we must conclude that he has right to die and a doctor must help him to die without pain and suffer. The goals of medicine are save, take care, also at the end of life, also helping to die. Physicians must be trained to help to die. To allow euthanasia the *physicians' curricula* should be improved, because physicians are trained to carry out actions against disease and death, to save lives, to care people: they must be trained also to attend dying people in a better manner, when nothing technically can be done, and to attend people who want to die.

The patient is the ultimate responsible person for his own life. Respecting the patient's autonomy also means respecting his values, also giving him the information of the process of his disease. Physicians and patients establish a moral contract. Physicians must inform patients about the time, the treatments, and expectations of recovery and future quality of life. This information process must be done with the adequate vocabulary according to the patient's capacity. The relationship between Physicians patients is so important that it would be recommendable for Physicians to learn communicative skills, which aren't taught at Universities.

Information and communication often fail because the doctor is not aware of the different levels of knowledge patients have about disease and their conception of death. Sometimes it is even a mater of different cultures. The physician must always take care of the patient's welfare and respect his customs. And here Physicians need pedagogical tools and, of course, ethical attitudes.

Physicians should be with the patient during the decision making process; it's not only a matter to respect the patient's decision: a good decision will need information about benefits, risks, processes. Autonomy is the capacity to make decisions and it requires knowledge and responsibility until the end of life.

As professionals in health organizations, with the leadership of civic ethics and its content (truth, justice, human rights and duties), we ought to make compatible the different ethics: the personal, the professional and the corporative ones. Dilemmas will surely arise: people have different interests, different cultures, and different scale of values; solutions will be found from the horizon of human rights. But if a person has good reasons, his reasons, to die, we should respect this decision and help him to carry out in the optimal conditions.

3. On duty to live

3.1 Autonomy: Personal preference or normative concept?

Who should decide the end of life? The same person who lives, only this person can decide about this subject because his life is a private property. The individual has the last word about his life. He is the only moral authority in his life, also even for religious people: God is a moral authority because they want so.The choice of living or dying is a very personal decision that should be respected when person is competent, autonomous.

Our relation with life and death depends on our personal moral. Now we are discovering that it is possible to live without autonomy (Alzheimer, dementia, etc). It is our responsibility to guarantee that no people suffer and it is our obligation, if possible, to guarantee their quality of life. But if a person, before he loses his autonomy, decided not to live without autonomy, we have the duty to help him to die.

But it is not the same to take a decision from autonomy than from arbitrary preferences. If we are talking about ethics, we are talking about normative concepts, not about arbitrary elections. Autonomy is something more than mere preferences. In this sense, from our point of view, Kantian concept of autonomy is better than the Anglo-Saxon one in order to reach a normative foundation: life is more than quality of life; life is something more than choosing pleasures

We are talking about Ethics, not about morals. Ethics is moral philosophy, a critical and rational reflection about morals. Nowadays we need to engage in this reflection because we are living in a multicultural world, a morally plural world, where morals are changing depending on new technical challenges that evolves moral values. We must think which options are not respectful, which options are respectful and which among these are better because of their arguments.

Kant, the author who made the concept of autonomy fashionable, reminds us that everything has its price, while people have their dignity. And this dignity causes in us the moral feeling of respect, from the Latin *respicere*, that means watchful look (in German, *Achtung* means both attention and respect). To respect people means to pay attention to their needs. Kant reminds us that dignity should be something sacred: humanity is worthy of respect, because humanity is an End in itself and implies rational competence, self-determination and responsibility.

To allow euthanasia is a matter of law and ethics; so we should think about life and the duty of live, not only about the pleasure of life. If we are rational beings, we should give reasons to live and to die: We have responsibilities and duties to ourselves and to others. Legalizing euthanasia requires social pedagogy about these subjects.

Regarding the duty to live -we argue that ethics, as a philosophical discipline-, it makes sense to propose universal obligations. Ethics is the discipline that reminds us the duty to make life something valuable and worthy, that is, the duty to construct a character, a meaningful life plan, an *Ethos*.

To conceive life as a mere preference (as is the case for many utilitarian or hedonistic philosophers and from a negative concept of autonomy as self determination), misunderstands the concept of autonomy, because it deprives ethical, normative obligation. It is even difficult to understand the very existence of a discipline, ethics, dedicated to studying the criteria of what is a good, fair, decent life without a fundamental duty to live. If everything is a matter of mere choice, of mere preference, without having to give explanations for the decisions that someone makes, we talk of aesthetics, not of ethics, nor therefore, of bioethics.

Regarding the reduction of autonomy to mere personal preference (the Anglo-Saxon notion of autonomy) , we are insisting that, in the question about euthanasia, the person must be competent and make decisions about his life and death only in the context of a disease that progressively robs his autonomy. If everything is based on the Anglo-Saxon concept of autonomy (as a right to self-determination), the decision making is reduced to mere preferences of an individual, the pleasure of living or not. But in that case, we could fall into "the slippery slope". Actually, an individual who has lost interest in life and wants to die, he could ask the doctor to help him die. In this case the ethical reason to end his life is an exercise of self-determination, but not precisely autonomy in Kantian sense, e.g. to continue to exercise autonomy and no finishing with it. In our opinion this is the fundamental argument from which we defend the ethical legitimacy of euthanasia. In this case, we find someone who despises life: is this also respectable from a normative Ethics?

From Kant, we said no; we think that there is a duty to live, to fight for life until the end. We can consider right the decision to die only in circumstances of progressive loss of the autonomy (Alzheimer, dementia, etc.) and in circumstances of a "total pain" caused by the disease. Thus, we want to go beyond Kant and his refusal to commit suicide and defend the possibility of the right to die, but we are precisely following Kant, that is, his concept of autonomy. So we agree with Kant's ethical foundation of the duty of living and his concept of autonomy: worthy life it is not a matter of preferences.

The lack of interest in the life of a person because he is getting bored, or because his life has no meaning, but there is no disease or progressive loss of autonomy, undermines the principle of making one's life a meaningful project. It is a duty to live, we must seek a meaning, beyond the pleasure that life can generate. Beside the right to live and the right to die, there is also a duty to live with dignity until the end.

4. An agenda for the future

Euthanasia cannot be legalized without ethically thinking before what is at stake, and what is at stake in the issue of euthanasia is all of the following:

4.1 The dignity and quality of life of people. We need a social pedagogy to live and to die

The patient autonomy paradigm puts the person in the centre. To talk about of the principle of respect for the autonomy of the person means that he is the ultimate moral authority, he is who has the last word; he sets the pace, about his life ant death. The use of advanced directives and informed consent documents must be enhanced. These tools are much more than documents and papers; they are the logical result of the dialogue between the patient and professionals. They will be the proof that the respect to patient's autonomy has taken place.

Euthanasia requires competences and legislative changes. Regarding competences, it must be reminded that professionals cannot infantilise either mature minors or the elderly, who, despite their years, have not necessarily lost their maturity and who may feel humiliated. Professionals must always ask his permission, and when necessary, forgiveness if they are not right. However, autonomy often remains only in the speech, in the theoretical level; but the unique "autonomous" are usually the physicians, they are not serving the patient's autonomy, but for best performance of the professionals or institutions at which they work.

With regard to legislative changes, the citizens' participation in decision making must be improved, not only regarding their own individual health, but also on proposing public health policies.

Even though bioethics should be a civic, secular ethics which respects personal options, it is difficult for several governments to maintain neutrality in its view of the world, as it should in a morally pluralistic society. Sometimes it even goes from secularity to secularism.

If in the welfare state the criteria were the supply and demand law and the populist policies; in the justice state the criterion must be the consent of involved people, that is, the citizens and the professionals.

4.2 Credibility and confidence in the professionals and health organizations: Medical professionals to serve people

The quality of professional and organisational service must be in accordance with human rights, and the right to healthcare is one of them; but quality of this service will also depend on the citizens' use or abuse. It must be responsibly, in line with their needs, accepting that the system must satisfy rights, not individual preferences. And if a quality service is to be achieved, we all must feel part of a shared world. The four areas of ethics must be reconciled: civic ethics; organisational ethics; professional ethics; and the last, the personal ethics (ethics of professional and of the citizen whose service the professional is on). If professionals and organizations health services want to gain people's confidence, they will need to begin to re-classify their decisions in the corresponding areas. This means not giving priority to personal preferences or the preferences of the "clientele" when making professional or organisational decisions, and weighing before-hand whether they are in line with the civic, organisational, and professional values.

Healthcare professions must focus on the person: he is the subject of rights. It must be reminded again and again to those who are serving the professions and health organizations, what their mission is, their ultimate responsibility.

4.3 The kind of world that humans construct, and the reasons to live: A normative solidarity

Life cannot be underestimated; human life is the only chance on Earth: we must make with our lives something worthy. It is a matter of justice and solidarity to promote the research of a good life. Nevertheless, we are not talking about solidarity by compassion; we are not thinking in a utilitarian solidarity: "I should cooperate because maybe, one day, I could be in these circumstances". No: it is not a contract; it is not a convenience or a matter of selfish interest. It's a matter of normative solidarity; it is a matter of rights, justice and respect to humanity wherever and ever. Life is the most important moral resource to do something worthy with it, also at the end of life. Anyway, it is also a way of dignifying life to decide the circumstances of death (Thomasma et al, 1998), when someone is loosing his autonomy, when to be able to decide is becoming more and more difficult.

5. Conclusions

This article has defended the following thesis on euthanasia:

1. The issue of euthanasia depends on personal moral. It is from the concept of quality of life where the person decides whether to continue living or not.
2. But it is a personal moral issue that must be supported by ethical reasons. This is not an aesthetic question of mere preferences, against the Anglo-Saxon concept of autonomy. We have therefore advocated a duty to live, to make life a meaningful project, from a Kantian concept of autonomy. It is in moments of loss of autonomy, not only of loss of pleasure, which it can be autonomously decided to not live longer. Precisely the autonomy that is being lost due to disease is the only cause that can legitimate to decide finishing life. This means that autonomy and ethics require biographical life beyond mere biological life.

3. Civic ethics does not speak of quality of life, which depends on personal moral, but of respect for the different options, and that's a matter of justice. It is fully consistent that an individual in his personal moral is against euthanasia and yet, from the civic ethic, the ethics of tolerance for morally pluralistic society, respects the choice by others with different personal moral in favor of euthanasia.
4. Medicine has its social legitimacy, its "raison d'être", in assisting people, but from the paradigm of autonomy and not from the paternalistic paradigm. Once people have made their choices from personal moral, physicians should remind from civic ethics the duty of hospitality, the duty of care to people in their concept of quality of life.
5. The doctor can be a conscientious objector. Of course the doctor, from his personal moral, can be against euthanasia. But his objection has limits: the physician cannot impose his own personal choice and must ensure always the care of the patient. If the objector doctor does not want to help the patient to die, he must find other doctors to do so.
6. Open societies are free societies, that is its precious value; the price to pay is the greater complexity of its management. And our complex societies need more ethical reflection; they need more reflection on what we owe to each other and what we owe to ourselves.

6. References

Aristotle (1934): *The nicomachian Ethics*, Cambridge, Mass (etc Harvard University Press.

Beauchamps, T.L. & Childress, J (1989): *Principles of biomedical ethics*, New York.Oxford University Press.

Engel, G (1980): The clinical appplication of the biopsychosocial model. *Am J Psychiatry*; 137: 535-544.

Kant, I (2002): *Grundlegung zur Metaphysik der Sitten*. Kants Werke, Akademie Textausgabe, IV, Walter de Gruyter & Co, Berlin, 1968. English translation: *Groundwork for the metaphysics of morals*. New Haven: Yale University Press.

Frankl, V (2000): *Man's Search for Meaning. An Introduction to Logotherapy,* Boston: Beacon; and Random House / Rider, London.

Mill, J.S (1989): *On Liberty*, Cambridge University Press.

Simón Lorda, P et altere (2008): Ética y muerte digna: propuesta de consenso sobre un uso correcto de las palabras, *Rev. Calidad asistencial*, 2008; 23 (6); pp. 271-285.

Thomasma, D.C. et altere (1998): *Askiing to Die*. Inside the Dutch Debate about Euthanasia, Dordrecht, Kluwer Academic Publishers.

5

Handling End-of-Life Care in Medical Decision Making: On a Bioethical View

Maribel Bont-Paredes, Carmen Malpica-Gracian and Carlos Rojas-Malpica
Universidad de Carabobo
Venezuela

1. Introduction

1.1 Life awareness

The world of life, is a world that precedes human existence, therefore it constitutes and projects us as human being, beyond men reflection allows to take it. Life itself was not men made, as a creative phenomenon it originated and per suited humanity. It is in its core substantially coated with dignity and respect, as well as that of the biological *materia*; in other words, body and soul are indeed equally precious (Cely, 2001, 2005; Gherardi, 2007)

Human life is one of the best emergencies of life itself, and holds within all its multifactorial harmonious complexity. So complex that it has become in abstraction of its own realization, in its auto-recognition thinking process. From life's fundamental nature emerged the spiritual essence of materiality and the profound giving of consciousness than allows the binomial energy-*materia* to appropriate of the existing reality. It corresponds to human kind the responsibility of humanizing life from our own cultures, by favoring thoughtfully reflexive processes with transcendental meanings on all forms of living existence (Cely, 2001, 2004, 2005; Gherardi, 2007)

Life could be defined as a sequence of moments that create the existence of a person, whose moral and cognitive development and evolution have been influenced by different socio-cultural factors that characterize the configuration and structuring of attitudes and personality, as being part of a society. Common sense implies the acceptance of dogmas that although could be interpreted in various individual ways, however are accepted and followed by most member of a community; as epitomized by experiencing birth and death (Cely, 2001; Gherardi, 2007).

Every human action is necessarily associated and related. This means that no one lives totally on its own; to enable the existence of each individual it must be articulated by needs and deliberation to other human beings and the natural surrounding environment, in a complex network of interactions. These connections respond to *Ecological* and *Ethological* links of reciprocity in manifold directions with chaotic and eventful energy exchanges of growing complexity that increases a higher new emergency in the *ethos vital* (Cely, 2001, 2005; Gherardi, 2007).

Nowadays *Bioethics* as a branch of applied ethics, new and required by the *society of knowledge of the third millennium*, proposes to take as a very serious matter all data that different sciences subsequently contribute with, from the beginning of life until its end, to distinguish this information with wisdom to all existence, doing so in the perspective of a *scientific humanism* which can attain responsibility for making moral consensus and prescribing binding actions to carry out this complex purposes (Cely, 2001, 2004; Albuquerque 2008).

The two dilemmas at the endpoint of life have represented enigmas that men have sought to penetrate along human history. Conception and acceptance of pain and suffering seems to be inexorably linked to the beginning and end of human lifecycle, since they distinct not only the peaks of biophysical life; but perhaps, also the advent of a new spiritual dimension, yet to be explored, comprehended and known (Gherardi, 2007; Cely, 2004).

Decision making for handling death and medical intervention has led civilizations to adopt different behaviors and cultural patterns at end-of-life, which have evolved over time, seeking to alleviate pain or suffering in cases where the patient's ill condition has taken to boundaries of where, may not be a health recovery.

With no doubt biomedical scientific and technological progress, has led medicine to participate and to intervene in this biotechnical development, using utensils and medical apparatus that enable the maintenance of life even in artificial ways.

The *principles of bioethics and medical ethics* arise to guide medical decision making and action taking, in a harmonious and concord approach, as a result of the agreement by consent between all members of a group or even among several groups. Behold, as occurs in *doctor-patient's interaction, coming out as result of this relationship reciprocally exerted in an affective and effective interaction deriving to a medical care technically desirable, in the management of those who are in a terminal stage disease* (Cely, 2001, 2004; Gherardi, 2007; Albuquerque 2008; León 1996; CENABI, 1999).

These dissertations about biomedical sciences and technology's contributions at *End of the Life Decision Making* (ELDM), demonstrates the need for a bioethical prosecution in the quest for these resolutions, under the scope that its complexities exceeds the competence of the medical profession, requiring the successful assembling of different disciplines; consequently there is an urgent need for consensus between medical doctors, ethicists, secular, lawyers, humanists and priests of various clergy, along with the whole society (Cely, 2001, 2004; Gherardi, 2007; Albuquerque 2008; León 1996; CENABI, 1999).

The different aspects related to the approach of life's end decision making, have to be analyzed from its various dimensions and in recognition of its integrations into a dynamical socio-cultural framework, as is life itself; having diverse perspectives involved within each other. This new complex approach allows a closer look to the reality in the process of dying, in which the convergence of all aspects of the phenomenon and their mutual relations, will allow to come closer to the multidimensional true existence (Cely, 2001; CENABI, 1999).

Bioethics brings a plural-dimensional view on reality concepts, creates an interwoven reciprocal and reflective connection that allows an altogether vision of dilemmas, re-evaluating humanity at its whole, to place it as a cardinal axis of dignity and into a higher purpose of human being. Emphasizing that all things that can be scientifically man made possible are not ethical or bioethical acceptable to accomplished (Cely, 2001; CENABI, 1999).

Death, once easy to identify by the cessation of breathing and heartbeat can be in our days, somehow more difficult to establish, as a result of the implementation of new technologies and procedures brought by biomedical sciences. The cease of organic functions, today only determines a state of "perceptible" death, as it may be resolved by resources of respiratory and/or hemodynamic support. Not even the irreversible damage of the neurorregulatory centers are enough to establish with accurate precision the time of death, when even under such circumstances, it is possible to maintain the visceral process unscathed.

As a result of this biomedical and biotechnology intervention, establishing the advent of death, nowadays appeals to a neurological refined approach, as in: *brain death*. This indeed is of complex concern especially in developing countries; therefore sanctioning death by this mean only, could become a decision mediated by increasingly sophisticated biomedical devices. Interestingly, it would be the sensitivity and appropriate management of this equipment which could authorize end of life decisions. In recent past, with a more human clinical approach and the help of few instruments, this pronouncement could be easily taken behold a closer interaction among the physicians as principal care takers, the patients and their families (Aguiar, 2003; Cely, 2005; Castillo, 2006).

However, the fear of ethical, bioethical and legal implications, actually frequently become a limiting condition upon therapeutic measures in patients who need end-of-life care; all of these immersed in a framework surrounded by social, economic and cultural contexts distinctive of each moment in time, which restrict, stipulates and determines the most appropriate approach through the course of action, being as well responsible for caring of life in the planet and of human survival (Aguiar, 1997; Cely, 2001, 2004;).

Different aspects of patients medical mediated death, have already engaged for decades scientific literature, with the emergence of new terminologies to distinguish the most frequent situations being discussed within the confines of human life. Declarations rights of the terminally ill patients have been bound-for to avoid any type of discrimination or abuse that could prejudice the patient's sense of individual dignity and self-respect (Gherardi, 2007).

Clearly, the circumstances of medical mediated death have provided legitimacy to the claims for a "*good death*", leading the way to a movement that aims to create a forum for discussion of the various aspects that should be considered regarding the ethical-bioethical problems at the finale of human lifecycle, as well known as "*Omega Dilemma*" (CENABI, 1999; Gherardi, 2007;).

Terminally ill patients going through the process of dying need to be appreciated in their own conditions and therefore rights. Which can be summarized as follows: right to the relief of pain and other symptoms; right to remain vigilant; right to be informed truthfully; right to exercise its decision-making capacity; right to maintain affective human contact; right to be respected in their religious beliefs; right to "die in due course"; in other words, to be marginalized of excessive medical practices aimed to keep them alive (Cely, 2001, 2004; Gherardi, 2007).

Nowadays new concepts as *Euthanasia, Cripthanasia, Dysthanasia, Orthothanasia, Tachythanasia and Assisted Suicide* are added to the terminologies used to refer end-of-life decision making within the terminally ill patient, brought by these novel spectrum of discussions being done by the reciprocal intervention of family members, legal representatives of patients, health care-takers and religious councils.

Currently in some Nations such as Venezuela, there are actually undergoing a legal reform of laws known as *Anteproyecto de Reforma del Código Penal Venezolano-New Project of the Venezuelan's Penal Code*, in which just few lawyers, members of the National Assembly have reviewed discussion, adoption and implementation of some of existing biotechnical interventions in medical-mediated death; which is described on text as the intentional physician's delivered purpose of ending a terminally ill patient's life, patient´s or family´s written consent and life testament; being both *active and passive voluntary euthanasia*, the two forms of execution.

As one would expect, in medical practice it is viable to identify different situations vulnerable of questioning and moral deliberation, in which are not always easy to complement the will of the patient, among the different treatment alternatives brought by the healthcare team, and at the same time, in the course of actions to be adjusted to the existing constitutional framework in every contextual location. In addition occasionally, some family members of the patients are those who inquire medical doctors to alleviate pain at all cost or in some way to bring to an end the suffering of their loved ones, regardless of the unwanted side effects.

However, *what is put into bioethical consideration are the possibilities of medical intervention and the legitimate moral behavior that will be decided during the process of dying,* a succession of events which would have its point of departure at the time of diagnosing an incurable disease and envisage of death, and its finishing point in the clinical representation of the "apparent death" (Castillo, 2006). How to confront suffering, pain or a disease which could inexorably bring to death, are subjective and absolutely auto-determined decisions by patients, among their family group.

Bearing agony and closure of lifecycle supported by medical conventional or palliative care is the reality that many of our Venezuelan's patients either alone or with the company of their families face every day; in a heroic attempt to keep alive, not letting feelings of discouragement overcome their hopes by the added hardships of poor public health care services. There are not enough well medical equipped health care centers for patients in need, or in most locations where not only the access to public facilities are complicated, but yet to obtain medical disposable material and equipment is not feasible either.

This scenery brings a more detail conflict into the bioethical discussion, reaching out-far the existing gap between developed and underdeveloped countries, which makes it impossible to mimic context of medical or legal situations; furthermore, embraces each national and regional context of its own proper deliberations. This is what makes bioethical dilemmas so significant and of a unique type, by considering in the consensuses of medical decision making a contextual reflection of a single kind. There are no "golden rules" to it, so all life human forces of every community parties need to be taken into account, within the introspection of their socials and cultural backgrounds (Bont, 2007; Castillo, 2006; León, 1981, 1996).

From an *spiritual dimension,* the topic of death can be tackled from the traditional dominant "*dualism*" of the west world, which sees the human being composed of two different reality matters, *body and soul,* irreducible one to the other, perishable the first and immortal the second. This anthropology, of Hellenistic and Christian origin, in which the majority of Venezuelans have been educated, currently receives deep questioning from sciences and contemporary humanities (Bont, 2007; Cely, 2004; Castillo, 2006).

In the other hand, the modern theological hermeneutics reinterprets the sources of revelation, to make them understandable to men and women of our days. Another view of this spiritual dimension would be the "*monist*", in which man is not divided between a body and a soul, but it sees as a "*substantive unit*", a single vital substance, as conceive by *Parmenides, Spinoza, Plotinus, Schelling, Hegel* and *Freud,* among others philosophers. For whom reality is the unity of the essence and existence. The essence is not behind or beyond the phenomenon, but for this same reason the essence exists, the essence is specified in the phenomenon; realizing that the phenomenon is life itself, life turned-as energy emerged from the Cosmos in the infinity of *ethos vital* (Bont, 2007; Cely, 2004; Castillo, 2006).

Being understood as well, men would be a very complex structure of embodied vital energy, forming part of the biota as a whole, coming through an intimate relationship and reciprocity with the abiotic. Being Humanity an inside-out of creation as nature's turned into the awareness of life, which means that we have become the consciousness of natures by itself (Cely, 2001, 2004).

The two anthropologies have their strengths and their weaknesses. With either of two anthropologies, *monist* or *dualist*, men will reach the same goal: *life after death*, in theological propositions that provide wisdom to human reasoning to grant ourselves with dignity inside an *ethos vital* that nourish our hope for a spiritual life without suffering anymore pain or perennial death, by the promise of a supra-dimension of eternal life.

Although different faiths believe also provide sense of binomial life and death. Religions, as part of the human spiritual dimension, are an attempt of civilized man to give an explanation to the emerge of life and its needed link relations, through enclosure devotion in a supreme being, endowed with all the wisdom, always eternal power, in its different forms of reflections, the only way to reach-out for salvation and allegory hope, beyond this earthly mortal abode (Cely, 2004).

The *Roman Catholic Church*, representing the predominant religion in Venezuela, raises the permissibility of not using extreme biomedical measures to sustain life and expressively supports the relief of pain in terminally ill patients, justifying the fact that when you cannot be cured, the therapeutic goal is to relieve symptoms and improve as possible, the quality of life of the patient. For that reason it sustains, that *palliative care* can be considered an extension of medical practice that, given the impossibility of doctors to cure any given disease, they must promote and uphold patients leading one's life based on faith, which is above all gifted with dignity by itself (John Paul II, 2004; Del Prete, 2008).

Christian Catholic anthropology interpretation supports respect for human life from its very conception known by the binding of the ovules and spermatozoids, through the fusion of gametes to produce a new organism, until life it-self with no extreme biomedical technology intervention comes to an end. In light of what the Scriptures say about the kind of care God wills that we provide to those who suffer and are facing death, rejecting such claims for active euthanasia and assisted suicide as neither compassionate nor caring (Bont, 2010; Cely, 2004; León, 1981).

Enlighten two major Biblical Principles to oppose euthanasia. The first is the *sanctity of human life*: Being a fault to voluntarily terminate a life, killing incurable physically or mentally ill patients, or commit assisted suicide, do to that life is taken only by God-given powers. The Christian faith cannot accept the argument that in such circumstances life has no value, so it must be finished (León, 1981; John Paul II, 2004).

The second principle attaches meaning to suffering. "God is omnipotent; when there is suffering on earth it is intended that this happens. God has an intellect greater than man, so it is sometimes impossible to the human understanding to fully comprehend God's purpose". To sum up Catholic Church, standardizes medical mediated forms of ending human life by the patient's voluntary decision, including passive euthanasia, with murder; considering them as a mortal sin. The reasons for this are based on the inviolability of human life and in human redemption suffering purposes, which lead men to Christ and heaven (Bont, 2010; León, 1981; John Paul II, 2004).

To what Paul VI express: "medicine is required to fight overcoming of death with all available resources, but when the battle is unavoidably to be lost, there is not necessity to use extreme resuscitation techniques. It is a useless torturing to maintain a person in a vegetative condition". **Euthanasia**, in its proper sense, is a synonym for **mercy killing**, which involves suicide and/or murder. It is, therefore, contrary to God's Law.

When the God-given powers of the body to sustain its own life can no longer function and doctors in their professional judgment conclude that there is no real hope for recovery even with life support instruments, a Christian may in good conscience "let nature take its course" (Bont, 2010; León, 1981; John Paul II, 2004).

Being Christian Roman Catholic, the dominant religious believe in Venezuela's social context, discussions over medical handling and management of life's end decisions, need yet a long way to go, especially if taken into consideration the constants disputes and confrontations undergoing between Government officials and cleric headquarters; leading this delicate topic to be devilish among general population, somehow as an intent of Government's legislators to overlook and contravene Human Rights principles. Never the less, what is indeed most preoccupying is the lack of interest of official congresspersons to come out in the open and let all community living forces to give their opinions and promote participation, in a clear effort for consensus over this essential dilemma of life; letting people know about de currently discussions that are held regarding the intension of lawmakers to reform the *Venezuela's New Project of the Legal Code* (Bont, 2010; Anteproyecto de Código Penal-República Bolivariana de Venezuela, 2000).

National lawmakers have not done up-to date proper researches or open discussions about arguments to sustain these modifications and to include for the first time in the country's history a new ruling, as in Article N° 217 *Dar muerte por piedad- Giving death by mercy.* Do to the novelty of the topic in our socio-cultural framework, its new applications and implications especially for terminally ill patients and physicians; this important matter has to be debate within a broad participation of Venezuelan's community members.

Foreign experiences as the ones quoted at current text project, are far from our socio-economic, cultural or religious reality, most of all if considering government's poor coverage of adequate medical services wide across the nation, particularly of intensive care units. Furthermore, there is a considerable gap between those who living in the same geographic region, but with different economic holding, have access to a barely satisfactory health service. There are many issues to bring about before lawmaking over this delicate topic. Lawyer who favor article support arguments on current changes in developed countries like Spain, Netherlands, Germany and the United States, this point of view lacks of profound academic knowledge or empirical practices to be properly sustained (Anteproyecto de Código Penal-República Bolivariana de Venezuela, 2000).

Some jurists consider that the whole writing of the article needs to be fully supervised anew, do to the insufficient clarification of the terminology implicit in it; which could lead to regretting misunderstandings on behalf of the medical care takers or even patients themselves. On the other hand, the Venezuelan Constitution as our maximum legal framework does contravene this proposal, as so does the *Law of Medical Practice* and the *Deontology Medical Venezuelan Code* followed by medical doctors. Never the less administering pain-killing medications is permissible, even at the risk of shortening life, since this does not entail the choice of death as either a means or an end (Piva & Pinto, 2003; Ley del Ejercicio de la Medicina en Venezuela, 1982; Código de Deontología Médica de Venezuela, 2003).

What is evident is the distance from general agreement that according to this matter we are about-of, for mediated medical end of life decision-making to be legally established, needing a meticulous debate yet to be done. Before, Government must guarantee all society members the benefits of being capable to receive appropriate, contemporary medical attention, distributed with justice and equitability in every nation's state, regardless of any social-economic or religious faith barrier.

Complex thought and paradigm projected on the phenomenon of human care in dying, allows integrating different methods for relating scientific knowledge in problem-solving, which is based on dialogue and consensus of diverse perspectives to view in and out the dilemma, considering *Social and Clinical Bioethics* and the *Bioethical Principles* of autonomy-respect for person, non-maleficence, beneficence and justice; on the common understanding by all parties involved, that is indispensable the adequate relief of pain, the emotional support on suffering, winding the patient's and family's anguish with affective and spiritual accompaniment.

1.2 Methodological framework: A new comprehension

Based on complex thought proposed by *Edgar Morin*, which serves as groundwork to the investigative episteme, researcher finds support in the *paradigm of complexity* from postmodernism, seeking to embrace and comprehend reality of patients and medical doctors at end of life decision management. On complex view the main purpose is to dialog in an interactive reciprocal relation among subjects participating in the phenomenon of study, rather than just determine or measure what happens under those circumstances. The investigators deepens on terminally ill patient's death as a phenomenon of interest within a creative, genuine and holistic intention, in which might emerge novel theoretical constructs, than through reflexive thought and into practice permits a better medical management at end-of-life (Morin, 2003, 2004; Orcajo, 2000).

The research is constructed considering postmodern anti-method, and method is structured on its way, to end-up on the conjunction of two investigative momentous, one of qualitative expression and a second one in quantitative terms. Guided by complex thought researcher adapts the method as a strategy resulting from the interaction between reality and its comprehension with the paradigm; in which each decision and procedure regenerates the method, not being applied as a pre-determined rigorous and unequivocal pathway to follow; allowing researcher to create new interpretative understanding and innovate strategies, relying on singular analytical and reflective investigative momentous connecting knowing, comprehension, and medical practice intended for intellectual enrichment and proper management of end-of-life decision making among *doctor-patient's interaction* (Leal-G, 2005; Morin, 1999, 2003).

In postmodern comprehension the enormous fullness that surrounds us, encompass and challenges our capacity of knowledge, which can't be established on a single rigid pathway method; perhaps, is the innovative result of such an effort, the only thing that truly appeals the attempt of learning new things by applying novel methodologies (Martín-F, 2006).

Researcher's view on a complex paradigm, is allowed to open to intuition and *amusement* (which is about freedom of thought and imagination), as the *muse* (from Latin *Mūsa)* or a source of inspiration that guides the meaning and essence of the exploration, using logical thinking in the investigation procedure, as well as letting passion inspire reasoning at the pursuit of learning the best way to come closer in reality's interpretation; this gnosis allows researcher to be an active participant subject in the development of the entire investigative process. This challenges the valuable sense of investigators, in the approximation of the living-dying phenomenon in a genuine, warm, imperative and provisional nature as is life itself. Giving this model its uniqueness, exhibiting its particular way, this is also fundamental in the generation of new overcoming knowledge (Leal-G, 2005, Martín-F, 2006).

Complex thought is a style of thinking and approaching reality. In that sense the complex thought generates its own strategy, indivisible of inventive participation of those who develop the research. Rationality is not the only mental process that guides the search and construction of an emerging understanding (Martín-F, 2006).

It is also necessary to take into account that method and paradigm are inseparable. All methodical activity is based on a paradigm that directs a cognitive practice. Since the complex thought proposes a paradigm that interacts, articulates and understands, at the same time that can develop its self-criticism (Leal-G, 2005; Martín-F, 2006; Morin, 1999, 2003).

In a primary stage of research, the author recognizes the need to provide an original scientifically valid construct in close relation to the contents of the Venezuelan socio-cultural and economic contexts; into the different manifestations of faith and spirituality as part of our life experience. Taking into account the current review carried out by the *Asamblea Nacional de la República Bolivariana de Venezuela-National Assembly of Venezuela's Bolivarian Republic*, about the *Código Penal- Legal Code* (Anteproyecto de Código Penal Venezuela, 2000).

The *first quantitative language momentous* approaches the phenomenon focused on an empirical-analytical basis research method, according logical positivism as the epistemological cornerstone, methodology research design is exploratory, transect of not-experimental, with the main object of exposing the importance of the medical practice decision making et end of life based on the opinion, degree of information and training of doctors working in areas of Surgery, Internal Medicine, Intensive-Care Units, Oncology and Anesthesiology of the *Servicio Autónomo Hospital Central de Maracay-Autonomous Central Hospital Service of Maracay,* in Aragua's State and the *Hospital Central de Valencia-Carabobo "Dr. Enrique Tejera"- Central Hospital Service "Dr. Enrique Tejera" of Valencia-Carabobo* (CHET); representing the 2 biggest middle states Medical Centers in Venezuela (Bont, 2007; Hurtado & Toro,1997; Hernandez & Fernandez 1991).

From primarily empiric process of data, the population of study from which our sample is drawn was represented by 185 doctors, to whom were applied an anonymous questionnaire, of not probabilistic selection sampling (opinatic and volunteer sample), being finally constituted by 123 subjects, who agreed to freely participate in research throughout written informed consent. Obtained data was tabulated and coded in Excel in comparative tables, which subsequently formed sectorial diagrams (pie charts) in the same program, for statistical analyzing. The collected data then was triangulated to become innovative figures representations of reality in terminally ill patient life decision making.

Depth perception of phenomenon led investigation to a *second qualitative language momentous*, within an inductive method, to come close and reconstructs the significance that terminally ill patients as subjects of study had regarded to the conscious decision making and action taking at the end of their own existence, which was accomplished through profound interviews by means of an intentional 5 patient's sample.

Throughout qualitative language in which *herméia and phenomenology* recreates, actions are intervened in order to understand them, the author strives to give a general sense in the interaction of parties to get a proximate vision if it all. Hermeneutics in its desire of interpretation causes a constant return and sway from whole meaningful sense to each element interacting, as a perfect complement of *complex thought* (Martinez-Miguélez, 2004; Spiegelberg, 1975; Morin, 2000).

Researcher's strategy seeks for an interpretative perspective, mainstreaming as is *phenomenology and hermeneutics,* in which the purpose is to embrace what patients are going in the course of a comprehensive and explicative perspective of events, *finally* inserting this experience into learning about the caring in terminally ill patients. Allowing when necessary, emotional assistance from religious or spiritual leaders of patients' creed.

Textual data analysis theoretical considerations obtained from the primer quantitative investigation, as result of the medical experience in decision making at the end of human life, is also integrated as part of the second qualitative textual document evaluation. Being able to concatenate the product of the first momentous as an initial element in the second momentous of comprehension and redefinition of terminally ill patient's reality.

Under this intention researcher conducts in-depth interviews with no limit of time and in several meeting moments (when necessary), with each patient selected as a *key-informant* with a clinical diagnosis of malignant neoplasm (cancer); afterward all informants' data collected is transcribed into a handwritten designed history profile, which is later transcribed in digital computerized *Word* format, to finally make a digital format makeover to a *primary document,* in the ***Atlas/ti*** textual data analyzing software (Muñoz, 2003; Glaser, 1992).

In the means of the study, the *process of dying* is understood to begin from the moment a person losses health condition associated with a medical adequate diagnosis of incurable illness, that subsequently evolves on dying within days or weeks, which imminently entails patient's envisage of death.

Theoretical approaches to health care ethics have evolved in response to societal changes; evolution of health care can be traced form the "Hippocratic ethic" with emphasis on duty, virtue, and gentlemanly conduct, which emerged from relatively homogenous societies where beliefs were similar and the majority of societal members shared common values; through the "principlism" and into the current "antiprinciplism" movement. The theoretical model proposed in this research brings into reflection from a bioethical perspective an intercurrence of facts and the participant's role at end of life decision making in medical death intervention, as the third millennium of humanity unfolds into biotechnological advances and challenges. Not rejecting principles but choosing to frame the use of values as standards to make them useful in a bioethical discussion. To construct this model, the author relies on broad and different referents theorists, who have sustained its investigative activity during the past years.

Principles are too far removed from the concrete particularities of everyday human existence; therefore principles do not represent a theoretical approach. The anti-principlism movement has risen with the expansive technological changes and the tremendous burst in ethical issues accompanying these changes.

1.3 Interaction of the research perspectives: Theoretical bioethical model

As to the profile of physicians whom participated by consent agreement and filled out the questionnaires in this research were of 123 out of 185 medical doctors. Sample's data analysis demonstrated that majority correspond to *females of 35 years old, with 15 years on average of graduated as medical doctors in Venezuelan Universities.* All working at the moment of consultation in Public Community Healthcare Centers, in the fields of *Surgery, Internal Medicine, Critical Care Medicine, Oncology and Anesthesiology* of the *Servicio Autónomo Hospital Central de Maracay-***SAHCM** *in Aragua's State (Autonomous Central Service Hospital of Maracay)* and of *Ciudad Hospitalaria "Dr. Enrique Tejera" of Carabobo's State-***CHET (Central Hospital Service "Dr. Enrique Tejera"),** representing the 2 biggest and most important public medical centers of the middle region in the country.

When asked about the knowledge of the content of **Article N° 217** *Dar muerte por piedad-Giving death by mercy* of the preliminary draft partial reform *of Venezuela's New Project of the Legal Code,* 90% of the surveyed doctors claimed to ignore it; 8% knew the undergoing reform and 2% did not response. As shown in this study most physicians surveyed had an important deficit of information or knowledge about the advance intention of Venezuelan Government on adding a new paragraph to our *Legal Code: article entitled "Giving death by mercy".* Discussions are currently carried out in the *Asamblea Nacional de la República de Venezuela-Republic's National Assembly,* which has a transcend impacts on medical decision-making and action-taking at end-of-life (Anteproyecto de Código Penal de Venezuela, 2000). On this discussion about *active and passive voluntary euthanasia* legal forms, the most significant disagreement among the entire medical community is whether if the Government is also supporting all forms of medical suicide participation, including the executive ones.

At the same time it was unclosed the insufficient information physician surveyed (74%) had about the improvement done in 2003 to the *Código de Deontología Médica de Venezuela-Deontology Medical Venezuelan Code,* which included new definitions on medical concepts, supporting medical guidance in handling end-of-life care for terminally ill patients. The result of this research is undoubtedly preoccupying taking into consideration that the medical staffs participating are working directly in areas such as Surgery, Internal medicine, Intensive Care Units, Oncology and Anesthesiology, having to deal day by day with medical mediated death.

On the other hand, 85% of physicians manifested to have cognitive theory *criteria for terminally ill patients.* And when they were asked about the behavior willingness to apply euthanasia to terminally patients 48% surveyed doctors responded affirmatively, the same number responded negatively while 4% decided not to respond. Also 54% of surveyed physicians claimed to theoretically know all different *types of euthanasia* that could be applied in terminally ill patients, while 41% thought they had lack of information; 5% did not provide their answers. Out of the data qualitative analysis it was shown that 69% of doctors declared to know the definition of *assisted suicide,* whereas 31% were not familiar with this concept.

This poor groundwork of theoretic approach has a direct negative impact on their knowledge and skills in medical practice; also established when taking into consideration the lack of interest expressed by medical doctors to know about our *national legal regulations;* possibly leading to the default in concepts and performance related to medical decision making at end-of-life, as demonstrated in this study; compromising the ethical and medical judgment and actions when managing patients in terminally ill stage disease. On the other hand, based on the results of this study, doctor's surveyed have a considerable level of acceptance regarding the accomplishment of *direct active voluntary euthanasia,* while a broad number of participants were favorable *to facilitate death without pain to the terminal patients*, being this another form of *active voluntary euthanasia*, but since there is no intention to cause death is *indirect*.

The above shows the importance for the subjects of study to relief pain in dying patient, what resembles the *Hippocratic Oath* and the Oath's evoking *Dr. Luis Razetti*, distinguished founder of Venezuelan Medical School and author of the *Código de Deontología Médica de Venezuela-Deontology Medical Venezuelan Code*. These Oaths are adopted as a solemn commitment in medical practice by physicians graduated at all Universities in Venezuela. There for *with regards to the relief of pain and caring of the terminally ill patient known as Orthothanasia* is favored by the majority (Aguiar, 2003; Castillo, 2006)

In relation to the *abolition of lives that doctors considered as a burden on society (Cripthanasia)*, the vast majority disapproved its application; from what we could deduct that medical participants in this research have highly appreciation for patients as persons and the dignity of the human life. This attest that surveyed physicians have the theoretical knowledge under which they cannot presuppose that upon medical reputation doctors have the moral or legal authorities to determine the value of a life worth living, thus taking into their own hands the action of killing another human being (León, 1975, 1981).

Concerning the possible practice of physicians in *Assisted Suicide*, a high percentage of respondents were in disagreement; But it should not be underestimate that 25% accept to facilitate the means and resources available to patients in terminal stage to help them die.

It is worth to highlight that these numerical results extracted from the quantitative phase of research about physician's cognitive and practice skills, are consistent with those related to theoretical bibliographic background that they acknowledged to possess; bringing out the importance between gnosis and behavior/*noemata* and *noesis* in decision's skill management, especially in medical assertive perform among life's end.

This amalgam between the theoretical constructs and humanistic principles within a reflexive attitude by physicians, leads to an *assertive medical practice*, impregnated with the value of humanist thought and the fondness for life, which comes evident in the *discernment and performing* of the health care team as a whole, especially for physicians who work at critical medical areas, where they have to deal with the process of perilously decision making, stating that train should be restrictively preceded by an adequate and followed theory learning process; assuring that when practitioners need to, they can relay-on a strong body of knowledge to guide them throughout the empirical experience.

These integrated complex way of approaching end of life decision making in terminally ill patients is of special significance, highlighting the expected linkage between the *awareness of self-been of a persons* within their reflection on values and principles, that become as projections connecting noema and noesis for a *right-doing*. There is a higher level of consciousness lead by the analysis of theoretic construct which puts into context the fact of doing something with a superior humanistic purpose favoring the wellbeing of others, respecting Human Rights and the sense of spirituality on human conduct; favoring the *knowing how-to do* expressed as a proper approach on professional behavior.

From de interrelation of the 2 investigative quantitative-qualitative perspectives accomplished throughout the research emerges an innovative approach of the *physician-patients-family auto-organizational systematic interaction*.

2. Universe of cosmic dimensions, sub-dimensions and their emerging elements

Out of this *retroactive-recursive integrated universe*, there are 3 main **macro-dimensions** to be discerned:

1. One related to the *patient*, with a macrocosm and microcosm patients related sub-dimension.
2. A second **macro-environmental dimension**, in which 2 sub-dimensions intervene as well, represented by the **patient's family and friends** and those who also work as part of the **healthcare team of support,** represented by nursery staff, lab personal, technicians and other hospital attendants who share the healthcare of patients.
3. A third one related to the *physician*, as the leader of the healthcare team; relating their macrocosm and microcosm.

Discourse and dialogue analysis of interviewed subjects allowed recognition of 2 sub-dimensions: *patient's microcosm and macrocosm dimensions,* in the spectrum of terminally ill patients. *Patient's microcosmic dimension* reflects their interpretation of new reality, referring to the inner world of patients as a gravely ill subject, facing the odds constrained by health deterioration, forcing the consciousness of life's end, which in turn has an impact in patient's *quality of life.*

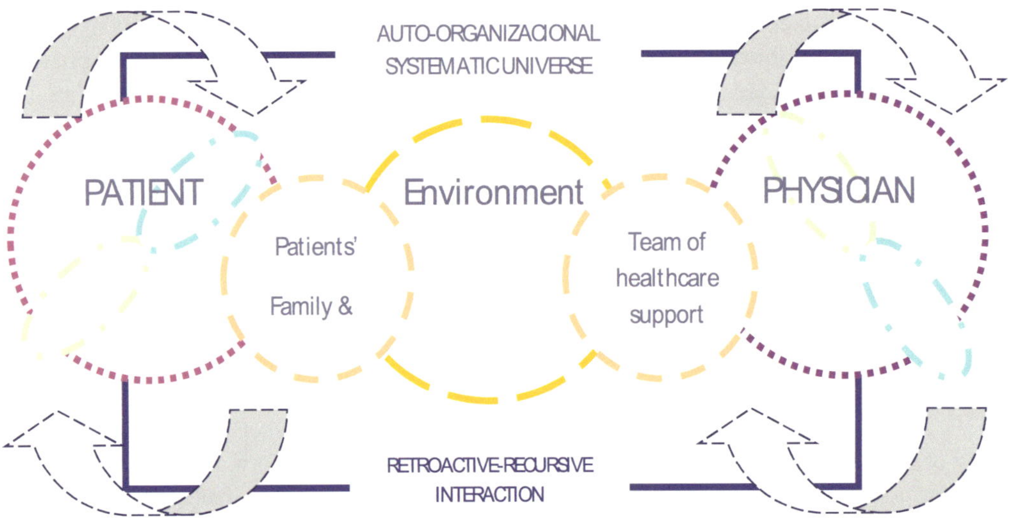

Fig. 1.

This sub-dimensional recognition proposes an inner reciprocal interaction about one self's thinking regarding *the health of the body-the health of the soul*. In this personal way of insight patients will re-elaborate a new adjusted project of life, expressed in actions and re-construction of their *lifestyle.*

Through the understanding of the contents of the patient's human consciousness, known as *noema*, researchers can achieve a better understanding of a person's way of thinking and actions, which are projected as *noesis*. The contents and their projections are do to the dynamics of life and individual development. Therefore, by this approach it is possible to establish a relationship between a patient's cognition and what will later be their behavior in the process of adjusting life to a burst dynamic of changes in a survival environment. This deep cognitive reflection cannot be done in everyday life conditions, the notion of death, loneliness and departure are otherwise rejected, out of one´s thoughts.

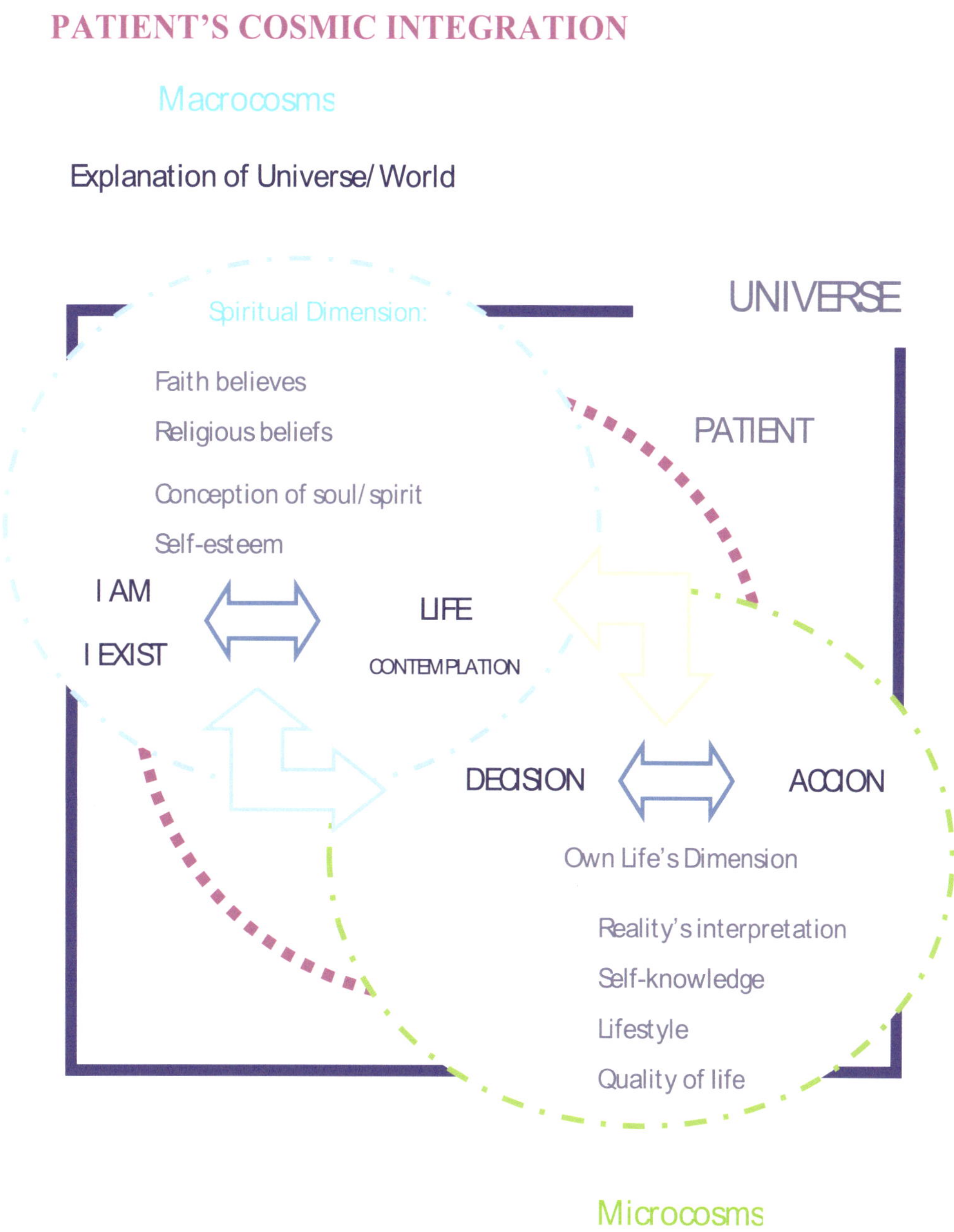

Fig. 2.

Upon this *self-knowledge*, subsequently patients may materialize their modes of action, to establish behavior to confront life's threaten circumstances re-balancing vital energy's state of mind-soul-body, aimed to re-establish their health conditions and quality of life as possible; or instead, successfully adapt to a new circumstance for survival.
In this sub-dimension were identified as emerging elements *fear, repentance, guilt, depression and denial* as negative elements, to the conscience of the incurable disease, the diagnosis of cancer or death's despair.
This is a process in spiral that changes permanently, which is given by a continuous, unfinished course of multiple interactions between the patient, his own capacity of internalization/learning, surrounding environment, self-spiritual and existence development and growth, with the main objective of achieving their personal fulfillment based on the moral values that the person possesses.
All these recurrences allow the creation of a network of intimate exchange and multidirectional (*retroactive-recursive*), complementary between the *microcosm* of the patient and the *macrocosm* (such as an *auto-eco-organizational process*), with their *eidetic* content (from the Greek eidetic: eidētikos, which means "relating to or subject to such imagery"), eminently contemplative that define the spiritual world of the subject.

1. First dimension: Terminally ill patient's dimension

a. **Microcosm:** dimension on their own health-disease process.

- Interpretation of reality
- Management of emotions
- Self-knowledge
- Quality of life in terminally ill patients
- Patient's Lifestyle

INTEGRAL BIOETHICS
PATIENTS' RIGHTS

b. **Macrocosm:** patient's individual spiritual dimension of life.

- Faith believe
- Religious beliefs
- Patient's own conception of soul/spirit
- Patient's self-esteem

Microcosm of patients' interview is based on their own perception on health-illness process, sustained on emotions management, self-understanding of reality, self-knowledge and expectancy of lifestyle and quality. In which *negative self-patterns as guilt, depression, fear to die, pain/suffering and self-meaning of cancer will contrast forces with positive conduct elements as acceptance and peacefulness.*
The *macrocosm* patient's sub-dimension emerges from the way in which patients from their own moral and ethics principles seek an explanation of the universe at whole, and of Cosmo's creation, constructing a frame of reference in the concepts and dogmas of their spiritual world.
In their own ways as individuals decipher and seek to understand the meaning of life, insofar as it relates to an immensurable-inexplicable and infinite supreme order, which is expressed through beliefs and convictions of faith, giving it the properties of divinity and Holiness to his own life and life-extended forms in other creatures that accompany men on planet and into the fullness of the universe.
Since this auto-perception of the macrocosm individuals creates their contemplative eidetic content, which they will have to pay worship and veneration; in view of these imaginaries

intellect constructs patients are to be founded in a superior belief, leading to the contemplation of the universe's creation, which gives the appraisal of their own existence in the world and their mission in life, consequently influencing their *self-esteem*.

Throughout this reflective process patients look for an explanation to their existence and all that is provided in their about, although still not understandable in some circumstances. But that in turn, allows the person to project itself beyond its biological and organic existence, becoming integrated to infinity, be no more death, in an always eternal supra-dimension.

In this sub-dimension the patient sustains *faith believes*, which consequently have an impact on *his lifestyle and quality of life*, to reinforce the interdependencies between the conceptions of the microcosm and the macrocosm of the human systemic universe, auto-organizational and dialogic, of complex associations in necessary instances, obligatory combined in human existence, required in the development and process of the phenomenon of life and its terminal process in death.

"*I am, I exist and feel, I am undividable linked with what is, exists and feels to my around and also belongs to an eternal dimension*", is a statement expressed in the context of the interviews conducted in the research, in which the terminal patient seeks to find a greater meaning than of finite biophysical worlds, provided within a non-perishable sensorial and existential dimension. Every intentional act has noetic content (or a noesis - from the Greek nous, "mind"). This noetic content, to which the noema corresponds, is that which gives meaning or sense to an intentional act.

Discourse analysis of interviewed patients allowed recognition of sub-dimensions in the spectrum of terminally ill patient, given by microcosm-macrocosmic patient's dimensions and understanding of reality based on their own perception of the health-illness process, sustained self-board of sentiment, self-understanding of reality, self-knowledge and expectancy of life; in which positive and negative self-patterns emerge as contrasting emotions and feelings to conduct their actions in the process of dying.

There were defined as elements of *microcosmic patient's dimension* in which interact the patients' faith conviction, religious upbringing, personal conception of soul and self-esteem, to balance patients' willingness to collaborate with treatment, to have confidence and relay on healthcare team work.

2. Second dimension: Interactional environmental dimension

a. Trans-disciplinary Healthcare team: *retroactive-recursive system*

- Justice and equity in health services for all patients in need
- Effective Social Security ⟺ **SOCIAL BIOETHICS**
- Intergenerational Social Security Plans for terminally ill patients
- Suitable treatment
- Care for patients with human kindness.

In this categorization of items, this dimension refers to the care and treatment given to patients with a terminal illness by the healthcare team, led by physicians, but involving nurses, bioanalysts, lab and technical assistants; even including administration, maintenance and protection of safety personnel, of Healthcare Centers.

The *reification of the individual* is considered by the patient, as the impersonal behavior, cold and distant towards them and their family. Not conceiving the idea that a patient could be treated as an object or a damaged "thing". The terminally ill patients interviewed referred be treated and of feeling like an artifact, like if their sickened body was interpreted by the caregivers as a damaged machine with an irreparable injury.

The terminal patient referred to feel *discriminated* upon doctors and nurses misbehavior. As well, they expressed to suffer financial fragileness and vulnerability *without an effective or reliable social security service*, with a sense of *hopelessness* do to the lack of economic resources to fill the needs of their treatment expenses. This increases the sacrifices that they have to do, to pay for procedures and treatments required.

One of the emerging elements in this sub-dimension also was the *accompaniment*, which is why each person who has contact and handles the terminally ill, are perceived by the patient as *companions* in their process of dying.

Fear is a predominant element in speeches, as a result of the feeling of death and separation from their loved ones, which is intensified if the patient does not dare to ask doubts to doctors, therefore to evade reality or because he does not feel confidence and empathy with caregivers.

In addition, patients recognize as important the following elements: 1. - simple and loving communication 2. - manage of symptoms and adjuvant treatment 3. - pain treatment and sedation 5.-accompaniment and a human warmth attitude related not only to the company of family members, in this case is extremely important to understand that the *doctors along with the healthcare team, are a group of affective and emotional support for the patient and their loved ones. Unable to cure, the health-team can accompany and support the patient and their family group.*

b. Family and Friends Group of Support for Terminally Ill Patients

- Economic livelihood
- Care and affection
- Solidarity
- Travels and other needs for transportation

This sub-dimension emerges in relation to the support of family members and friends of the critically ill persons, in which sickened patient's finds *support and solidarity* in order to understand the decline of lifetime; in them they'll seek for harbor to their feelings and the comfort to manage the emergency situation.

They will be inclined to look for the family member that offer a sense of security and trust under such circumstances, and even will go to those who he thinks might offer *financial support*, to the huge costs of their disease. In some cases it was referred by patients with low incomes and no social security uphold end-up selling their few belongings in order to find required money to pay for expensive treatments; demonstrating the devastating economic consequences of life threating sickness in those who are out of the social security system, needing to provide themselves even with the most simples dispensable medical materials such as disposable syringes and cotton.

Patients refer *nostalgia*, sense of loneliness and loss. They felt sadness because they were far from home country/home town, or dear somewhere, their house, family and friends. Speaking about their sentiment of melancholy, which came along with the memories of old times or people to whom they once felt linked emotionally, but that are not in present days, and perhaps the imaginary possibility or hope to be reunited again at a unknown dimension.

As patients get closer to an end, some of family member who accompanied them, tend to retrieve exhausted by suffering and sense of *impotency*. Loved ones need to deal with sentiments of regrets and helplessness, as they watch their relative die.

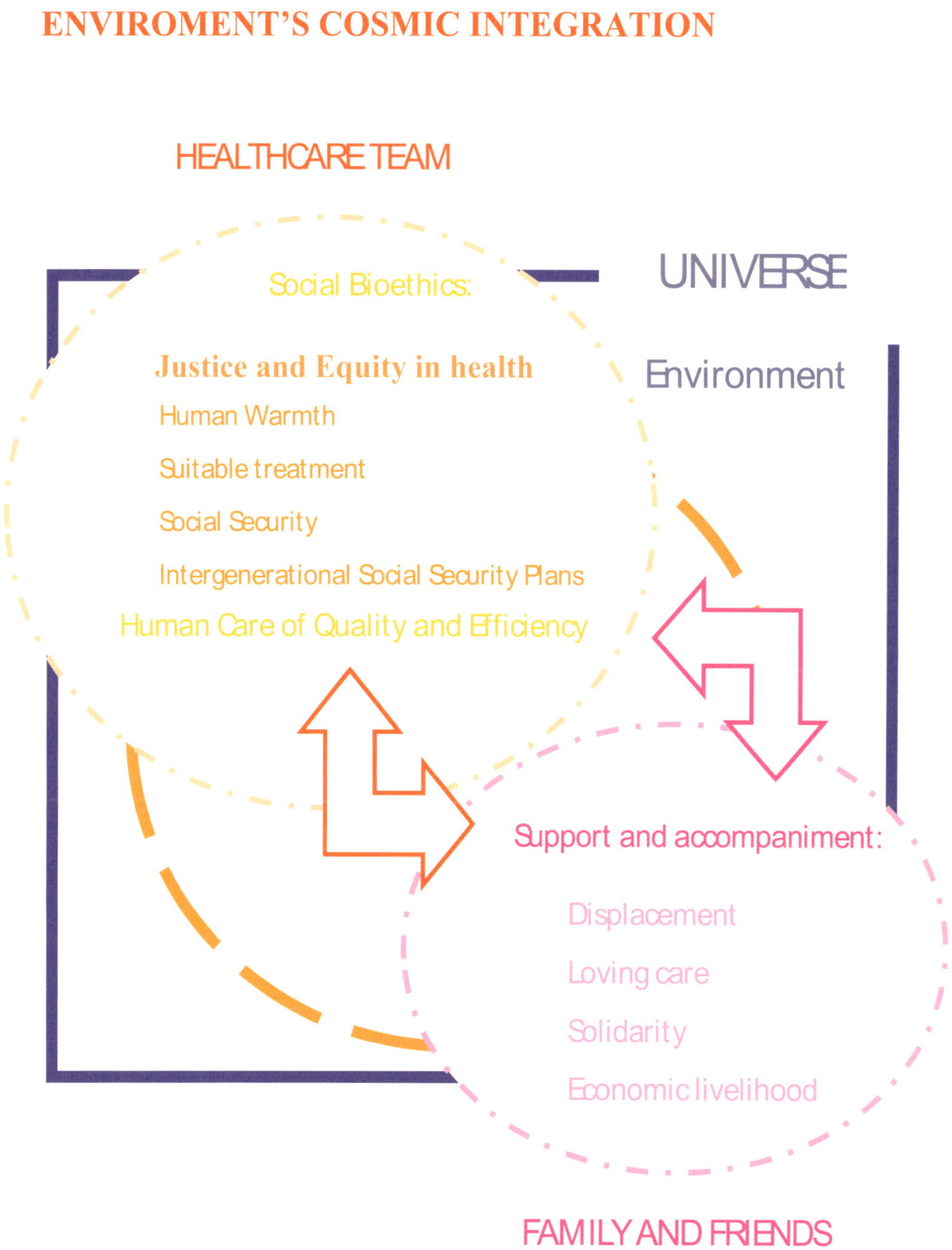

Fig. 3.

Displacement refers to the need of relocation which is undergone by the patient, at first by getting out of private home or city of residence, moved by the hope to find other medical opinions and secondly, being able to have access to better resources in health services in the infrastructure facilities of other institutions, gaining access to procedures and treatments, which may not able to have in own location. This place shift creates primary a sudden change in the family and physical environment of the patient, which implies a detachment of their near loved ones, and having to get used to other home surroundings or to the development within this new community; secondly, with all the economic adaptation and unexpected modifications generated.

The heated discussion about life's end was paradoxically exempting increasingly needs and cries of the terminally ill patients. Little by little, as their lives were quenched, their voices were extinguished and silenced in stealth of their finale, as so their pain and fears. *The life support machines replaced the caretakers in the accompaniment of the dying.*

The excessive maelstrom of biotechnology's advances burst leaving behind the consideration of peoples Human Rights, principles and values, which should encourage civilized communities in the realization of a good modest life worth living for, what in consequence has a negative impact on a deserved worthy death (Universal Declaration of Human Rights-Declaración Universal de los Derechos Humanos, 1948).

In an attempt to be heard, groups of terminally ill patients across the glove and professionals dedicated to take care of them, as in palliative care, aiming to ensure the correct medical exercise concerning the terminal sickened, with the support of international organizations, proclaimed their rights: *Patient's Right.* Patients' rights vary in different countries and in different jurisdictions, often depending upon prevailing cultural and social norms; for instance WHO in Europe proclaimed *a declaration on the promotion of patients' rights in Europe*; in Latin America the Fundación pro Derecho a Morir Dignamente have declared: *Terminally ill Patient´s Rights.* Specifically in Venezuela there is Fundación Hospice Venezuela-Hospice Foundation Venezuela, in which they provide guidance for terminally ill patients. (Fundación Hospice Venezuela, 2009; Fundación pro Derecho a Morir Dignamente-Derechos del Paciente Terrminal, 1991; World Health Organization-Patient's Rights, 1948; WHO-European consultation on the rights of patients, 1994)

Still these rights were not enough, the medical scientific community highly mechanized imposed their dominance in the units of intensive care with new and sophisticated equipment and procedures; while this was the reality in some developed countries, not for underdeveloped ones, these new facilities just opened even more profound inequities in health care service, between these nations and those immersed in poverty.

3. Thrid dimension: Physicians´ dimension

a. **Microcosm of physicians:** Dimension that reflects the attitude of doctors on health-disease process of terminal patients.

- Human Rights and Terminally ill Patient's Rights.
- Respect for person's Autonomy
- Beneficence ⟺ CLINICAL BIOETHICS
- Non-maleficence
- Justice
- Ethical and Deontological aspects of Medical Doctors' Practice.
- Approach between scientific and humanistic medical's sense.
- Attachment and self-conviction upon JURIDICAL NORM:

VENEZUELA'S BOLIVARIAN REPUBLIC CONSTITUTION

VENEZUELAN'S PENAL CODE and its amendment.

b. **Macrocosms of Physicians:** Spiritual dimension of medical specialists.

- Religious belief: dealing patients with affection and compassion.

- Conception of the Soul-Spirit
- Confession of faith: attachment to the values and principles of owns religion

In the **physicians' dimension** again there were acknowledged 2 sub-dimensions, one **microcosmic physician's dimension** in which the professionals' own understanding of Humans Rights, Medical Ethics, Bioethical Principles and legal framework regulations, will lead his conduct favoring respect for persons opinion, patients' autonomy, benevolence and most proper communication and using best techniques available for the right treatment of terminally ill persons, in the sense of a **Clinical Bioethical interaction** inserted in the **knowing how-to do**

Once again we see that in the way as a subject confronts the tensions that exist in the mode of conceiving his process of health-disease, in this specific case referring to the medical specialist, their position will be clearly expressed in their speech, conduct and actions (*noema-noesis*), *with which they will have to deal and resolve the conflicts of life, especially before a big dilemma, such as death, seen through his patients.*

The projection of these noema in noesis will let glimpse the conception of its principles, values and the attachment to the legal regulations, as well as, their correct medical exercise in accordance with the professional conduct and ethics. From the microcosm doctors joint their technical knowledge (*knowing*), with his technical skills *knowing-how*, this will define their biotechnical *knowing how-to do*, in their professional environment.

It is based on their own preconceptions about the *health-disease process*, as the specialist will feel motivated to enrich its values, principles and duties, supporting them on *Human Rights, Social Bioethics and the Principles of Clinical Bioethics, and Medical Ethics and Deontology.*

From *Social Bioethics* guided by the *Principles of a Clinical Bioethics* and *Human Rights*, they strengthen the links between the parties involved in the medical-patient interaction, and will favor consensus decisions, allowing doctors gradually abandon paternalistic behavior traditionally imposed on patients, looking forward to encourage, direct and support them in the taking of autonomous, reasoned and informed decisions, of great importance into the finitude of life.

On the other hand, *macrocosmic physician's dimension* is related also to personal religious convictions, spiritual contemplation, life divinity and on physicians' own perspective of existence, which leads to a beneficent human patient relationship submerged in kindness, solidarity and good willingness into *physician-patients-family auto-organizational systematic interaction.* It's of special significance to accent the connection expected between *self-being* with oneself values, principles and spirituality belief, which together with the theoretical consciousness content will be expressed in high quality professional's technique combined to the individual capacity of analysis, allowing a greater understanding in the *knowing how-to do.*

In this sub-dimension individuals combine the principles of faith and spirituality with which doctors contemplates the existence, in which religious beliefs will be fundamental mainstay to define actions, leading him to the *knowing-how,* as a result of the balance between knowing and doing from the humanistic point of view as in result, into a humane compassion behavior interaction, with quality and warmth inside their individual technical knowledge (*knowing).*

In their macrocosm Galen will seek for *dialogue and the emotional warmth in relationship* with patients and their family members, encouraging linkages to strengthen solidarity, trust, honesty, harmony, flexibility and interaction. Is this sub-dimension doctor's will project their personal skills using of simple, clear verbal language providing adequate information to patients; as well as, they shall assume the importance of affective and proximate gesture language to patients and their relatives.

Never the less, throughout the investigation patients perceived that *physician-patient relation* was classic and *paternalistic*, with a lack of effective and efficient communication between both parties. From physicians' conduct towards critically ill patient, it's manifest that based on their own knowledge of *medical ethics, deontology and principles of Clinical Bioethics*, the specialist who works in areas such as *Surgery, Internal Medicine, Critical Care Units, Oncology and Anesthesiology*, will feel motivated to enrich their moral values and principles to encourage the adequate conduct behavior and technical approach in proficient healthcare (Hernandez, 2001; Malpica, 2008).

There was documented by the hermeneutic-phenomenological interpretation of facts, that terminal patients' awareness of incurable disease, as negative-depressant conduct behavior can be more bearable when *patient's family and close friends* support them by companionship, economic uphold and solidarity throughout these crucial circumstances. As well as the *team of healthcare* based on *Social Bioethics and an Integral Bioethics* ensure that each person in need will receive an optimal adequate treatment for their illness, with dignity, without discrimination of social status, age or gender.

By systematic triangulation of all data information gathered the author proposes to reconstruct an approximation theory which enunciates that, in the process of decision making and action taking at end-of-life in terminally ill patients, physicians should take into consideration with each person first of all Human Rights, patients' own values and believes, respecting their opinion as well as that of their families or surrogate representative, according to preserve everyone's right to a dignified moment of death, being offered and receiving technically countable efficient resources in a caring and comfortable environment. Furthermore, doctors working in critical areas using life-support measures should make a constant update of the concepts and emerging procedures involved in the application of vital support effort; at the same time as taking awareness of changes done or yet close to come in the legal framework on our underdeveloped Latin-American countries, to provide patient appropriate and timely media in the process of dying.

It is in this multiple humanistic movement towards life, in the reflection of *Human Rights*, through the caring of life and all its living components over the world, in which is validated an upcoming concept of *Integral Bioethics*. Without losing a specific perspective to be applied in every contextualized circumstance, as we have to deal in Venezuela. In view of the fact that *Bioethics* exhorts and promotes inclusion, solidarity, of profound depth in social, tolerance and respect, is that we can assume the center of attention in the use of new biotechnologies advantages, guiding their profits towards a vital preservation of the environment, heartfelt admiration for biodiversity, protection of life and living (Lolas, 2008; Sass Hans, 2008).

3. Conclusion

Systematic generation of a theoretic approach from triangulating data as conducting research, follows construction of theory, enunciating that at end-of-life ethical and bioethical decision-making health care givers, led by physicians, must consider and respect the values and personal opinions of patients and family members to shelter terminally ill patients into the lifecycle dying process; therefore, medical doctors working in critical areas practicing life support measures should make a continuous update of theoretical concepts and emerging technical procedures involved in the appliance or not of vital support, considering the current ethical, socio-economical and legal framework in Venezuela and present-days changes, preserving in mind the *maxima* moral cognition and behavior to offer patients opportune-adequate means in the process of dying.

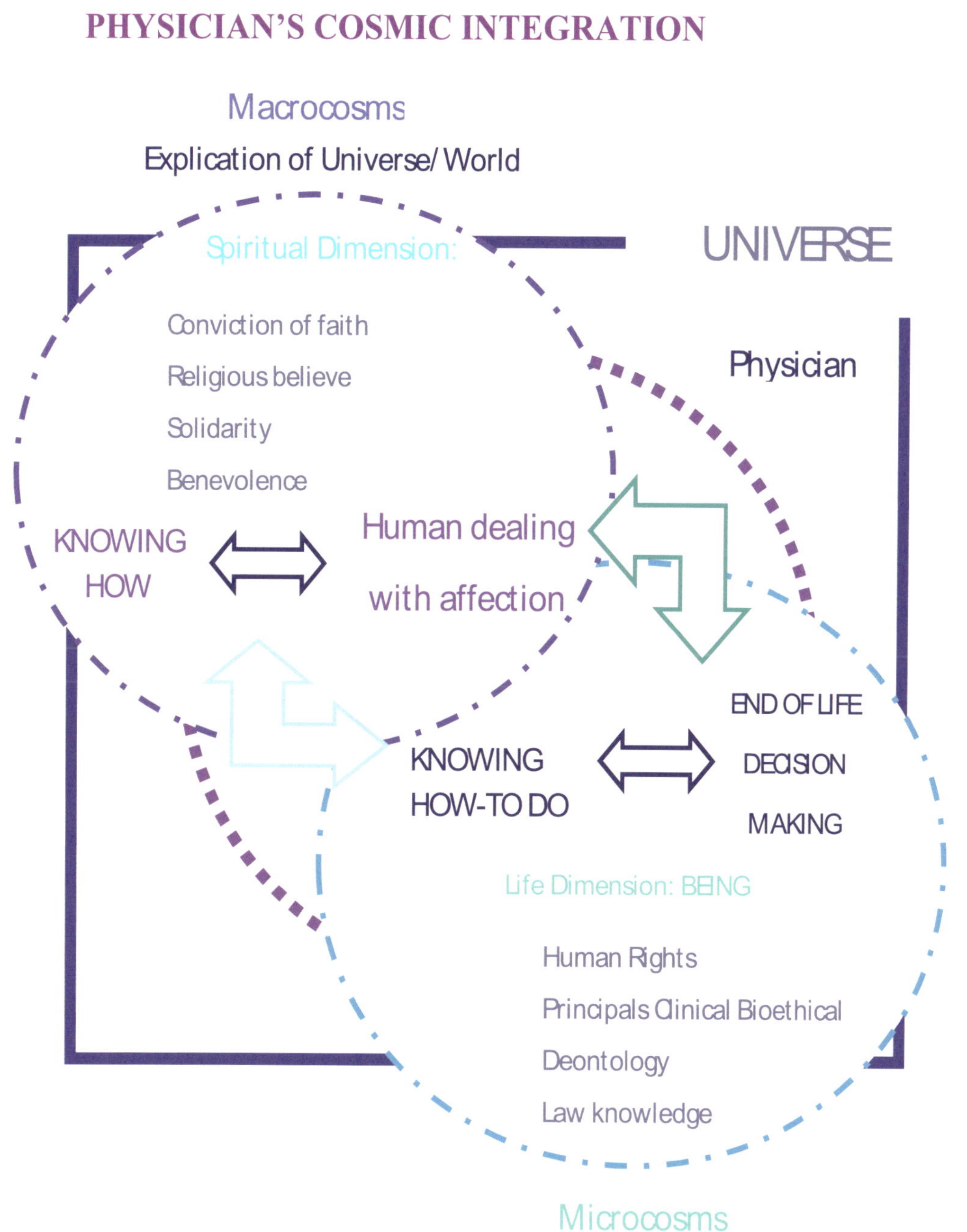

Fig. 4.

Model offers insight into how medical doctors think about the dilemma omega as care givers of terminally ill patients, provides a way to assort, real situation decision-making, by recognizing that adult development is linked to educational and work experiences and it is not just a reflection of socioeconomic status or degree of theory academic knowledge of physicians; by extent, working experience and degree of education may provide the stimulus for further moral development in health care gives. Highlighting the importance of the interaction between cognition-as how individuals think about moral dilemmas and behavior-what they would actually do in a particular decision situation. It emerges from this new complex and holistic thinking that given the impossibility of curing, might the ending be "caring" as an assemblage of coordinated actions of the health care team members, led by medical doctors, in a transdisciplinarity effort accompanied by the nursing and bioanalysis staff.

4. References

Aguiar Guevara R. (1997). *La culpa y su prueba*. Primera edición, Editado por Aguiar-Guevara & Asociados, ISBN: 980-07-4112-7; Baruta, Caracas-Venezuela.

Aguiar Guevara R. (2003). Eutanasia: mitos y realidades. Primera edición, Editado por Tamher Editores, ISBN: 980-12-0242-4. El Silencio, Caracas- Venezuela

Albuquerque de Oliveira A. Bioética y Derechos Humanos. In: *Primer Curso de Bioética Clínica y Social para América Latina UNESCO y Red Bioética*. (2010). Access 04-10-2011. Available from: http://www.unesco.org.uy/shs/red-bioetica/fileadmin/shs/redbioetica/revista_1/Albuquerque.pdf

ANTEPROYECTO DE CÓDIGO PENAL-REPÚBLICA BOLIVARIANA DE VENEZUELA (2000). Gaceta Oficial N° 5.494; 20. Access 04-18-2011. Available from: http://www.tsj.gov.ve/informacion/miscelaneas/anteproyecto2.html

Bont M, Dorta K, Ceballos J, Randazzo A & Urdaneta-Carruyo E. (2007) Medical decisions at end of life: importance based on personal opinion, degree of information and training of doctors working in Aragua and Carabobo States. *Revista de la Facultad de Ciencias de la Salud-Salus*, Vol. 11 N° 3, pp. 30-36. ISSN: 1316-7138.

Bont M, Dorta K, Ceballos J, Randazzo A & Urdaneta-Carruyo E. (2007) Euthanasia: a historic hermeneutical view. *Revista Comunidad y Salud*, Vol. 5 N° 2, pp. 34-43, ISSN: 1690-3293.

Bont M. (2010). Bioethical-legal and spiritual dimensions at ending of human life decisions. *Revista Comunidad y Salud*, Vol. 8 N° 1, pp. 46-57, ISSN: 1690-3293.

Castillo-Valery, A. (2006). Aspectos bioéticos del final de la vida. In: *Bioética*. Primera edición, editorial Disinlimed, ISBN: 980-6142-95-0, Caracas-Venezuela.

Cely Galindo G. (2001). *El horizonte bioético de las ciencias*. Quinta edición. Fundación Cultural Javeriana de Artes Gráficas, ISBN: 958-683-087-X, Bogotá D.C.

Cely Galindo G. (2001). *Gen-Ética: Donde la vida y la ética se articulan: El mundo de los Transgénicos*. Primera edición, 3R Editores Colección Bioética, ISBN: 958-80-1779-3, Bogotá D.C.

Cely Galindo G. (2004). *Ethos vital y dignidad humana*. Primera edición, Fundación Cultural Javeriana de Artes Gráficas, ISBN: 985-683-705-X, Bogotá D.C.

Cely Galindo G. (2005). *Bioética: Humanismo científico emergente*. Primera edición, Fundación Cultural Javeriana de Artes Gráficas, ISBN: 958-683-752-1Bogotá D.C.

CENABI-CENTRO NACIONAL DE BIOÉTICA. (1999). Ética Médica Aspectos conceptuales y ético-morales de la muerte. In: *La Muerte y la Medicina Actual*. Editores Alfredo

Castillo Valery & Elizabeth Piña de Vásquez. UCV-Centro Nacional de Bioética, modulo 5, ISBN: not known *exclusively for educational purpose*, Caracas-Venezuela.

CÓDIGO DE DEONTOLOGÍA MÉDICA. (2003). Aprobado en CXXXIX Reunión Extraordinaria de la Asamblea de la Federación Médica Venezolana. Access 04-11-2011. Available from: http://www.federacionmedicavenezolana.org/fmv2010/DEONTOLOGIAMEDICA.pdf?phpMyAdmin=e30ec5ecaf76b23604b3d58660ccf494

FUNDACIÓN PRO DERECHO A MORIR DIGNAMENTE. (1991). Derechos del paciente terminal. Access 04-18-2011. Available from: http://www.dmd.org.co/pdf/donce.pdf

FUNDACIÓN HOSPICE VENEZUELA. (2009). Derechos del paciente terminal. Access 04-18-2011. Available from: http://hospicevenezuela.blogspot.com/2009/09/derechos-del-enfermo-terminal.html

Gherardi CR. (2008) Ética del final de la vida. *UNESCO y Red-Bioética*. Access 06-06-2008. Available from: http://portal.iner.gob.mx/bioetica/macros/GenericDocumentWithPhoto.jsp?contentid=2115&version=1&channelid=1

Glaser B. (1992). *Basics of grounded theory analysis*. Mill Valley, C.A. Sociology Press. Access 09-15-2008. Retrieved from: http://www.groundedtheoryonline.com/

Hernández-Sampieri R, Fernández-Collado C & Baptista-Lucio P. (1991). *Metodología de la Investigación*. Primera edición, McGraw-Hill Interamericana de México S.A. ISBN: 968-422-931-3, México-DF.

Hernández N. (2007). *Modelo Teórico de Desarrollo de Habilidades Profesionales para la Función Profesor Investigador Universitario* Primera edición, Editado por la Universidad de Carabobo, ISBN: 987-980-12-2660-4, Valencia-Venezuela.

Hurtado-León I & Toro-Garrido J. (1997). *Paradigma y Métodos de Investigación en Tiempos de Cambio*. Primera edición, Talleres Gráficos de Clemente Editores C.A, ISBN: 980-328-413-4, Valencia-Venezuela).

Juan Pablo II. Carta Apostólica: *Salvifici Doloris*, Sobre el Sentido Cristiano del Sufrimiento Humano. (1984). Accessed 04-18-2011. Available from: http://www.vatican.va/holy_father/john_paul_ii/apost_letters/documents/hf_jp-ii_apl_11021984_salvifici-doloris_sp.html

Leal Gutiérrez J. (2005). *La Autonomía del Sujeto Investigador y la Metodología de Investigación*. Primera edición, Centro Editorial Litorama, ISBN: 980-12-1254-3, Mérida-Venezuela.

León Cechini, A. (1975). La muerte y el morir. *Rev. Tribuna Médica de Venezuela*. N° 501. Tomo XLII, N° 5, 1er Número de Marzo, ISBN: not known, Caracas-Venezuela

León Cechini, A. (1981) *Eutanasia. Academia Nacional de Medicina* Primera edición, Editorial Científica Médica, ISBN: not known; Caracas-Venezuela.

León Cechini A. (1996). Eutanasia y suicidio asistido. In: *"Primeras Jornadas Nacionales de Bioética"*. Editorial Científica Médica ISBN not known, Caracas-Venezuela.

LEY DE EJERCICIO DE LA MEDICINA. Congreso de la República de Venezuela. (1982). Gaceta Oficial N° 3.002; extraordinario del 23 de Agost, access 09-15-2008. Available from: http://legal.com.ve/leyes/C106.pdf

Lolas F. (2008). Bioethics and animal research: A personal perspective and a note on the contribution of Fritz Jahr. *Rev Biological Research*, V 41. N° 1, pp. 119-123, ISSN 0716-9760.

Malpica-Gracián CC. (2008) *Modelo Inacabado para Comprender la Bioética Integral en los Estudios Médicos Venezolanos.* Primera edición, editado por la Universidad de Carabobo, ISBN: 978-980-12-3318-0, Valencia-Venezuela.

Martin-Fiorino VR. (2008). Primeras Reflexiones sobre Investigación. Centro de Investigación de Humanidades y Educación CIHE Universidad Dr. Rafael Belloso Chacín. En Maracaibo. Zulia, access 04-15-2011. Available from: http://www.urbe.edu/publicaciones/redhecs/pdf/2-conferencia-victor-martin-fiorino-julio2008.pdf

Martínez Mígueles M. (2004). *Ciencia y Arte en la Metodología Cualitativa.* Primera edición, Editorial Trillas S. A. ISBN-968-24-7011-0, México.

Moran D. (2000). Introduction to Phenomenology. Routledge Publishers, ISBN-13: 978-0415183734, access 04-18-2011. Available from: http://www.amazon.co.uk/Introduction-Phenomenology-Dermot-Moran/dp/0415183731#reader_0415183731

Morin E. (1999). *El Método. La Naturaleza de la Naturaleza.* Quinta edición, Ediciones Cátedra, S. A. ISBN: 84-376-0267-X, Navalcarnero, Madrid-España.

Morin E. (2003). *Introducción al Pensamiento Complejo.* Título original: Introduction á la pensé complexe, traducción: Marcelo Pakman. Sexta reimpresión, Editorial Gedisa, S. A. ISBN: 84-7432-518-8, Barcelona-España

Morin E, Ciurana E & Motta R. (2003). *Educar en la Era Planetaria.* Primera edición, Editorial Gedisa, ISBN: 84-7432-835-7, Barcelona-España.

Morin E. (2004). La Epistemología de la Complejidad. *Gaceta de Antropología,* N° 20: 02-20. Access 04-19-2011. Available from: http://www.ugr.es/~pwlac/G20_02Edgar_Morin.html

Muñoz-Justicia J. (2003). *Análisis Cualitativo de Datos Textuales con ATLAS/ti. Versión 2.4.* Editorial Universitat Autónoma de Barcelona, Computerized Educational System, España.

Orcajo Á. (2000). *La Postmodernidad o las Fracturas de la Ilusiones.* Tercera edición, Editado por la Universidad de Carabobo, ISBN: 980-233-262-3, Valencia-Venezuela.

Piva, Gianni & Pinto, Trina. CONSTITUCIÓN DE LA REPÚBLICA BOLIVARIANA DE VENEZUELA. (2003) Editado por Livrosca C.A. Caracas, access 04-19-2011. Available from: http://www.gobiernoenlinea.ve/docMgr/sharedfiles/ConstitucionRBV1999.pdf

Sass Hans-Martin. (2008). Fritz Jahr's Concept of Bioethics. *Kennedy Institute of Ethics Journal.* The Johns Hopkins University Press; V. 17 N° 4, pp. 279-295. ISSN: 1054-6863. Access 09-15-2008. Available from: http://muse.jhu.edu/journals/kennedy_institute_of_ethics_journal/v017/17.4sass.pdf

H Spiegelberg, Herbert Spiegelberg & E Spiegelberg. (1975) *Doing Phenomenology: Essays On and In Phenomenology.* Publisher: Springer, ISBN: 9024717256. Access 09-15-2008. Available from: http://books.google.co.ve/books?id=wu12ClbDsl0C&printsec=frontcover&source=gbs_slider_thumb#v=onepage&q&f=false.

UNIVERSAL DECLARATION OF HUMAN RIGHTS. (1948) Adopted and proclaimed by the General Assembly of the United Nations 217 A (iii), on December 10. Access 04-20-2011. Available from: http://www.un.org/en/documents/udhr/index.shtml

World Health Organization. Patient's Rights. (1948) Access 04-22-2011. Available from: http://www.who.int/genomics/public/patientrights/

World Health Organization. A declaration on the promotion of patients' rights in Europe. (1994). Accessed 04-21-2011. Available from: http://www.who.int/genomics/public/eu_declaration1994.pdf

6

Euthanasia, Dignity, Autonomy - A Reflection on Medicine

Dominique A. Lossignol[1] and Cristina Dumitrescu[2]
[1]*Head of the Supportive and Palliative Care Unit, Institut Jules Bordet Free University of Brussels, Brussels*
[2]*Medical oncology, Institut Jules Bordet, Free University of Brussels, Brussels Belgium*

1. Introduction

The purpose of this chapter is to present a reflexion on euthanasia using personal experience and philosophical references. Our goal is to present some aspects of this topic but not to say what to think or what to do. We hope it will give the debate a good introduction[1].

In what follows, the term euthanasia must be understood as being the act of ending, at his request, the life of an adult (or emancipated minor), who is able to decide for himself, suffering from a serious incurable condition (illness or accident) and experiencing constant and unbearable physical or psychological suffering. This request will be repeated with calm, and without any external pressure. The act will be carried out by a third party, in the case considered here, a doctor. It is important to specify that the doctor can refuse to carry out euthanasia and that in addition no one is forced to participate if it is against his morals or conscience.

The Belgian law of 28 May 2002, published at the same time as the law on palliative care and the law relating to patients' rights, imposes more obligations (1). The most pertinent ones concluded in giving the patient all information, particularly in relation to palliative care, obtaining the opinion of a second or even third doctor (in the case of unforeseeable short-term death), and making sure that all persons designated by the patient have been met beforehand. The legal text does not specify the practical medical methods (this is not its role), but these are accessible and have been published many times. It is useful to specify that the legal text avoids the notion of medically assisted suicide, and that the stage of the condition ("terminal phase," "palliative phase," "end of life") has been removed. By adapting the second proposal, it echoes opinion issued by the Belgian Bioethics Consultative Committee on 12 May 1997 (2). As a reminder, the essential question posed by the BBCC was: "Is it appropriate to legislate on the subject of euthanasia?" which resulted in 4 proposals: A complete decriminalisation of euthanasia (The practice of euthanasia is freely accepted), a *"a posteriori"* regulation (The act is declared after its completion), a *"a priori"* regulation (A commission decides before if the act is legally acceptable) and a complete *Status quo* (no change of legal framework).

---

[1] Some references are taken from book written in French or translated from other languages in French.

Since its implementation, the Federal Commission for Evaluation and Control has published the conclusions detailing the declarations of the doctors who have carried out euthanasia. All the data are available (3).

We shall not go into details about the history of the Belgian legislation on this theme, but it should be remembered that we had to wait many years before the subject could be debated in Parliament, that it was needed a conversion of the majority so the historic veto be lifted. The debate was rich, contradictory, pluralist, with both sides being heard and many different opinions expressed, resulting in the present-day text. This text was based, should it be noted, on legal proposals such as those of Roger Lallemand or Edouard Klein (invariably rejected...) or on the texts of Professor Yvon Kenis, co-founder of ADMD (Association for the Right to Die with Dignity), who wrote about the legal proposal: "It is not ideologically oriented, as it takes no position about the direction of life or about the hereafter. It deals only with real cases of unbearable suffering and denounces the prejudice whereby death must be preceded by a long and cruel agony. (...) Should one not sacrifice the duration of life for its quality that a patient wishes to retain until the end?" Such foresight and such sense of the issue could only demand respect.

Although some oppose euthanasia and palliative care (similarly to the therapeutic obstinacy), this Manichean position is absurd both semantically and in practice. How can we say that medicine is capable of alleviating all physical, mental or moral suffering? In Belgium, where, should it be noted, all euthanasia must be the subject of a declaration to a Control Commission, it can be observed that most of the patients having requested and obtained euthanasia had previously benefited from palliative care. A recent study by a VUB (Vrije Universiteit Brussel) team confirms that decisions, taken within a multidisciplinary framework regarding euthanasia and assisted suicide, did not restrict the practice of palliative care (4). Evidently, this will not doubt its qualities, but its limitations. We have many times received patients, referred by doctors working in palliative-care units, who maintained their request for euthanasia despite the efforts and undeniable competence of our colleagues. These patients recognised the quality of the care, the support, the listening, the appropriate monitoring of pain in these units, but could not tolerate to be made to feel guilty, either because their request was refused in the name of precepts to which they did not subscribe, or because a so-called "controlled" sedation was proposed to them as an alternative. This solution eludes both the patient's request and the real meaning of the action that is carried out. In effect, far from being "controlled," this sedation only prolongs the agony and if death occurs prematurely, some health professionals mention the double-effect phenomenon (result of an act that was not part of their intention). Of course, there are circumstances in which it would be better to sedate a patient in order to spare him a painful death, such as in the case of terminal dyspnoea or the threat of a haemorrhage. This ties in with both compassion and ethics. This is well described in the book "Principles of biomedical ethics of Beauchamp and Childress[2], (5). By contrary, if this sedation is proposed as an "alternative" to euthanasia, it is an intellectually inappropriate process that is aimed merely at appeasing the practitioner's conscience. To deliberately sedate a patient in the name of his comfort is not a harmless act. We know the risks involved in the administration of sedatives in the context of precarious medical situations. The side effects and complications inherent in

[2] This book is a reference in terms of ethics and is highly recommended.

this practice are most often irreversible. To claim that, in this case, the sedation is "controlled" displays a lack of honesty, as death very often occurs within 72 hours (6), (7). From all the evidence, the "palliative filter" that some would impose on all patients requesting euthanasia is neither a medical nor an ethical guarantee...

The other fear advanced by opponents is that of by-products, of the "slippery slope." This would be nothing more or less than mass killings, carried out for social reasons (the poor), economic reasons (the elderly), or medical reasons (the very ill, the disabled, the mentally ill), implying that by legislating, and by legalizing euthanasia, the legislature would enable health professionals to feel free to act without constraint. By all evidence this is hugely contrary, as if a law would supplant all moral reflection, all ethical analysis. In effect, it is like saying that doctors generally work without "conscience" and that only the law ("which forbids euthanasia") protects patients from arbitrary decisions taken by their doctors while at the same time these detractors, opposed to all legislation, claim for example that no doctor wants to carry out euthanasia. This is another undisputed manifestation of the manipulation of opinion and bad faith, based on lies. Neither Belgian nor Dutch experiences, which provide official data, have led to the by-products mentioned. On the contrary, since 2002, there has been no "explosion" of euthanasia or similar acts, in Belgium. All patients had a long and hard medical past, thus demonstrating their will to fight as long as possible against the disease. (For more details, see reference 3)

The approach adopted by Jean-Yves Goffi (pp 29-42) on the theme of the "slippery slope" is among the most interesting (8). For him, those who fear this ineluctable by-product "in fact demonstrate their inability to perceive the imperceptible, and their argument is made at the cost of a certain number of confusions regarding arbitrary attributions of causal relationships." Their systematic references to Nazism is furthermore an error in evaluating the problem and the erroneous attribution of the same term ("euthanasia") to two completely different situations, namely a political choice on the one hand and an individual choice on the other. Should we say that the Nazi Party usurped many symbols and themes, turning them away from their initial function.

J-Y Goffi continues by clarifying "that we must revise downwards the claims of the argument (of the slippery slope), which is reduced to recording the fact...that the use of certain concepts in ethics is particularly delicate and can lead to abusive interpretations."

For our part, we would add that this "Newtonian" vision of risks (slope, etc.) is related to a heuristic sense of fear and has no place in rational medical practice. It eludes the moral sense of patients and doctors and at the same time condones the adherence of the masses to genocidal behaviour.

The work of J-Y Goffi certainly deserves paragraph, both for its originality and for its relevance. His chapter "Euthanasia and virtues" is in this case a very good demonstration on the subject, tackling it by means of virtues, of consequentialism, of aretism (virtue ethics). He concludes, but without really concluding: "In exceptional although inevitable circumstances, death can become a desirable end; and the most virtuous attitude consists of assisting others to pursue this end.").

Finally, it must be repeated that from what we know of the issue, carrying out euthanasia is not an ordinary act and is never done emotionless. No doctor desires to carry out euthanasia, but when his patient's request is clear, when the issue is declared as unbearable for the patient, helping him to die without suffering, sparing him a painful and pointless agony, assumes such a human dimension that refusing to carry out this act would be still, much more painful. Refusal is in our view a desperate exhibition of the doctor's existential anguish much more than a proof of respect for deontology and ethics. The only valid argument advanced is an argument with moral value, very often with religious connotations. But then, what value does it give to the suffering of the patient? How far must this suffering go so that the patient would be listened? For how long?

A question remains unanswered: is it conceivable to consider that patients die without dignity when the euthanasia they requested is refused. In our opinion, undoubtedly yes. As long as a patient makes a request for euthanasia that complies with the legal framework (conscious and competent patient with incurable condition, suffering that cannot be eased, repeated request), to refuse him in the name of personal moral or philosophical principles without proposing a solution that satisfies the patient (suggesting another doctor for example, as set forth by law) consists of no longer recognizing the patient's dignity and of protecting the doctor's conscience, which takes precedence for him over the wishes of his patient. Although no doctor is constrained to carry out an euthanasia, to place the person who requests it in an impasse is an attack on respect for this person and his independence, using him as a tool for one's own morals, for one's own conscience, "denying" personal dignity. This argument is, in our view, fundamental for considering the act of euthanasia not only as a respectful act, full of humanity, but also as the unconditional recognition of the dignity of the patient.

In a context of medical practice, respectful for the patient, the ethics in force take priority over the doctor's personal morals, even if these are overturned. Despite the difficulty in transgressing certain moral concepts, in particular religious ones, health professionals must refer to the ethical values of the moment, considering that the decision to be taken is the "least bad" one for the patient. Paula La Marne (pp 116-117), in the conclusion of her book on "*Ethics and the End of Life*," writes: "Nothing can prevent someone from choosing his death, provided that this choice is firm and clear, and that the doctor is sure of this." (9) She insists on the importance of developing palliative care, and mentions the fact that patients requesting death are rare. But the notion of "rarity" is not synonym with insignificance. To help one, two or five patients has no countable value in my eyes. These are major events in the life of a doctor, events that cannot be neglected and that are more than simple statistics. It is at these moments that clinical experience, but also wisdom and respect for others, cannot be subjugated to a current of dominant thought, to diktats that suppress dialogue. The words used by Bernard Baertschi are clearly along these lines: "...euthanasia appears to be an ultimate means of satisfying the aims of moral enterprise: leading a happy life, or at least preventing it from becoming radically unhappy or even worse infra-personal." (10)

We have met many patients who have spoken of their suffering, of their wish, not to go beyond a certain limit that they have fixed, who have asked us "calmly and repeatedly" to be present at the last moment and to help them to leave with dignity, *their* dignity. For all these people, we think that we have acted in the best way possible with the feeling that the act carried out was what had to be done. At this moment, concepts of dignity, independence and ethics were all present, but free of any passion or sterile rhetoric. In medicine, there is no "right time" to start asking questions about the meaning of what one is doing. It is a reflection of each moment which certainly becomes richer over time, but which can never be carried over to the next day. A little experience is worth much more than any blind certitude.

2. Dignity - morality

An universal term, of which we speak a lot, but for which, when you think about it, there is no definition that really satisfies or at least for which there is no disagreement depending on points of view.

Dignity is sometimes linked to virtue, to a certain social class ("dignitaries"), sometimes to an attitude, to a bearing ("a noble and dignified allure"), sometimes to respect for the autonomy of the person ("retaining self-esteem despite adversity"), sometimes to the inherited quality of the individual ("the fact of being simply a human being"). Among these different concepts, how do we interpret the notion of dignity in medical practice? For some, like Ruth Macklin, the notion of dignity appears even useless or at least should not be evoked in medicine. In an article published in 2003, she writes that it is a bad use of the term, in the place of "respect for individuals and their independence, which concerns essentially obtaining the informed consent, respecting the confidentiality, and the need to avoid abusive discrimination." While radical, this argument should not be accepted as it is and should even be reassessed. (11)

One can, according to Roberto Andorno, distinguish between an inherited, "static," intangible, immutable dignity that is present in the "being," and a "dynamic" dignity, which is present in the "acting." (12) In any case, it can be seen that dignity remains an absolute concept that exists only because of what derives from it and therefore, because of its universal character, is unalienable whatever the circumstances.

Consequently, expressions such as "a life worth living" or "a dignified death" are in themselves meaningless as dignity cannot be lost; this can depend only on the person (independence, respect).

It can be understood that as a concept, dignity can be limited to one of these aspects alone and that a reductive approach leads to confusion. We must therefore be clear about the terms. In the opinion of Bernard Baertschi, it is possible to tackle the question as follows: dignity is a question of "morality" (what one does), a "personal" question (what one undergoes), and a "human" question (what one is). On the other hand, indignity is evidently related to humiliation and using people as tools. All these elements coexist in everyone, but without any one affecting the others. This ranges from self-esteem to the image that one projects of oneself to others. There is often a moral sense that will give either a respectable image, or a feeling of shame or remorse in relation to what one has done: theft, lies, insults. There is the personal dimension, which can be noble, but can also cause a feeling of debasement as is the case with mutilating or degenerative conditions, in the case of pain or when a patient is placed in a situation of inferiority with clear comparative strength: i.e. patients infantilised. These two dimensions do not relate to the third, the one that is most often the issue during ethical debates and that is at the centre of the Declaration of Human Rights.

This is the human sense of the concept of dignity, which cannot in principle be lost, unlike the first two. That said, it is evident that there are no clear boundaries between moral sense, personal sense and human sense; on the contrary, the existing interconnections justify the term dignity as a concept. Thus an act that is undignified in the moral sense of the term will detrimentally affect human dignity: the act of one who lies or steals, or who uses others as a means in human experimentation without consent, or torture. However, nothing that anyone does or undergoes deprives him of his human dignity; but the latter may be violated or ridiculed.

A person physically and/or morally violated or ridiculed will feel humiliated, used as a tool, according to Kant's first imperative: "Act so that you treat humanity as well in your person as in the person of all others always at the same time as an end, and never as a means." This philosopher in his time discarded the foundations of contemporary morality and his works remain references for the occidental philosophy, particularly with regard to the human person, even if one could reproach him for imposing only reason as a fundamental element of morality. Kant 's "Categorical imperatives" remain the bedrock of many arguments.

Using people as tools and humiliation thus represent major attacks on human dignity and are by their nature unethical. Can such attacks be observed in medical practice?

Recent history has shown us the degree of ignominy that certain doctors have attained, especially during the Second World War: experiments without the aim of progress, without improving treatment, brutality, refinement of torture, contempt for humans in the name of a nauseating ideology.

We think that one must consider dignity, in the sense of not using humans as tools or humiliating them, as an essential element enshrined in medical practice. These are nuances permitted by rhetoric, but in the particular case of a patient, these nuances appear highly relative. The feeling of humiliation in fact relates more to an attack on self-image - "personal dignity" - than an attack on "human dignity," but for the person concerned there is no difference. He feels unbearably affected, which is how one measures that which degradates or injures. To tell him that his "dignity" is intact, that there is no reason to feel humiliated, is at the same time a semantic error and above all a clear lack of common sense.

However, some would argue the contrary by claiming that one must make a distinction between relative (or moral or personal) dignity and absolute (human) dignity, as an alteration of the first does not affect the second, even going so far as to evoke camp prisoners to justify their suggestions: "...their immense eyes that truly express beauty, the dignity of the human being that no offence, no cruelty...can reduce." These same arguments are sometimes used to claim that palliative care provides the only response that is humanly "dignified" in response to the "anguished claim for the right to die with dignity"! (13) It can be understood that this semantic game is not innocent, that it can serve as fertile ground for opponents of the decriminalisation of euthanasia and moreover that it is manipulative, removing the patient from the debate without telling him.

In medicine, the respect must go beyond the patient's independence, sparing him the shame, the humiliation, the feeling of being used as a tool, that is by recognizing his dignity as conceived by him.

Dignity has a multidimensional value, which is part of the individual history of a person who cannot be understood by one of its aspects alone. By being rhetorical about a concept, the latter ends up being empty of meaning. In other words, we must consider the patient individually and assist him without imposing on him moral standards that do not stand up to reality and bring difficulties and conflicts when taking decisions.

3. Independence - self-determination

Absent from the Hippocratic Oath (it is interesting to note on this subject that Hippocrates did not take into account the patient's point of view when drafting his oath), the patient's independence is however part of the ethical code. This independence defines our capacity to choose our lifestyle, our behaviour and our values, but cannot be at the cost of moral and ethical reflection. To respect individual independence is to respect the basis of free, informed, advanced consent, essential before any experimentation (the Nuremberg Code, the Declaration of Helsinki, the Belmont Report), is to ensure that the patient is involved in decision-making processes, that he understands the information given to him.

The doctor cannot decide for the patient, even if the latter does not make the best choice from a medical point of view. A patient suffering from pancreatic cancer in an inoperable stage may, for example, refuse chemotherapy even if encouraging results are presented to him, and prefer exclusively palliative care. Treatment must be oriented in accordance with the patient's objectives and priorities. The situation can be more complex in the case of an unconscious patient. If the latter was not able to make his wishes known beforehand (advance declaration), the doctor has to judge whether the care provided will bring relief, or even an improvement, of the clinical situation. Bioethical principles are then to be taken into account while obviously avoiding therapeutic obstinacy, which can be condemned as an unethical attitude. If arrangements have been made beforehand, they must be respected.

In the case of a weakened patient, made vulnerable by illness or an accident, the situation also requires many precautions, mutual confidence and confidentiality. The patient goes to his doctor in the hope that the latter will act in his best interests and will respect his dignity. This is the case of patients suffering from a progressive disease of which certain complications may alter their judgement capacity.

One can see independence as a risk of harming, if circumstances impair the patient's full judgement, if his *freedom* to judge is no longer really so, hence the importance, in good time, of dialogue and expression of the wishes of the patient, who has furthermore been duly informed of his condition. It remains the question of free choice, of due abandonment of the paternalistic position of medical ethics in favour of an autonomist model. (14) (Marzano pp 23-24)

In a very complete work on ethics and the end of life, Paula La Marne (9) evokes the principle of independence by clarifying that this is the indispensable, reasonable condition of dialogue with the patient, the latter clarifying his conceptions of a valid existence in relation to his body and maintaining his life. The doctor's benevolence, however noble, should not have a bearing on the patient's freedom, which is nothing more or less than a fundamental right. "The duty of compassion (*Agape, brotherly love)*, etc.) on the doctor's part encompasses respecting the patient's choices (respecting his independence). It is the patient who has the last word," she writes in chapter II concerning "Face to face with therapeutic obstinacy and euthanasia."

In order for there to be independence, there must obviously be appropriate information, ensuring free, informed and conscious consent on the part of the patient. Consequently, the patient may choose what he sees fit: treatment, intervention (specific or experimental), or refusal of care.

The patient's independence is more a starting point than an end point, thus condemning all paternalism. The ever more frequent use of "information forms" in clinical studies, protocols or interventions is one of the most obvious manifestations of this. It remains to clarify what takes precedence depending on the case, taking into account that the doctor must respect the patient's dignity as well as his independence (his self-determination), without forgetting the three other main principles of bioethics, namely: doing good, not doing bad, and (distributive) justice, as presented by Beauchamp and Childress.

4. And to continue...

In particular, it will be necessary to demonstrate that carrying out euthanasia, within an established framework as set forth by (Belgian) law, is neither an exception nor an ethical transgression.

Opponents of euthanasia advance arguments rooted sometimes in

1. religious precepts ("Thou shall not kill"), sometimes in
2. Kantian categorical imperatives and deontologism, sometimes resting on
3. the slippery slope argument (see above), or even on the fact that
4. carrying out euthanasia is in total contradiction of practising the art of healing ("Killing a patient is immoral," "I didn't do my studies for *that*," etc.), that it contradicts
5. the Hippocratic oath "Do not prescribe or counsel a lethal product" Art. 4), that
6. euthanasia is suicide in disguise.
7. A law will give an absolute power to the doctor.

While one can understand these arguments, again they must be considered at a supra-personal level, which places the opponents in a decision-making impasse, obliging them literally to abandon the patient in need. We think that for each of these arguments, it is possible to demonstrate that they have been advanced wrongly or at least that they lie in the field of meta-ethics. So as not to lengthen the text, we propose to deal with each of them in the discussion by setting against them the counter-argument that I consider most relevant.

1. The adage advanced is of course respectable, but it has never prevented anyone from killing his neighbour, nor prevented conflicts, nor of course religious wars. And here also, the word "kill" is loaded with meaning and does not relate to clinical reality. Moreover, we find in the founding texts writings that mention assistance to die with compassion...
2. As mentioned earlier, the act of acceding to a request for assistance to die in a precise context is not in contradiction of a Kantian imperative. I will repeat in particular that not respecting a patient's wishes is in itself an attack on his dignity.
3. The "slippery slope" is an argument that has its limits and in this case is advanced wrongly. To mention the risk of the slippery slope is indirectly to demonstrate the inability to react faced with what would be ineluctable. Belgian experience demonstrates that there is no slope and that nothing slips...
4. Assisting a patient until the end of his life is an integral part of care. Preferring "natural" death to medical aid that guarantees comfort is dubious. Imagining that nature will be more moral that health professionals shows a lack of grasp of the subject. In addition, the semantics used are among the most biased: "Put to death," "Kill," "Terminate," etc.)
5. The reference to the Hippocratic Oath is habitual but forgets that this text has been "transgressed" for a long time (abortion, surgery, etc.). Likewise its text must be read as a set of ethics for life and not for death. Furthermore, the recourse to "poison" concerns essentially suicide, condemned by the Pythagoreans, and not assistance to die.
6. Analysis of actual cases experienced shows that a request for euthanasia is clearly different from suicide, in its conceptualisation by the patient, in what motivates the decision, and in its execution.
7. Because of a law, discussion about end-of-life is now open without clandestinity and a law will never erase or avoid professional conscienciousness.

These various points are not exhaustive and should be subjected to more in-depth analysis, but that lies outside the scope of this work.

5. Veil of ignorance...

Every day brings its new set of declarations. On reading the "collective" work of Luc Ferry and Axel Kahn (16) one cannot help but be struck by the lack of acuity and even intellectual honesty with regard to the subject of euthanasia. Coming from such respectable and influential people, this is worrying. Ferry speaks among other things of a "supposed humanitarian act that consists of killing..." Kahn considers that "euthanasia is a transgression of the law," and that "the "Leonetti law" avoids transgressive euthanasia." Although in meta-ethical matters one must above all analyse statements logically and reflectively, abstaining from all moral judgement, such comments are in my view highly debatable and very far from an approach in line with cases actually experienced (casuistic ethics, etc.).

After reading this work, we wondered whether one could not apply John Rawls's famous theory of justice and the fiction of the veil of ignorance to reflect on the question of the decriminalisation of euthanasia (17). Of course, Rawls is thinking first of all of the functioning of institutions and the practices of contemporary societies. However, why not do the exercise of searching on the one hand for what represents an equal right for everyone to access the broadest set of fundamental liberties (compatible with a set of liberties for all) and on the other hand how to respect social and economic inequalities, and make it such that they are not an obstacle to personal choices.

Still with Rawls, and considering his 1992 "u-turn," the "consensus by overlapping" would also enable the various moral principles found in our plural societies to be brought together. As pointed out by Ludivine Thiaw-Po-Une (pp 1063-1071), "moral disagreements do not result from the irrationality of some or other persons. They are rather the inevitable result of the exercise of reason in conditions of liberty."

To resort to the fiction of the "veil of ignorance" does obviously not mean, "To veil one's face."

Référence D before to conclude

6. Conclusions

We will say for the moment simply this, that to help a patient to die without suffering, respecting his philosophical, religious and spiritual choices, is an integral part of the role of the doctor and that to refuse the help requested at any level whatsoever is at best an error but above all a lack of respect for others.

Euthanasia raises and will continue to raise many questions relating to ethics, spirituality or even ideology.

Although it is not possible for everyone to adhere to the same single attitude with a universal value, it is however inappropriate to disdain the reflective work already accomplished.

The subject tackled concerns everyone even if is the act only of "some" in practice. In addition, on this matter it is obviously not the numbers that count.

Euthanasia must not be considered in terms of Good or Bad, Moral or Immoral, but in terms of what is right, both for the individual and for society, and it is there that the ethical approach comes into its own.

Finally, it would be useful if the opponents would familiarise themselves with the reports by the Federal Commission for Evaluation and Control before launching into alarmist speeches, mentioning by-products, clandestine euthanasia, elderly people fleeing abroad, etc.
Although medicine cannot do without morality, ethics, deontology or law, it should be noted that it inevitably has the nature of philosophy, in its complexity but also in its relevance. Although one can philosophise without being a doctor, it nonetheless seems inconceivable to practise medicine without philosophical reflection.

7. References

We highly suggest the reader to go through books and web sites. Although some mentioned pages are of interest, they will not replace a deeper reading.

[1] Moniteur belge - 22 juin 2002(p 28 515) See : http://staatsbladclip.zita.be/moniteur/lois/2002/06/22/MoniteurBelge.html
[2] Avis N°1 du Comité Consultatif de bioéthique de Belgique 12 mai 1997.
[3] Commission fédérale de contrôle et d'évaluation de l'euthanasie : Rapports aux Chambres législatives. Service fédéral de la Santé publique : www.health.fgov.be/AGP/
[4] Van Den Block L et al. Euthanasia and other end of life decisions and care provided in final three months of life: nationwide retrospective study in Belgium. BMJ 2009; 339 b:2772 (online first).
[5] Beauchamps T, Childress. Principles of biomedical ethics. (6th edition)Oxford University press, 2009.
[6] Lossignol DA, Obiols M, Mancini I, Body JJ: Supportive care, sedation and euthanasia. Support Care Cancer, 1999, 7, p 163.
[7] Lossignol D, Englert M, Hanson B. Deux années d'euthanasie dépénalisée en Belgique: comparaison avec les Pays Bas. Premier bilan d'une unité de soins palliatifs. Rev Med Brux 2005 ; 26 :145-152.
[8] Goffi J-Y. Penser l'euthanasie. Question d'éthique, PUF, 2004 (pp 29-42).
[9] La Marne P. Ethiques de la fin de vie. La bioéthique en question. Ellipses, 1999 (pp116-117).
[10] Baertschi B : Dignité, instrumentalisation et humiliation. Rivista per le Medical Humanities, 2008 ; 7 : 83-89.
[11] Macklin R: Dignity is a useless concept. BMJ 2003; 327 : 1419-1420.
[12] Andorno R : La notion de dignité est-elle superflue en bioéthique ? www.contrepointphilosophique.ch/ethique, mars 2005 (consulté le 27 février 2009).
[13] Marmet T (et collectif) : Ethique et fin de vie, Pratique du Champ social, Erès, 1997 (p58).
[14] Marzano M. L'éthique appliqué. Que sais-je? (2è edition) PUF, 2008 (pp 23-24).
[15] Ferry L, Kahn A. Faut-il légaliser l'euthanasie, Odile Jacob, 2010.
[16] Rawls J. A theory of justice, Cambridge, MA: Harvard University Press, 1971
[17] Thiaw-Po-Une. Questions d'éthique contemporaine, Les Essais, Stock, 2006 (pp 1063-1071)
[18] Lossignol D. Une réflexion sur l'amour, la médecine et l'euthanasie : Je connais ce que j'aime et j'aime ce que je connais mais est-ce bien vrai ? Rev Med Brux, 31 ; 5-13, 2010

7

Everything Under Control: How and When to Die - A Critical Analysis of the Arguments for Euthanasia

Josef Kuře
University Centre for Bioethics & Department of Medical Ethics, Masaryk University, Brno Czech Republic

1. Introduction

The aim of this chapter is to provide an analytical overview of some of the arguments used in current discussions of euthanasia.[1] Before doing this, however, several introductory remarks are necessary. First, the scope of the topic will be defined, as not all discussions which are related to "euthanasia" interpreted in a very broad and unspecified sense will be included. The second remark concerns the semantics to which the term "euthanasia" in this chapter refers. The third remark will deal with the methodology applied in this study.

The debates about both the morality and legality of euthanasia have been a significant phenomenon of the last decades of the twentieth century and one can expect that they will remain a source of powerful controversies well into the twenty first century. Within these debates, euthanasia is often replaced by "(physician-)assisted dying" (Quill & Battin, 2004; Young, 2007), or extended to an "assisted death" (Lewis, 2007; Lewy, 2011), a broad term under which both euthanasia and assisted suicide are subsumed. The general term "assisted death" is not understood as euthanasia in the sense used both by legislation in the countries in which euthanasia has been legalized and by its debaters who use this quite precise notion of euthanasia. Finally the term "assisted death" is not conceived in the sense as the term "euthanasia" as being used in this article. The use of the broad notion of euthanasia leads to the fact that many diverse situations are discussed under the term "euthanasia". So John Keown identifies the problem when he notes that "much of the confusion which besets the contemporary euthanasia debate can be traced to an unfortunate imprecision in definition. Lack of clarity has hitherto helped to ensure that much of the debate has been frustrating and sterile." (Keown, 2002, p. 16). For its similarity with "assisted death", euthanasia is being frequently discussed within similar but distinct contexts such as assisted suicide, medical futility, life sustaining treatment and (other) end-of-life decisions (Bauer-Maglin

[1] The proposed title for this article was originally "Euthanasia *pro et contra*: Analytical synopsis of argumentations for and against euthanasia". Its aim was to provide a synoptic and comparative analysis of both types of arguments used for support or refusal of euthanasia. However it soon became clear that such an approach transcends the format of one book chapter. So instead of a very short analysis of all arguments for and against euthanasia, only five leading arguments *for* euthanasia have been critically scrutinized.

&Perry, 2010; Onwuteaka-Philipsen, 2003; van der Maas, 1991). It is obvious that the decisions in clinical medicine- both in palliative and intensive care- encompass a much broader spectrum than just the issue of euthanasia (Battin et al., 2007; Kinzbrunner & Policzer, 2010; Wanzer & Glenmullen, 2007; Wennberg, 1989). As such, if two people are discussing whether 'euthanasia' should be legalized or criminalized and by the same word they understand two quite different things, their discussion will be fruitless and meaningless; they will be addressing each other without being able to reach any common ground, instead developing two distinct monologues.

Although for euthanasia and assisted suicide the same or similar arguments can be used, for the purpose of this book it is held that euthanasia and assisted suicide are two diverse entities -from both a moral and legal point of view (Watts & Howell, 1992; Beech, 1995). Consequently in discussions on issues raised by those two concepts, two distinct notions should be used. To this effect, the debates on both assisted suicide and physician assisted suicide and the arguments used in this context will be not included in this chapter. The scope is demarked by the topic "euthanasia", although the same or similar arguments are used in assisted suicide debates as well.

Despite the fact that in some current debates taking place under the term "euthanasia", "assisted suicide" is discussed, "euthanasia" in this chapter is semantically understood not as a notion common for both "euthanasia" and "assisted suicide". The term "euthanasia" within this chapter means that one person brings about the death of another person because the first person believes that the life of the second person, who has asked for euthanasia, is so miserable that it would be better for him/her to be dead. More precisely, *A* kills *B* upon the request of *B* for the sake of *B*. The motive of *A*, who commits the act of euthanasia, is to benefit *B*. In contrast, assisted suicide is basically a suicide: *B* kills *B*; *A* is solely providing help, not taking the life of *B*. Albeit the help provided by *A* is an essential element in the death of *B* (*B* probably would be not able to kill him/her self without this help of *A*), *B* still has the possibility and freedom not to complete the act and not to kill him/her self. *B* remains the author and originator of his/her act even though his/her free volition may be diminished.

Thus the term euthanasia is here understood as a deliberate act of termination[2] of the life of *B* by *A* upon an explicit request of *B*. In addition to the benefit of *B*, a set of other criteria must be fulfilled so that one can use the term euthanasia in a precise sense: (a) person *B* must be suffering the terminal stage of an illness or undergoing unbearable suffering (the Rotterdam criterion for euthanasia); (b) person *B*, having an enduring, voluntary and competent wish to die, has expressed repeatedly this wish; (c) the act of euthanasia is performed by a physician. The last condition is naturally not a necessary condition - euthanasia can be conducted by anyone - however the fact that a physician is conducting euthanasia is of relevance as far as the medical profession is involved in the administration of euthanasia. The last condition is not often mentioned in the argumentations *pro et contra.* Since euthanasia in the countries where it has been decriminalized is administered by members of the medical profession, the participation of a physician in euthanasia is a relevant circumstance. The second condition introduced (competence) means that the term euthanasia is understood to refer to so-called "voluntary euthanasia", i.e. a competent person makes a voluntary request (the repetition of this request serves as a guarantee of the

[2] The term "termination of life" (instead of "killing") has been used as a neutral description, which is open to diverse value-laden interpretations, including "taking life", "killing" or "homicide".

consistent and authentic will of the person wishing to die). It would be counterproductive to set a framework for the analysis of arguments of euthanasia if such a term were to include various imprecisely specified forms of assistance in dying. Therefore, for the purpose of this chapter, the term "euthanasia" will refer to "active voluntary euthanasia". So-called "passive euthanasia" will not be included here in the term "euthanasia" even though one can repeatedly find such references in literature - fortunately less and less often. If euthanasia is defined in the above mentioned sense, then there is no point talking about "passive euthanasia". We should not mix "killing" (an active action) with "allowing to die" (the deliberate lack of application of treatment that would only increase suffering and prolong dying, but not involving administration of drugs which causes termination of life).[3] Thus to refer to "killing" (active euthanasia) and "allowing to die" (passive euthanasia) by the same word (euthanasia) is semantic nonsense. Provided the term "euthanasia" is used within the introduced semantic framework, euthanasia can only be active by nature.

The other two types of euthanasia, namely "non-voluntary euthanasia" and "involuntary euthanasia" are not *prima facie* included in the following argument survey; one of the main arguments for euthanasia (autonomy) would not be applicable to both types.[4] Non-voluntary euthanasia, the termination of the life of a non-competent person by someone other than that person or termination of the life of a person who is not able to express his/her will may be supported by a compassion argument, but not in conjunction with the autonomy argument. The question as to whether someone can authorize another person to make the decision about euthanasia on their behalf by making a request to be killed (the third person *C* is requesting euthanasia for person *B* and the physician *A* terminates the life of *B* upon request of *C* who has been authorized by *B*) is quite different from the question mentioned above (*B* requests euthanasia from *A* and *A* conducts euthanasia upon request of *B*). The issue of substituted judgement used in intensive care, where person *C*, as health care proxy, makes a decision for person *B* is quite different from the substituted judgement in the context of euthanasia for many reasons. First the rationale for the substituted judgement is to follow the authentic will of a non-competent person in health care and his/her individual (value-based) preferences regarding a particular treatment in the given clinical conditions as much as possible. Furthermore in intensive care a decision about treatment *has* to be made (one of the therapeutic options has to be decided upon and realized) in difference to non-voluntary euthanasia where there is not an objective necessity to conduct the act of euthanasia; *a fortiori* if the authentic will of the patient is not known. There is no imperative to follow the unknown will of the person in the case of euthanasia. In addition, in many cultural contexts, providing treatment (or either withdrawing or withholding treatment) in a non-competent patient is adopted not upon the request of one single person (health care proxy) but by all persons involved (i.e. relatives and the whole therapeutic team including nurses, psychologists, social workers and other non-medical staff).

So within the following analysis of arguments, the focus is on active voluntary euthanasia. All sub-forms such as euthanasia of minors (e.g. terminal stage of cancer in small

---

[3] The "passive action" of allowing to die can include not only passivity in the sense of diverse avoiding of treatment (e.g. withholding or withdrawing); it can also include "active actions" such as the psychological or spiritual accompaniment of a dying person or the support by those close to the patient.

[4] "Non-voluntary euthanasia" and "involuntary euthanasia" will be included mainly in the role of counter-argumentation.

children) or euthanasia of (extremely immature) newborn children with abnormalities has naturally to be discussed, however some of the arguments would have a different and modified form, taking into account the particular context (e.g. parents as decision-makers), but maintaining a certain congruence. A distinct argumentative framework would be appropriate for involuntary euthanasia, also for killing a person despite an explicit expression of his/her opposition towards euthanasia. Such a framework is not elaborated in this chapter.

The last introductory remark refers to the methodology of this chapter. During the last few decades several studies that (also) deal with the arguments concerning euthanasia have been published.[5] They provide a valuable source of diverse views on euthanasia. The majority of studies about euthanasia have been written as manifestos which serve to support one side of the controversy. They are often intended as tools to be used by either the opponents or by the proponents of euthanasia, being akin to instruction manuals or catechisms: if you are against/for euthanasia, therein are to be found the arguments you can use in debates to support your position. In difference to many monographs on the ethics of euthanasia, this text strives to provide a critical analysis of the arguments *for* euthanasia only. An analytical and comparative synopsis of both types of arguments remains beyond the scope of this chapter.

Various numbers of arguments for and against euthanasia are listed within current literature. Similarly, different categories of arguments are used in euthanasia debates - for instance arguments based on rights, philosophical arguments (the universality of moral rules vs. tolerable exceptions), practical approaches (regulation of euthanasia by law) or religious belief (only God can give and take life). It is practically impossible to list the arguments for euthanasia as pure arguments *for* euthanasia, while at the same time giving another inventory of arguments *against* euthanasia, as if both lists were mutually exclusive and reciprocally independent. The opposite is true. Many of the *pro* arguments can simultaneously be *contra* arguments and vice versa. So the resultant categorization of arguments derives from the precondition that the individual arguments can be assigned as to their prevalent use as arguments *for* (e.g. autonomy) or as arguments *against* (e.g. slippery slope). It has to be noted that some other arguments are so truly "ambidextrous" i.e. the base of the same argument can be used both for and against euthanasia, that assigning them according one camp is fleeting at best. Some aspects of the arguments can be utilized or even manipulated in different ways or have an inverse complement in the form of counterargument - for example autonomy as one of the primary arguments for euthanasia can be challenged by one of the serious counter-arguments, namely that of competence (to which extent a terminally ill or unbearably suffering person is competent to make an autonomous choice).

The only alternatively appropriate option would be to go through the individual arguments and analyse them without labelling them as predominantly *pro* or *contra* arguments. This approach could be regarded as unbiased (or less biased) but at a cost where the individual arguments would be almost neutralized with regard to their stance on euthanasia, with the outcome and justifying power of the arguments being lessened

---

[5] Beauchamp, 1996; Behnke & Bok 1975; Bernards, 1989; Biggar, 2004; Brody, 1989; Cohen-Almagor, 2001; Dworkin, 1993; Dworkin et al. 1998; Engdahl, 2007; Gentles, 1995; Grisez & Boyle, 1979; Harris, 2005; Keown, 1995, 2002; Leone, 1999; Medina, 2005; Moreno, 1995; Morgan, 1996; Oosthuizen et al., 1978; Rachels, 1986; Roberts & Gorman, 1996; Snyder 2006; Torr, 2000; Wekesser, 1995; Young, 2007a.

considerably or disappearing altogether in the analytical critique. This would be contrary to real life application of these arguments used in euthanasia debates not as neutral arguments but as either *pro* or *contra* arguments. So the chosen general differentiation of arguments has to be taken rather as an auxiliary framework than as the final definitional scope. The following figure shows a matrix of the arguments,[6] based on the prevalent dichotomy *"pro et contra"*.

PRO	*CONTRA*
Autonomy	Competence
Right to die	Inviolability of human life - a human right
Unbearable suffering	Sanctity of life doctrine
Compassion	Prohibition of killing (Hippocratic tradition)
Human dignity	Risk of abuse
Patient's best interest	Slippery slope
Quality of life	Quality palliative care - as a/the alternative to euthanasia
Health care costs	Patient's good[7] - as an counterargument to the pure economical calculation
Legalization	The compromised role of the physician
Transparency	Vulnerability - social pressure

Fig. 1. Synopsis of arguments for and against euthanasia

Some of the arguments complement each other (e.g. autonomy and competence). Other arguments, located on the same line, illustrate the respective sides of a viewpoint. The added value of such a matrix is the emphasis on complexity. In euthanasia debates, arguments usually have an either/or, either for or against structure. This matrix seeks to "interweave" diverse arguments, putting them into a fabric of dualities. For instance, proponents would argue for the decriminalization of euthanasia in the following way: let us regulate what is being done anyway, regulated euthanasia is better then the grey zone in which it is occurring today. But the legalization of euthanasia would also affect the public role of the physician, who would become both healer and killer in the same person, with the potential to put vulnerable patients under social pressure. And these aspects have to be considered as well.

2. The arguments for euthanasia

According to the methodology described above, some of the main arguments for euthanasia will be analyzed. The remaining *pro* arguments will be scrutinized less intensively. It has to be highlighted that all arguments have their objections and counter-objections; so all of the *pro* arguments can simultaneously be used as *contra* arguments. Therefore, while dealing with the objections to the *pro* arguments, the *contra* argumentation is in fact scrutinized inherently.

---

[6] For purposes of this study, only the first five leading *for* arguments have been examined.
[7] Misbin, 1992; Sullivan, 2005.

The following structure of analysis of the arguments has been adopted:

1. Introduction
2. Description

The argument will be characterized by its most relevant features, and presented in a simplified version. The aim here is to provide a fair and well-balanced presentation of the argument (including diverse ways in which it is used).

3. Contextualization

The aim is to provide information about the background of the argument, placing it into a broader context, showing from where the argument is derived.

4. Presuppositions

In euthanasia debates, the precondition(s), as departure point(s) for the arguments are rarely stated. The aim is to clarify what the argument presupposes, what its preconditions are or which ethical theory are related to it.[8]

5. Analysis

In connection to the second step, an analytical and comparative explanation of the arguments is provided (how the argument is used in euthanasia debates); a critical analysis of both the argument and its objections is given.

6. Evaluation

The argument is assessed as to its strong and weak points, to its explanatory and justificatory power and coherence. The role and usage of the argument in euthanasia debates is addressed.

7. Conclusion

Within this structure the first five of the arguments listed for euthanasia have been critically analyzed. The analysis of the remaining five arguments have only (for the reason given above) been outlined.

2.1 Autonomy

2.1.1 Introduction

Autonomy is frequently given as one of the main arguments for euthanasia (Achille & Ogloff, 1997; Begley, 1998, 2008; Brock, 1992; Quill et al., 1997; Smith, 1989; Tulloch, 2008), usually in conjunction with the right to die (Dworkin, 1993; Finkel et al., 1993; Ogden, 1994; Smook & de Vos-Schippers, 1990). As per its proponents' arguments, a ban on euthanasia imposes a considerable restriction on the options of an individual to govern his/her life, denying a competent individual's ability to shape his/her own death. Opponents' arguments are based on different interpretations of autonomy and its role in the life of individuals: self-determination regarding one's own death (euthanasia) would be a false autonomy. Other opponents argue that the positive principle of autonomy (and self-determination) cannot outweigh the prohibitive (and therefore negative) principle of not killing. The essence of the euthanasia controversy is the tension between the values of life and individual liberty.

[8] The vocalization of the presuppositions is of significance for mutual understanding in euthanasia discussions. Otherwise these starting points, often based not only on certain ethical theories but on personal beliefs, or on various dogmas and ideologies which (even as non-identified) play a pivotal role in the debate, if not revealed cannot be addressed, rendering the debate both more difficult and superficial and inconclusive.

2.1.2 Description

Autonomy is certainly one of the essential values of Western societies and is therefore worthy of protection. The autonomy argument states that a person, while asking for euthanasia, expresses his/her personal choice, realizing his/her autonomy. The request for euthanasia is part of the human freedom to terminate one's own life (Dworkin, 1993; Russell, 1975). Thus the euthanasia request of a competent individual is a basic freedom to define the framework and conditions of his/her life, more precisely it is a decision about how that life should be lived and ended. To ask for euthanasia means to end one's own life in a prearranged way, without loosing control over one's own process of dying and death. From this point of view, euthanasia is the execution of control over one's life and death. Therefore euthanasia can and has to be practiced and has to be legalized, because the legalization of euthanasia protects and promotes the autonomy of an individual. Euthanasia not prohibited by law or legislatively decriminalized is an essential element for the execution of autonomy. On the other hand the criminalization of euthanasia results in a restriction of autonomy. The legalization of euthanasia also eliminates unnecessary or inadmissible barriers to the right to die.

The legalization of euthanasia argument has at least two forms, the two prime ones we will call liberal and libertarian respectively.[9] Within the liberal approaches, individuals can express their autonomy by asking for euthanasia. However the physician, also having his or her own autonomy, is not obliged to administer euthanasia since the autonomy of the patient is not paramount to the physician's autonomy. The moderate liberal approach tries to weigh the detrimental side-effects of the legalization of euthanasia vis-à-vis the benefit one can see in promoting autonomy (The Danish Council of Ethics, 2006). Such an approach would assess the importance of legal euthanasia for personal autonomy. All the necessary regulatory tools would have to be applied to avoid the abuse of autonomy by the heteronomy of others (including the abuse of legalized euthanasia in the form of non-voluntary or involuntary euthanasia). Within a liberal framework, euthanasia is tolerated either as a form of individual preference (despite the fact of being a criminal act, euthanasia in practice is not legally prosecuted and such a "grey zone" is in practice tolerated) or as a form of societal free choice (the decriminalization of euthanasia - the model in the Netherlands, Belgium or Luxemburg). (Gomez, 1991; Muller et al., 1994; Thomasma, 1998). Thus the genuine autonomy of the individual requesting euthanasia in a specific clinical situation is crucial.

Within the libertarian approach, decriminalization of euthanasia is an imperative of autonomy; euthanasia has to be legal, individuals have the right to request euthanasia, physicians have the duty to administrate euthanasia and in some radical approaches, individuals have not only the freedom but even a moral duty to request euthanasia in situations where the suffering is unbearable, the quality of life too low and dissatisfying and the dignity of person hurt, when in short to die is better than to live. Thus the demand of liberty would predetermine a call for euthanasia. The initiation of the use of force by one individual against another is contradictory to libertarian understanding. The libertarian approach would postulate the suspension of laws banning euthanasia. This radical (ideological) form of duty to request euthanasia (in certain situations) would be close to

[9] This terminology is not usually used in euthanasia debates and it can rightly be criticized. For the purposes of this study, the terms liberal and libertarian have been used instead of saying 'less liberal' and 'more liberal'.

authoritarian and totalitarian thinking. Ironically, these extreme perspectives on both sides are very close each other.

2.1.3 Contextualization

As a prerequisite to the concept of autonomy one of the central features of liberal political philosophy can be found: a commitment to respect the dignity of persons. This states that it is not sufficient to do good for patients and to forestall their harm. Doing good could endanger their dignity (Childress, 2000). Therefore the primary concern is that the persons are respected in their dignity; dignity is the base for autonomy, or in other words, dignity is expressed in the form of autonomy. From the respect for persons as the first principle, it follows that a person has the right to make his/her own life shorter in order to maintain a certain quality of life (shorter but better), while keeping or protecting dignity. Thus making life shorter is a necessary means of making it better as a whole (Velleman, 1999). James Childress describes this typical feature of Anglo-American thinking in the following way: "Autonomy does not imply that an individual's life plan is his or her own creation and that it excludes interest in others. The first implication focuses on the source, the second on the object of autonomy. Neither implication holds. Autonomy simply means that a person chooses and acts freely and rationally out of her own life plan, however ill-defined. [...] Thus, personal autonomy does not imply an asocial or a historical approach to life plans. It only means that whatever the life plan, and whatever its source, an individual takes it as his own". (Childress, 2000, p. 149). With regard to death and dying, personal autonomy in the form of shaping one's own life and imparting sense and meaning to it is even more relevant than in everyday life. "The way people die is of great importance to individuals' overall perception and understanding of their existence." (The Danish Council of Ethics, 2006). We do not have any better alternative to autonomy in Western societies but we have diverse societal and cultural contexts in which autonomy is realized.

2.1.4 Presuppositions

Autonomy is regarded as not only for one of the primary values in Western societies but also for one of their fundamental rights. However the debates on autonomy and euthanasia presuppose that we have some notion (*Vorverständnis*) of what autonomy and self-determination mean. Autonomy is certainly not a univocal concept in philosophy, having two main and significantly diverse expositions in European thinking.[10] The prevalent notion of autonomy in euthanasia debates can be encapsulated as the following: I want to be the author of my life whose decisions have to be dependent on my will, I want to be the subject not an object (Berlin, 1969). One of the most influential concepts of autonomy in bioethics is the one of Principlism: "Personal autonomy is [...] self-rule that is free from both controlling

[10] Autonomy in the continental European tradition can be represented by Immanuel Kant (*Grundlegung zur Metaphysik der Sitten*). The notion of autonomy in the Anglo-Saxon tradition is based on authors such as Jeremy Bentham, John Start Mill or Isaiah Berlin. For Kant, autonomy is (a freely accepted) commitment to the universal law given by the maxim of the will (autonomy is expressed by the Categorical Imperative). For Kant, autonomy is the highest (and the only acceptable) principle of morality; any heteronymous morality has to be rejected. In contrast, autonomy is for Mill an individual free choice, free from any social or political control or constraint. Autonomy for Mill coincides with liberty and independence (*On Liberty*). For Mill, autonomy is an issue of (subjective) liberty; for Kant, autonomy is an issue of (objective) reason.

interference by others and from limitations, such as inadequate understanding, that prevent meaningful choice." (Beauchamp & Childress, 2001, p. 58). However beyond the Western hermeneutics of autonomy, different presumptions could be identified in other cultures.
Autonomy follows from liberal theories which put the individual, fundamentally free and rational, into the centre; the individual not state legislation knows better what is good for his/her life. The individual, not state institutions, has to decide in which way to die. The autonomy argument is based on the liberal notion of freedom: as long as one is not causing harm to another he/she can (and has to) exercise his/her freedom. Autonomy in euthanasia debates presupposes the following structure of argument: If an action does not violate the moral rights of another individual and promotes the good of the person concerned, then that action is morally good. Since euthanasia does not violate the moral rights of others and promotes the good of the persons concerned (of everyone involved) euthanasia is morally good. Thus euthanasia is not only an action which could or should be tolerated, it is much more so an action which has to be performed, promoted and protected.
The sense of autonomy comes from the notion of positive freedom. Not only must I not be coerced by someone (negative freedom) but as an individual I want to be my own master: "I wish my life and decisions to depend on myself, not on external forces of whatever kind." (Berlin, 1969, p. 131) Once the right of a person to make his/her life shorter (and better) is recognized, the second presumption consists of being in favour of deferring to an individual's judgement regarding his/her own good. This presumption means that an individual has the right to life and to die in his/her own way, by his/her own convictions about which life is better for him/her. (Velleman, 1999). In contrast "making someone die in a way that others approve, but he believes to be a horrifying contradiction of his life, is a devastating, odious form of tyranny" (Dworkin, 1993, p. 217).
The next condition of autonomy is the freedom to choose between several options for an action. The patient (moral agent) has a preference for performing the elected act (*preference autonomy*). From this point of view euthanasia is a preferred autonomous choice, for instance the patient prefers euthanasia to palliative care and to suffering. The principle of autonomy as a basic faculty of self-determination presupposes that every moral agent is an autonomous agent. This means that not only the patient has his/her autonomy but so does the physician. To be autonomous agents is a precondition for the defence and protection of self-interests. Therewithal the principle of autonomy presupposes more than that an individual is an autonomous agent, but also a rational agent able of decision making and of (moral) action. The autonomy argument assumes that the individual is fully capable of autonomy.
In summary autonomy presupposes capacities such as understanding, reasoning, deliberateness, freedom of choice and self-governance.

2.1.5 Analysis

As has been demonstrated, the core concept of the autonomy argument is based on freedom: one wants to be the author of his/her life, who in turn shapes his/her death and dying, while making an autonomous choice as to how to die (rational self-governance). A request for euthanasia is an expression of the fundamental value to have one's own life and its circumstances under one's own control. The contrary would be a fatalistic belief that delegates the right and duty of control over one's own life and its course to some external power. Some people would argue that to repudiate control over one's own life is irresponsible, while on the other hand to realize autonomy regarding the final stage of life is regarded as a form of responsibility. A petition for euthanasia would be an act of proper responsibility, being both within the faculty and quality of a person who attempts to influence the design of his/her life by making efforts in accordance with his/her best convictions. In his analysis of the right of self-termination, David Velleman, he himself suffering from cancer, argues that the person living his/her life is therefore the best judge of the value that its continuation would afford him/her – despite the fallibility of his/her judgement. A person's judgement, being usually more reliable than anyone else's, and based on his/her values, tends to be self-fulfilling because it can respond to its own set of values. The justification for deferring to a person's judgment about serving his/her own good goes beyond her reliability as a judge. Respect for a person's autonomy requires that we defer to the well considered judgment about his/her own good even when we have reason to regard that judgment as erroneous. Thus, if an individual is capable of making the autonomous choice of asking for the termination of life which he/she deems to be not worth living, then he/she has the right to be guided by his/her own judgment. (Velleman, 1999). The question of whether the person asked to provide euthanasia has therefore a duty to conduct euthanasia will be discussed later.

Preference autonomy has been introduced as one of the conditions for autonomy. However many authors argue that preference autonomy is a necessary but not sufficient condition for an autonomous action, emphasizing the relevance of preference building. The preference is very much influenced by society, by its dominant morality and by societal expectations, and by the stage of psychological and moral development of the concrete person. So preference autonomy could easily mislead the real and authentic preference of the person asking for euthanasia. Thus for some authors the determining condition for autonomy is *dispositional autonomy*: the autonomous agent is able to reflect on his/her preferences, and be able to change his/her first-order preferences (Holm, 1998). "If disposal autonomy requires preferences that are fully self-chosen and authentic in the way described by Camus, Sartre, and other French existentialists, very few persons would ever be autonomous." (Holm, 1998, p. 270) It can also happen that a person is autonomous in one area, while not being autonomous in another area. The autonomous person who has self-governing capacities sometimes fails to govern him/herself due to temporary constrains caused by illness, depression or other conditions that restrict his/her options (Beauchamp & Childress, 2001). Autonomy can also be understood as an ideal, something very important and worthy to possess that however, not everybody achieves in his/her lifetime. In euthanasia debates the autonomy argument is used as a non-idealist moral requirement, rather one based on real situations. So as the decisive criterion for autonomy the following determiner has been proposed: autonomous is a person who is substantially autonomous; then autonomy is understood as *substantial autonomy* (Beauchamp & Childress, 2001, p. 60). Autonomy in these debates is also a faculty of a mature person who has the basic understanding of the circumstances of his/her life, who chooses and acts intentionally and who, free of constrains, is determining his/her life and death.

With regard to some of the psychological concepts of personal development (J. Piaget, E. Erikson, L. Kohlberg), autonomy is taking various faces and roles during one's life. In relation to developmental psychology, autonomy can also be understood gradualistically: autonomy is something what we progressively acquire, develop and lose. Then the question of to what extent a dying person has real autonomy is reciprocal to the question of to what extent has this person lost his/her autonomy (understood as full autonomy, as dispositional autonomy or as substantial autonomy). Thus any claim of autonomy (autonomous choice) is valid only if the person concerned (patient) still posses the necessary degree of autonomy. In some clinical situations such as a terminal or pre-terminal stage, there is a high probability that the person does not possess full autonomy; the question which has to be clarified is whether there exists a dispositional or substantial autonomy.

There are at least two main objections to the autonomy argument. The first objection, departing from the fact that not all persons in all situations have full autonomy, concludes that at a normative level with regard to life and death not everyone can be presumed able to make such an autonomous choice (some persons may have the full capacity of autonomy but on the policy level it is not feasible to distinguish full and partial autonomy and to discriminate persons, therefore the more practical conduct is to repudiate the autonomy argument as such). The second objection, departing from the fact that someone who is dying or in the (pre)terminal stage of disease (and life) is not a fully autonomous agent, invalidates the autonomy argument for a dying person.[11]

The counter-objection to the objection which states that true autonomy of a dying person is not possible at all or rarely possible is the following: Even if the choices of many persons asking for euthanasia are psychologically and socially shaped and conditioned, they must be respected as real choices. (Battin, 2003).

The other objection to the autonomy argument states that one cannot impose on another person a duty to do what the other person does not (subjectively) agree with or what is (objectively) morally wrong, even if the choice of the requesting person was made freely and rationally. (Battin, 2003). The counter-objection bases itself on the lack of sufficient proof that euthanasia as such is morally wrong and on the presumption that a well thought out decision done in accordance with the values, preferences and conscience of the person concerned, though being possibly wrong, is the best one can do and therefore it morally obliges the person concerned to act accordingly. Another counter-objection is based on the presumption that no one is obliged to do what the other person requests, especially in cases when there is a conflict in moral assessment regarding the requested action. (Battin, 2003). The autonomy principle does not insist that a free, well-considered choice of an individual must be respected. The person who is asked to perform euthanasia also has her autonomy which can prohibit or allow the requested act of euthanasia to be performed; in some cases the performer's autonomy, guided by compassion, could even oblige the person to conduct euthanasia (with or without being requested).[12] The next objection to autonomy states "that a decision about one's own death is something fundamentally different from other life decisions and life choices" (The Danish Council of Ethics, 2006). Therefore it cannot be meaningfully said that a person's own death is a subject of a free and autonomous choice. The next objection is built on the fact that "the concrete circumstances surrounding the choice scenario in the form of the role played by the doctor, society and the next-of-kin mean that the request for euthanasia will have arisen partly or wholly out of a situation in which autonomy cannot be practised, either because the person is not competent or because of direct or indirect pressure from their surroundings."[13] (The Danish Council of Ethics, 2006). So the aforementioned circumstances in such a case, either partially or fully disqualify the autonomy argument and its legitimacy for euthanasia.

---

[11] The competence of a dying person would be a part of the counter-argument.

[12] The compassion argument is discussed below.

[13] Social pressure as a negative consequence of legal euthanasia is a strong objection to this argument.

Finally there is a fundamental objection to the autonomy argument: Based on the previous analysis of autonomy in the context of an autonomous request for euthanasia and despite the broad consent that autonomy is an essential value to person's life, it is not obvious that legalization of euthanasia would automatically promote the individual's scope for practising autonomy as authentic self-determination. (The Danish Council of Ethics, 2006).
Therefore, critics would re-qualify autonomy as something that not only has to do with self-conception (as architect of one's own life) but also with self-identity, interpersonal recognition and the vulnerability of a dying person.

2.1.6 Evaluation

In euthanasia debates, arguments based on autonomy often erroneously presuppose that we all use one and the same concept of autonomy; autonomy in these debates is predominantly identical with autonomy in the sense of Anglo-Saxon liberal political philosophy. However, there is a significant difference between the meaning (and history) of autonomy in moral philosophy and the appropriation of the term in euthanasia debates (Schneewind, 1998). This difference is frequently overlooked in euthanasia debates.
Furthermore, an autonomy argument based on dignity (or related to dignity) implies a diverse notion of dignity (for example dignity characterized by empirical features as it is the case in philosophical Empiricism or dignity as it is understood in philosophical Personalism). Therefore some autonomy arguments are rather collateral discussions than a *dia*-logical enterprise.
A specific category is built by the arguments based on an ideological concept of autonomy (Ells, 2001). Eventually the relationship between the meaning of autonomy in moral philosophy (ethics) and its usage in euthanasia debates is highly selective and tenuous (Jennings, 2007). The prevalent concept of autonomy used in euthanasia debates is the concept derived from Berlin's negative liberty: negative liberty here being a necessary condition for autonomy, sometime identified with autonomous action. This approach mirrors the liberal individualistic culture of the Anglo-Saxon world, while relating less to other cultural settings and their respective philosophical traditions. Autonomy, a prerequisite for moral standing and basic moral values, has been criticized in particular by many European and other non-Anglo-Saxon authors, by feminists (e.g. Ethics of Care) and Communitarians. These authors criticize the emphasis on autonomy as a product of American society (different from values such as vulnerability or solidarity, as emphasized in the European tradition), the masculine tradition in moral philosophy, which neglects feminine moral experiences (the fact that less women than men ask for euthanasia) and its stress on atomic individualism (Communitarians).
Respect for the autonomy of the individual has always been given as the principal argument for euthanasia, understood as an active medical intervention to intentionally terminate life at the explicit request of the patient in the Dutch debates (Gunning, 1991; ten Have & Welie, 1992, ten Have, 2001). However, there have been a number of cases occurring without the explicit request of the patient (ten Have, 2001), without respect for the autonomy of the individual. So the theoretical autonomy argument is being invalidated by some instances of practice.
Autonomy indisputably should be considered a necessary but not a sufficient condition for a moral life (Callahan, 1984); what is needed as well is a broader perspective that includes interpersonal relations and interdependence (Christman & Anderson, 2009; Gaylin &

Jennings, 2003). These aspects are usually neglected in euthanasia debates that adopt autonomy as its main argument.

2.1.7 Conclusion

Despite the fact that no single concept has been more relevant in contemporary bioethics than the concept of autonomy and that the autonomy argument has played a pivotal role as the principal argument for euthanasia, autonomy can be used in euthanasia arguments in both support for and rejection of euthanasia. In this context the competence of the patient requesting euthanasia must be recognised as one of the main counter-arguments.

2.2 The right to die

2.2.1 Introduction

Beside autonomy the right to die is usually given as the most common argument for euthanasia (Cavan, 2000; Dorman, 2010; Ferguson, 2007; Stefoff, 2009; Sunstein, 1997; Yount, 2009). In recent times, many studies dealing with the right to die have been published and the ethics of the right to die has been reflected upon.[14] In some cases euthanasia even is directly equated with the right to die (Humphry & Wicket, 1986; Jussim, 1993; Wilshaw, 1974; Woodward, 2006). Euthanasia is not only the expression of a fundamental freedom but also a right one has. This right is understood as a moral right which can be claimed as a moral warrant or as a legal right supported by law which can be claimed in the legal sense. The simplified version of the argument states that every person has the right to die (whatever "right" means here). This right includes the power to specify the conditions and circumstances of one's own death and dying so the right to die includes autonomous determination *when* and *how* the person wants to die. Opponents argue that the right to die does not exist and therefore cannot be claimed.

2.2.2 Description

The usual form of this argument is based on the moral fundament of the right to die (Feinberg, 1992). This moral right can be expressed as the right to control one's own body and life and consequently to determine at what time, in what way, and with whose help one will die. The other form of the right to die is the right in a legal sense, a right which either exists (or should exist) as a specific right or can be derived from other rights such as from the right to life.

In the debates about the right to die (euthanasia) one important distinction has to be made, namely between the positive and negative right to die (right to self-determination). "A positive right of self-determination implies that a person can *demand* to have euthanasia carried out, providing the criteria for being able to request euthanasia are otherwise met." (The Danish Council of Ethics, 2006). Thus the positive right of self-determination implies that there is an objective duty to conduct euthanasia if requested; *B* requesting euthanasia imposes an obligation to perform euthanasia on *A*. While a negative right does not imply any *entitlement* to demand to conduct euthanasia. "Legalization here would merely mean that euthanasia is an action that is not illegal. No

---

[14] Bernards, 1989; Blocher, 1999; Cosic, 2003; Haley, 1999; Moreno, 1995; Ogden, 1994; Rebman, 2002; Russell, 1975; Scherer & Simon, 1999; Tada, 1992; Uhlman, 1998.

one is *obliged* to comply with the request for euthanasia, but it is legal to carry out euthanasia if the individual meets the qualifying criteria for having euthanasia carried out." (The Danish Council of Ethics, 2006). There are diverse practical implications if euthanasia is understood as a positive or negative right.

2.2.3 Contextualization

Historically the right to die has been recognized after World War II in the context of human rights development.[15] Several factors, such as advances in medical science (by technological means, life can be significantly prolonged or continued almost indefinitely), reduced sudden deaths, greater incidence of death from degenerative diseases, greater incidence of becoming elderly, dispersed families (atomic family) and increased institutionalization of the elderly have led to the recognition of the right to refuse (futile) treatment or to discontinue treatment (withdrawing) in medically desperate situations. Since the 1960s, the right to die has been supported by human and civil rights movements that have emphasized the right of self-determination, individual empowerment, bodily integrity and the right to control end-of life decision-making. In the 1970's and 1980's, the right to die was used as an equivalent to voluntary passive euthanasia based on the patients' right to refuse treatment.[16] The right to refuse treatment (and to die) being the precondition for the right to die being understood as an active termination of life (killing)[17] (Matthews, 1987). Some authors associate the right to die with the right to physician assisted suicide but not with euthanasia (Sunstein, 1997).

Two different settings of the right to die can be identified: a moral claim and legal claim. These two settings and two different forms of right are often intermixed in euthanasia debates. Therefore which type of reasoning used should be distinguished in euthanasia debates. There are at least four different types of reasoning based on the right to die: moral reasoning (euthanasia as a moral right), legal reasoning (euthanasia as a legal right), euthanasia as a positive right and euthanasia as a negative right.

---

[15] The key declarations for the furthering of human rights development, which have been the background for euthanasia as the right to die, were The UN Declaration of Human Rights (1948), The European Convention of the Protection of Human Rights and Fundamental Freedoms (1950) and The International Covenants on Economic, Social and Cultural Rights and on Civil and Political Rights (1976).

[16] The "Patient's Bill of Rights" (which includes the right to reject medical treatment even if such refusal causes death) was adopted by the American Hospital Association in 1973. The American Society for the Right to Die (the former Euthanasia Society of America) has promoted the legalization of a living will (1974) which includes refusal of treatment (called "passive euthanasia"). The Patient Self-Determination Act (1990) has implemented the right to die (refusal of treatment) by legally requiring all health care institutions to provide patients on admission with information regarding their rights to make decisions about medical treatment (to accept it or to refuse it); this right (to die) has been confirmed by the U.S. Supreme Court (1990) based on constitutional liberty rights.

[17] In this chapter only the right to die in the context of the right to be killed (active voluntary euthanasia) is discussed. The right to die as the right of a competent patient to refuse (futile) medical treatment even if it results in death (letting die) is not covered here as the right to euthanasia. The argumentations about passively hastening death, forgoing life-sustaining treatment as they have been discussed since the Karen Ann *Quinlan* case (1975), as well as the forgoing of artificial nutrition and hydration and legalisation of physician assisted suicide have not been included. The focus is on actively hastening death by (active) euthanasia.

2.2.4 Presuppositions

The right to die presupposes that such a right exists and that this right can be exercised by a competent (autonomous) person who is terminally ill or who is suffering unbearably. The basic presumption is that in order to exercise the right, two conditions have to be met: an external and internal one. The first condition lies in the absence of any external pressure on the person exercising this right. The second condition is defined by the lucidity of the person concerned. This internal condition means that the person (patient) is fully competent with a clear intention regarding euthanasia.

The right to die derives from the idea that humans should be as free as possible and as little suppressed as possible; unnecessary restrains on human rights are in principle bad. In contemporary euthanasia debates this link between right and freedom can be found very often, although not always in an explicit way. So the "right" argument and can be transformed into a "freedom" argument (autonomy) and vice versa. It is important to emphasize that one can acknowledge the right to die without necessarily agreeing to its legal codification.

2.2.5 Analysis

Within this chapter, if the right to die has been defined as the justifiable claim of a competent, terminally ill person to avoid excruciating suffering by embracing a timely and dignified death; then euthanasia is a moral right based on ordered liberty.

There are diverse constructions how to derive the right to die (which does not exist as such in the form of a positive law) from the existing legal provisions. Some argue that the fundamental human right to life equally includes the right to die. So the right to die does not have to be created or acknowledged as a specific right. Insofar as human beings have the right to life, which is more than just a right to exist but also covers a minimum quality of life, then he/she has the right to influence the process of dying which, in difference to death, is part of life (active voluntary euthanasia) (Downing, 1970; Downing & Smoker, 1986; Wilshaw, 1974). Since dying, despite the tabooization of death and dying in our culture, is one of the most significant events in human life, one has the right to make his/her dying as good and meaningful as possible.

Another attempt to deduce the right to die is to derive it from the rights to privacy and freedom of belief. However this deduction, using a specific concept of privacy which also encompasses the right to die as the private issue (under the presupposition that death is inherently a private issue) is more debatable than the deduction of the right to die from the right to life.

Some people deduce the right to die from the worthlessness of life: on the grounds that life is not worth living one has the right to die. Opponents remind that such argument has been used for justification of eugenic euthanasia by the Nazis (*lebensunwertes Leben*). This deduction presupposes that life may be worth living in one case, being worthless in another. This results in the value of life becoming relative, depending on specific situations and changeable factors - as it was in the Nazi period.

From another background comes the utilitarian argument, justifying the abridgement of life (and the dying process as part of life) if the dying process is unpleasant and exceedingly painful. By shortening the dying process then both the unpleasantness and suffering of this process are reduced. In this way the right to shorten one's own life (dying) is established and justified. The utilitarian argument based on a reduction of unhappiness and suffering is very often used in euthanasia debates - not only to support the right to die (and the right to shorten one's own dying/life) but also in arguments based on compassion and suffering. The utilitarian argument of a reduction of suffering provides the justification for the right to die. So the right to die is not solely the right of an individual to self-determination but also a right which affects the social benefits of all persons involved (relatives, health care personnel); it also reduces their unhappiness and suffering. Despite its social utilitarianism, the right to die does not imply a physician's duty to kill the patient. As an individual right the right to die should be exercised solely by its bearer - that is to say by the person requesting euthanasia only. However the right to die (as an individual right) can be converted into a social right which empowers society to reduce unhappiness and suffering by administrating euthanasia without request.

In difference to suicide where a person is killing him/herself, claiming he/she has the right to do so (and he/she certainly has the right to do so in the sense that he/she is at the same time the bearer of such right and the one who is exercising that right), the person who claims the right to be killed as the bearer of such right is not the person who is realizing this right. From this follows that no physician can be forced to administrate euthanasia on a patient who claims the right to be killed since such a claim does not constitute a duty of the physician to realize this specific right that the patient is claiming. If the patient's right to be killed would be a standard patient's right within the reciprocity of right and duty framework (*A* has a right, *B* has a duty towards *A*), then physicians would have an objective duty to administrate euthanasia in patients who claim this right (or possibly even in patients who do not claim this right but who fulfil the criteria for realization of this right, e.g. intensive suffering, futile clinical prognosis) (Smith, 2006). The only exemption from such an objective duty of the physician would be one of conscientious objection. One should distinguish whether euthanasia as the right to die belongs to the introduced right-duty framework or not. To avoid the right-duty framework some authors suggest distinguishing between rights/liberties and privileges. As such, then the right to die would be a specific form of privilege. A privilege does not imply a duty for anyone else (Williams, 1977).

In some specific areas such as neonatal and child euthanasia, the right to die is especially problematic; as the origin, scope, justification and purpose of parental rights are unclear (Chervenak, 2006; de Vries & Verhagen, 2008; Lindemann, 2008; Moreno Villares, 2005; Schneider, 1988; Verhagen & Sauer, 2005).

2.2.6 Evaluation

The differentiation between euthanasia as a negative and positive right is crucial:

"If arguing for the legalization of euthanasia as a negative right, the practical implementation of euthanasia will depend on there being some people among those able/entitled to carry out killing on request under such a law who are willing to do so. If arguing for the legalization of euthanasia as a positive right, a legitimate request for euthanasia will result in individuals or institutions being obliged to accommodate that request. But the positive right can be graduated in terms of the authorities or persons in whom that obligation is vested. In one radical variant, it is possible to envisage all doctors being obliged to carry out euthanasia. A less restrictive variant might mean that the health services as such were obliged to arrange for euthanasia to be carried out, while leaving the individual doctor free to choose whether he or she wishes to perform euthanasia. […] A positive right of self-determination regarding euthanasia cannot be introduced without simultaneously acknowledging that, in certain cases provided for in law, society is duty-bound to take the life of a human being. A negative right of self-determination regarding euthanasia, on the other hand, can be introduced on the grounds that euthanasia, under certain circumstances provided for in law, is a matter for the judgement and conscience of the individual. The fundamental difference is that the first form of legalization, more so than the second, turns euthanasia into a communal, general matter, which must be acknowledged by society as a whole as being worthy of aspiring to ethically." (The Danish Council of Ethics, 2006).

Some authors reject the right to die argument on the grounds of benefit and harm (Velleman, 1999). The common religious counter-argument states that the right to decide when and how to die belongs to God. (Gill, 1998; Larson & Amundsen, 1998; Manning, 1998). The common secular counter-argument is doubly based on obligation. First the right to die does not imply a legal obligation of another person to conduct euthanasia. Secondly our rights are limited by our obligations. One may have a right to die however one has also obligations to other people such as our partners, family, friends, healthcare professionals (Finkel et al., 1993). The enactment of the right to die (euthanasia) would affect other people so we must consider the consequences such an exercising of the right to die would have on them (grief, sorrow, guilt, anger). The enactment of the right to die could affect the professional integrity of the physician who would conduct euthanasia. All these consequences have to be measured against our right to die and the individual rights have to be balanced against the good/consequences of the community and society in general. (Sullivan, 2005). Regardless of the fact that these consequences might seem to be practical (the dying process of a person suffering extremely has been made easier), one of the negative consequences is the risk of vulnerable persons' integrity being undermined, whereby the principal argument is switched from one of autonomy and right (voluntary euthanasia) to compassion (possible involuntary euthanasia).

The limitations of the right to die are provided not only by the obligations to society but also by the rights and duties of other persons who are requested to provide euthanasia. There is not an evident moral right to kill a person even upon his/her explicit request. Likewise there is not an objective moral duty to conduct euthanasia upon explicit request. It is obvious that a legal obligation to administrate euthanasia does not exist; the establishment of such a legal obligation would require a substantial transformation of our democratic society, based on fundamental rights and liberties.

2.2.7 Conclusion

The right to die is one of the main arguments for euthanasia. It is closely related to autonomy and to the principle of respect for autonomy. So in some discussions both arguments (right to die and respect for autonomy) are intertwined into the right to autonomy. However, there is no unanimous consent that the right to die exists (that it can be derived from other rights such as from the right to life), and the right to die argument can also be used as an objection to euthanasia, in that this right does not exist. Despite its moral or legal appeal it serves poorly as a medium for debate as common argumentative precepts are difficult to establish.

2.3 Unbearable suffering

2.3.1 Introduction

Unbearable suffering is one of the criteria required by Dutch and Belgian legislation on euthanasia. One would assume that the right to die argument is not a sufficient legal requirement for the decriminalization of euthanasia since there is no broad consent that such right exists or that it can be derived from other rights in a very convincing way. Similarly the autonomy argument alone is not strong enough an argument to justify legal euthanasia. No doubt every competent person has his/her autonomy, however to justify autonomous choice in the case of euthanasia would require some additional conditions. Otherwise any competent person would be able to request euthanasia - regardless of the circumstances they find themselves in - as a legitimate tool to terminate his/her life. The only validator would be a reference to his/her autonomy. So when legislators were specifying some additional conditions under which the autonomous choice could be decriminalized there was the evocative condition "unbearable suffering", which made sense, as all else being equal, no person in their right mind would prefer to die in a painful way or with immense suffering. So among the circumstances that could lead one to choose death for him/her self and/or for a loved one, unbearable suffering occupies the prime position. The expression "unbearable suffering" clearly states that not every painful process within health care entitles one to ask for euthanasia but only great ongoing pain and suffering which trespass one's faculty to tolerate it can be a legitimate reason to request euthanasia. Proponents of euthanasia defend the decriminalization of killing on request in well defined situations as a kind of last resort and under serious conditions.

It comes as no surprise that both proponents and opponents of euthanasia agree that the prevention and alleviation of people's suffering has been one of the noble goals of medicine from ancient times and that compassion is a valued emotion in general and in health care in particular. However, they heartily disagree about the extent to which the means can be justified by the end (alleviation of pain and suffering). (The Danish Council of Ethics, 2006). While proponents argue that the alleviation of terrible suffering in desperate situations justifies killing a person on her request, opponents do not tolerate alleviation of suffering by removal of its cause (a suffering human being), arguing that pain and suffering have to be controlled medically (pain killers, terminal sedation), but not by killing.

2.3.2 Description

The suffering argument can be briefly described in the following way: Once a person is suffering to an extent which is beyond her will and capacity to tolerate such a degree of pain and suffering, having become "unbearable", than he/she should not have to bear it. Moreover, all medical attempts to relieve this unbearable suffering have been unsuccessful and unsatisfactory to this person. Then the basic rule about impossibilities which do not establish moral commitment would apply: *ad impossibilis nemo tenetur* (no one is obliged to do what is not possible). Thus, as a last option, it is morally right to help this person not to suffer unbearably and on compassionate grounds to terminate her suffering and life.

2.3.3 Contextualization

With regard to suffering, it is a paradox of contemporary medicine that thanks to powerful technological advances the lives of many people have been saved but an additional suffering of many other people is being produced and prolonged. Despite the fundamental physicians' obligation to relieve suffering, little attention is explicitly given to the issue of suffering in medical practice; it is not unusual for suffering to occur not only as an implication of disease but as a result of its treatment. (Cassell, 2004).

Suffering is usually associated with pain. However suffering is not identical to pain. Pain, being caused physically (e.g. by injury or metastatic cancer), can be onerously assessed: one cannot see pain, but feel its manifestation. As clinical findings demonstrate, the amount of pain a person reports is not directly related to the degree of disease. There are important psychological factors which help to explain why people perceive, report and give meaning to pain in different ways. Pain, perceived as hurt, is a highly subjective experience, affected by mood, morale and other conditioners. (Skevington, 2002). In spite of the fact that the current pain therapy can provide continuous pain relief up to the very end of life in more than 90% of cases, these new therapeutic tools are not yet widely known and practiced by physicians. In addition, suffering is much more difficult to treat than physical pain. Severe pain can lead to suffering which cannot be easily controlled. Paradoxically a patient whose pain is managed well may still suffer. The suffering, as an individual sensation of discomfort and malaise, may continue for a very long period of time without any specific correlation to the physical pain. Heavy suffering can violate one's integrity as a person; the self may become unravelled, fragmented, and disintegrated by massive suffering (Ben Mitchell, 2010). There are feelings such as hopelessness, loneliness, alienation, pointlessness or unworthiness which may occur even if pain is being relieved properly, making suffering intolerable and unbearable.

While pain is more related to a physical condition, suffering can be caused by both physical and non-physical factors. There is no consonant approach to pain and suffering. While some authors sharply distinguish suffering from physically caused pain, other authors regard physically caused pain as one of the many forms of suffering. Some people believe that suffering is person-centric (Cassell, 2004a). That suffering, dissimilar to the physical symptoms, is a personal phenomenon which cannot be accessed by a third-person view; suffering as the personal (subjective) phenomenon cannot be objectified. Other people believe that suffering has different forms which, in addition, can be objectively described. Since there is no consensus about the nature of suffering, diverse hermeneutics of suffering would have diverse consequences in an assessment of suffering.

Within the biological model, suffering can result from disease; where pain is the source of the suffering. Suffering can also arise from the impact disease is having on the person's life. This type of the suffering will depend on the attitudes and objectives of the suffering person - to what extent the person is able to modify attitudes and to adjust objectives to the new situation. Finally suffering can also be found on the existential level; some people reduce the existential level to spirituality (Peck, 1997), however it should be noted that not only religious persons have their existential needs- more precisely "non-believers" can have existential questions as well and do not call them "spirituality".

It is important in arguments based on suffering to distinguish between physical, psychological, social and existential (which includes spiritual) suffering. With regard to unbearable suffering it is important to distinguish if suffering is understood as a personal phenomenon (that only the person concerned is able to determine the level of "unbearable suffering") or as an objective phenomenon (then "unbearable suffering" can be assessed by external criteria and by other persons). It is important to define "unbearable suffering". Dutch law states as a criterion merely "unbearable suffering", while Belgian law holds it to be "unbearable physical or mental suffering". Besides suffering, similar specifications of other conditions related to suffering but distinct, such as being in a terminal stage of disease are relevant to warranting euthanasia.

2.3.4 Presuppositions

The basic presupposition of the suffering argument can be found in the following axiom: unbearable suffering founds the (moral) right to ask for euthanasia. Justification of such a right can be found for instance in the European Charter of Fundamental Rights (2000), where Article 4 states that no one shall be subjected to torture or to inhuman or degrading treatment or punishment. It could be argued that to subject a terminally ill person to medical treatment which produces horrible suffering goes against the aforementioned article. The suffering argument usually assumes that unbearable suffering is the only condition required for euthanasia. So unbearable suffering is simultaneously a sufficient condition for euthanasia.[18] The person intolerably suffering induces compassion in the other person who then kills out of mercy.

2.3.5 Analysis

Suffering can be considered both an objective and subjective phenomenon. However the unbearableness of suffering is rather a personal phenomenon and therefore a subjective criterion. Once the suffering has become "unbearable" for an individual then this suffering is intolerable, insupportable and insufferable and only the suffering person can know at what point or when this state has been realised. No one acting as an external (and "objective") observer can assign the unbearably suffering person to tolerate such suffering. If we would regard the unbearableness of suffering as an objective criterion then this threshold could only be determined after a palliative care trial or after a committee or inquiry, after which some group would have authority to say "You are entitled to die" or "You are not allowed to die", which would be in contradiction both to autonomy and the right to die arguments. It seems that the praxis in the Netherlands tends to assume that the unbearableness of suffering is a subjective criterion which is validated by a longstanding declared wish to die rather than by some exact empirical tools. Furthermore it remains unclear if for instance the mental torment as documented in the Dr. Chabot case is included in unbearable suffering (Sheldon, 1994) or if suffering would also cover situations like "tired of life" which can be existential and very afflictive but not necessary qualifying as grounds for a euthanasia request (Sheldon, 2003). Surely it is easier to medically measure pain than suffering. The level of both pain and suffering can be measured - albeit such assessment is problematic if pain is not reduced to the physical entity and if suffering is taken in its complexity - while it can be taken for granted that "unbearable" suffering can be assessed by the individual concerned solely. Even two accounts of very heavy and awful suffering, which according to an external evaluation would be graded as almost the same could be perceived as "unbearable" for one person and as "bearable" by another person.

Proponents of euthanasia argue that unbearable suffering is more that sufficient reason to request euthanasia. Their other supportive arguments are compassion, respect for human dignity, the patient's best interest, quality of life, autonomy and the right to die.

Opponents of euthanasia refuse the suffering argument as such, saying that suffering, even "unbearable ", is not sufficient grounds for killing a person. Their counter-objections mostly refer to compassion in the sense of psychological support, efficacious relieve of suffering,

[18] "Suffering as a criterion for access to euthanasia is based on an approach that is taken for granted and regarded as self-evident" (The Danish Council of Ethics, 2006).

good palliative care and human proximity; to care in the sense of avoiding alienation, shame, helplessness, emotional and social burdens and dealing with needs, such as worthiness and being treated as a person- not as a non-person or as a no person anymore.
Some authors argue that the desire for euthanasia cannot be interpreted at face value. The meaning of the desire for euthanasia is not related to the reality of physical disintegration or physical and psychological suffering from the effects of disease such as cancer, but includes anxiety, fears, existential concerns and desires for respect, care, and connectedness interpreted within the context of the patients' whole lived experience. (Mak & Elvyn, 2005).
For some adherents of euthanasia, unbearable suffering is a necessary but not the sufficient condition for a patient's eligibility to request euthanasia. They argue that unbearable suffering is the minimal requirement and some objective criteria of the patient's conditions must have been met before the desire to die can be fulfilled. Such additional and more objective criteria, such as being in the terminal stage of an illness, can be medically assessed more exactly than the subjective evaluation of unbearable suffering.
Opponents of euthanasia point out the ambiguity of pain and suffering: "If the pain and suffering are by definition unbearable, then it seems clear enough that the decision to die is not freely chosen but is compelled by the pain. [...] Under the conditions of unbearable pain and suffering, then, if the concern of the agent is to alleviate the pain it seems to be a mistake to speak of voluntary choices. The natural conclusion to draw from this is that there can be no such thing as voluntary euthanasia, or, at the very least, that we have no means to ensure that the patient's request to die was not compelled." (Campbell, 1999, p. 243). Thus in situations where the decision to terminate one's own life is made while experiencing unbearable suffering, the possibility that such a choice was not made freely has to be taken seriously. Opponents also argue that effective pain control can alleviate the suffering. The counter-objection is focused on the fact that not all pain is manageable in terminally ill patients, stressing the difference between pain and suffering. Suffering is inevitably a solitary condition and always involves self-conflict, since, among others, the meaning is essential to suffering. (Cassell, 2004a). In addition, in cases where the disease is progressing and state of health worsening, even the best pain therapy can prove to be unsatisfactory, leaving the person suffering to an intensity that the other person, imagining such suffering, neither has suffered nor could possibly imagine suffering.
Proponents argue that it is more in accordance with human dignity to relieve suffering by termination of life then to incapacitate the patient with high doses of drugs (analgesics and sedatives) and to keep the patient in a state of unconsciousness so that he/she does not have to consciously suffer (palliative sedation, terminal sedation). Then if there is an option between existence with suffering and unconsciousness without suffering, it is more appropriate to choose death instead of continuing such an unconscious existence (or choose life alternating between suffering and sleep). They conclude that such a way of living (caused by medical intervention) is pointless, harmful and inhuman and such "medical suffering" should be avoided.
Some people, with reference to the fact that the full autonomy of a person requesting euthanasia may be doubtful, propose the use of a similar framework as the ones we use in other areas of end-of-life decision making, such as the withholding or withdrawing life support treatment for incompetent patients, in particular in the context where there is doubt as to the genuine autonomous choice of the terminally ill patient. This would involve a cascading process of assessment. Then the first condition would be a clear wish to die expressed in a qualified and authentic way repeatedly. The next condition would be the

assessment of the patient's unbearable suffering as a reason for choosing death. Then the external social controls would apply (medical evaluation done by the therapeutic team, proxy evaluation). When all relevant facts and circumstances are weighted and assessed and all persons involved agree then choosing death at a chosen time is better option than continuing unbearable suffering.

2.3.6 Evaluation

Suffering is an ambiguous phenomenon in our contemporary world. On the one hand there is a strong tendency not only to avoid suffering but also to negate it as such since suffering does not fit into the picture of a young, healthy, wealthy and successful person. In current Western culture, pain and suffering as symptoms of disease and illness, are perceived as contrary to a healthy life, corporeal performance and the cult of youth. On the other hand suffering is glorified by some popular (and in fact unorthodox) versions of Christianity which can be characterized as "dolorous Christianity" (Christ has suffered, therefore you have to suffer; the more you suffer the more you are loved by God). Suffering, denied or glorified, overlooks the positive aspects of suffering as part of our personal development. However it is neither easy nor appropriate to say to the person suffering unbearably, who does not see any sense of such terrible suffering and of her destroyed life, that suffering has its place in the process of personal development. Whatever the case, a lack and/or superficiality of analysis from the patient's perspective should temper calls to make euthanasia legal (Mak & Elvyn, 2005).

The argument "unbearable suffering" should not be taken in its "simplified version": they suffer unbearably, therefore let us legalize euthanasia. There are many hidden existential concerns of the terminally ill and horribly suffering patient's that should be addressed and discussed. And the patient's personal perspective has to be taken more into account.

Some authors are hesitant to address suffering as a determiner for eligibility to euthanasia as they criticize the medical world's objectification of patients. They believe our dominant biomedical model should be modified, improved and re-oriented to the patient's personhood (Mak & Elvyn, 2005). It is not only the patient's mental competency that is at the stake but also a new professional moral competency of health care personnel; such professional competency, not entirely fitting into the biomedical model, would ensure appropriate existential care, exploring the covert meaning of "a good death" and dealing with the authentic desires of patients rather than mechanically applying arguments of autonomy or suffering. As many studies demonstrate, the desire to die (due to unbearable suffering or due to personal preference not to have to go through the final, painful, hopeless and possibly meaningless passage of own life), in many situations, is not so much a request for death as a request for help (Lesley, 2006).

With regard to the medical practice of euthanasia in the Netherlands, "the ethical justification has been shifting from *respect for autonomy* to *relief of suffering*. But this has created a tension within the justificatory strategies regarding euthanasia. The two arguments are mutually exclusive. It only makes sense to talk about respect for autonomy if a physician *refrains* from making judgements about the patient's benefits." (ten Have, 2001, p. 477).

Another question which has to be clarified is about "suffering" and "unbearable suffering" as the only criterion for euthanasia (the autonomy argument is very problematic in a situation of terrible suffering). There are two approaches to this question: either unbearable suffering as a purely subjective phenomenon is understood in a broad sense, as any physical, psychological, social or existential suffering, and, once claimed as "unbearable" (and only the patient can decide whether his/her suffering has become unbearable) becomes the necessary and sufficient grounds for euthanasia (and any patient including psychiatric ones would have the right to euthanasia on the grounds of "unbearable suffering") or "unbearable suffering" is a necessary but not self-standing condition and some additional criteria such as terminal stage illness or consent of all persons concerned would need to apply.

2.3.7 Conclusion

The unbearable suffering argument is based on the patient's perspective and perception. Many feel that only the patient can assess his/her intolerable suffering. Unbearable suffering is in line with the right to die and with (one of the interpretations of) human dignity to ask for euthanasia in such a humanly devastating situation assessed as unbearable suffering. Regardless of whether one is able to determine where the suffering threshold is, and if that is therefore grounds for euthanasia, the issue of whether it serves as the sole ground for such also serves to divide opinion.

2.4 Compassion

2.4.1 Introduction

While the suffering argument stems from the patient's perspective, the compassion argument comes from the other person's perspective. Compassion is a kind of external response to that devastating suffering. One feels morally obliged to help, to relieve such suffering and to save the intolerably suffering person (Begley, 2008).

2.4.2 Description

The compassion argument is usually used in euthanasia debates as "mercy killing". Under the presupposition that no person should be obliged to endure interminable suffering perceived as pointless, and supposed that the intolerable suffering cannot be relieved by medical tools and the only way to avoid such suffering is by death of the patient, then such a death may be brought about as an act of mercy. (Battin, 2003). From this perspective, euthanasia is not to be applied based on an evaluation of the suffering by a second or third person (in order to determinate if the suffering is unbearable) but about the response of the health care professionals and family members, who draw attention to the suffering person and to the distress and misery of such a situation. As an act of humanity and showing mercy they terminate the life of the suffering person. The counter-argument is based on false interpretation of compassion and mercy: killing is not compassion. To show compassion in such a situation would mean to take care of the suffering person, but not to kill him/her (Schotsmans & Gastmans, 2009).

2.4.3 Contextualization

In animals it would be regarded as inhuman to allow a dog or horse to suffer not just a terminal illness but also conditions such as a broken leg in the wild. As such, one could use animal euthanasia as an argument, making it an *a fortiori* argument: if we euthanize animals on the grounds of compassion, all the more so we have to act with compassion towards suffering humans by providing a merciful death. As such, euthanasia is an expression of humanity.

2.4.4 Presuppositions

The compassion argument comes from the general belief that the desire to relieve suffering and feeling compassion are highly regarded human values which also include volitional elements. Compassion by definition motivates one to action. Another presupposition is based on the old medical tradition of beneficence. At present the utilitarian arguments similarly presume beneficence as the justification for euthanasia (Kohl, 1975; Rosenblatt, 1992). Compassion can also be a condition for legal assisted dying (Kay, 2006).

2.4.5 Analysis

Under the condition that there exist no effective means to relieve (unbearable) suffering, euthanasia may be justified as the only remaining option available, or even required by the principle of beneficence. The commitment to act with regard to the benefit of the patient is still one of the most relevant principles in medical ethics. Thus on such grounds of beneficence physicians would have to ensure that a peaceful and painless death is offered to patients who are suffering while dying in a horrible way. On such grounds physicians may be even obliged to administrate euthanasia due to the virtue of compassion, which seeks beneficence rather than to observe impassively and inactively as a patient dies in a horrible way with his/her painful death prolonged (Van Zyl, 2000). Such an "omission" could be qualified as contrary to basic human values such as sympathy and mercifulness.

The beneficence argument can be reinforced by utilitarianism. The killing of a patient may be contrary to the sanctity of life doctrine but as such is morally good because the consequence of such an action is good: suffering has been eliminated and the death has been achieved in a desirable way (painless and peaceful). Naturally this moral assessment of an action in accordance with its good or bad consequences can be applied not solely to physical pain and suffering but also to mental suffering such as feelings of unworthiness, loss of self-control and self-sufficiency or complete dependence on others for their assistance in daily activities starting with hygiene and food. Utilitarians argue "that frustration of being unable to perform everyday tasks for oneself, and the erosion of dignity as personal and previously private tasks have to be performed by someone else as one reverts to behaviour not experienced since infancy." (Draper, 1998, p. 184). The utilitarian argument of beneficence will be potentiated in situations where no alternative exists to the miserable death the patient is experiencing, when the suffering is ceaseless and increasing by its protraction and death is imminent. Then compassion would override that little of (very miserable) life which is lost by the act of euthanasia. The utilitarian argument of beneficence caused by compassion is an external criterion for euthanasia: the autonomous patient is not making the decision to die but another person, on grounds of sym-pathy (etymologically to suffer with), decides about the death of the suffering patient. By this argument euthanasia of incompetent patients (both of adults and children) can be justified. The common utilitarian argument would not usually justify involuntary euthanasia of a competent person. Once liberty is granted as one of the basic values, then the autonomy of individuals has to be respected. However, once the patient is no longer able to express his/her autonomy and freedom, his/her way of dying can be determined by feelings of compassion. It is very valuable if a person, moved by compassion, is seeking to act and to defeat suffering and if the sense of compassion is not limited to feeling alone. (Ramsey, 1997).

A specific target of the relief of suffering is that of terminal suffering. It could be argued that since virtually all pain can be treated pharmaceutically, compassion is not an applicable issue. However, 'virtually all' pain is not 'all'. Thus some pain and suffering remain to be treated though it cannot be treated medically and the usage of terminal sedation is justified. However terminal sedation as complete sedation is complete obtundation as well (the patient can no longer perceive and communicate) being almost the same as causing death, thus making their use questionable. Some people argue that pain and suffering as part of the dying process can be a valuable, positive and transformative experience leading to personal and spiritual growth. Nevertheless it should be said that there is no guarantee of such a positive, valuable and transformative experience. (Battin, 2003). Moreover experience of such terminal suffering is far more likely to become a very negative, horrifying experience.

2.4.6 Evaluation

Once compassion is taken as the competence which decides for the good of the patient, then the competence of the patient concerned doesn't necessarily have to be taken into account, thus compassion becomes the normative upon which decisions are made and for the incompetent patient, even in some cases for the competent one, more for the other person's self-esteem and peace of mind than for the good of the suffering patient, who did not express his/her wish to be terminated. Here the compassion argument is attacked by the slippery slope argument: from autonomous euthanasia to non-autonomous mercy killing. "The ethical acceptability of one person taking the life of another at the latter's request and based on a feeling of compassion will depend, as a minimum, on the situation involved being one of extraordinary suffering and agony that cannot be relieved" (The Danish Council of Ethics, 2006).

The ethical evaluation of compassion directly depends on the understanding of the moral significance of compassion. If compassion is ranked as a primary human virtue then the compassion argument plays a different role in the euthanasia debate than when compassion, with a focus on its unsteady and non-rational nature, is ranked as a secondary moral faculty.

2.4.7 Conclusion

The compassion argument is surrounded by many emotions which place it between compassion as the response to unbearable suffering (only the suffering person can say what suffering is not bearable) and mercy killing based not on the patient's perspective and request but on the feelings of mercy of the person who is providing a "good death"; the "good death" being interpreted exclusively by that other person.

2.5 Human dignity

2.5.1 Introduction

Human dignity[19] is an argument commonly used by both proponents and opponents in euthanasia debates. Its proponents use human dignity and the possible harm to dignity as an argument for euthanasia, mainly as a secondary argument next to the suffering and compassion arguments as the primary ones. For some people euthanasia coincides with human dignity in the sense that the administration of euthanasia is an expression of the respect for human dignity. (Humphry, 1992; Biggs, 2001). Consequently the law which

---

[19] For the meaning and history of dignity see Meyer, 1995.

specifies provisions for physician assisted suicide in the state Oregon is called the "Death with Dignity Act". Opponents argue that human dignity is contrary to euthanasia because it undermines human dignity, especially of elderly, disabled and dying persons. Obviously there is a diverse interpretation of human dignity beyond these controversies.

2.5.2 Description

The human dignity argument in euthanasia debates can be articulated in two simple but contradictory theses:

a. Euthanasia is in line with human dignity.
b. Euthanasia is a violation of human dignity.

The first thesis supposes that human dignity has to be protected and harm to dignity should be avoided. Since the enormous suffering of a dying person would wound the dignity of that person, it is justified to protect human dignity by the act of euthanasia - either on grounds of autonomy and right to die (voluntary euthanasia) or on grounds of compassion (non-voluntary/involuntary euthanasia).

The second thesis is similarly based on the preservation of human dignity, using a contrary argument: euthanasia is contrary to human dignity; euthanasia cannot be performed because not only the dignity of the person requesting euthanasia would be violated but also the dignity of the person who performs euthanasia (regardless of whether it was requested or not).

2.5.3 Contextualization

Human dignity is usually given as the philosophico-anthropological essence of human rights (Schachter, 1983). Thus one of the goals of human rights is to protect human dignity (respect for the inherent dignity of the human person). Consequently the right to die is not only a positive or negative right of self-determination but also a tool by which human dignity is protected. (Swarup, 2009; Cohen-Almagor, 2001). Once a person reaches the conclusion that his/her dignity would be affected by great (or unbearable) suffering and inhumane dying then the person has to take steps to protect his/her human dignity. There are plenty of historical examples of such scenarios starting with Stoa (*autothanatos*), when the person suffering in an indignant way was obliged to avoid or to end such a devaluing and dehumanizing situation by suicide.

This becomes contextualized in the form of medical futility, whereby clinical situations arise in the form of reduced therapy such as withdrawing and withholding life-sustaining treatment or termination of artificial hydration and nutrition and the relevant decision-making processes. It creates a paradigm of medically futile treatment which technically can be administrated and continued but also, from the patient perspective, such reduced treatment is justified by the respect for human dignity: it would be against human dignity (and against the patient's best interest) to produce suffering and to prolong dying if there is no other perspective than the imminent death of the patient. Since there are areas within medical practice that are already governed by measures for the protection of human dignity (e.g. advance directives) (Cantor, 1993), this protection has to be extended to other areas of end-of-life decisions such as voluntary euthanasia (Hillyard& Dombrink, 2001).

2.5.4 Presuppositions

There are two completely different philosophical presuppositions in euthanasia debates about human dignity which are very rarely revealed and addressed. One presupposition assumes that human dignity is by its nature a changeable faculty which can be developed during the life of human being. Thus human dignity is an empirical entity which can be assessed and measured by external criteria such as level of consciousness. So while for some people human dignity is given by birth (or even before); the newborn child already has its human dignity, other people assume that human dignity has to be acquired in the course of a lifetime (after birth), when the person has developed abilities of perception, awareness, self-interest etc. As an example of this philosophical assumption Peter Singer and his approach can be given. Within this understanding, human dignity is something what we gradually acquire, develop and lose. Thus the human dignity of a terminally ill or terribly suffering person who is devastated by his/her biological and physiological condition is "on retreat" because the person is in the process of loosing his/her dignity or may have lost it to a various extent.

A different presupposition is grounded in the metaphysics of the person, which understands human dignity as a constant entity which human beings possess continuously: to be human means to have human dignity. So dignity does not belong to some aspect of a person but to the person as such, being that which is essential to the person (Ramsey, 1997). In this sense dignity is not what one has (diverse faculties and capacities) but what one *is*. Human dignity as a whole can be harmed (for instance by killing) but not taken away or lost. Thus both newborn child and dying person have the same human dignity which cannot be diminished or augmented.

2.5.5 Analysis

There is no doubt that as human beings are mortal, everybody wishes for a "death with dignity". However there are huge controversies about the meaning of dignity and its implication for dying. So for one group, "death with dignity" means legal reform which accommodates active voluntary euthanasia as an appropriate response to a perceived need for the option called "death with dignity" (Paust, 1995). While for the other group, "death with dignity" amalgamates with palliative care, hospice and spiritual care which have to replace the request for euthanasia; death with dignity seems a mutation of the original concept of human dignity and therefore euthanasia being indignant.

For the first group "being dignified is having a sense of the importance of one's life or achievements and appearing and behaving, before oneself and others, in the light of these. To lack this sense of importance or to fail to (or be unable to) present oneself in accordance with it is undignified. This lack of dignity is properly a humiliating thing for the subject, and connected to lack or loss of self-esteem, or even of the sense of self-worth." (Ramsey, 1997, p. 48). Then to live such a diminished life or to suffer such diminishment or impoverishment is sufficient to conclude that such life ought to be ended (Quill, 1993; Ramsey, 1997). Thus personal dignity is part of personal liberty which includes the ability to choose to die more or less quickly; dignity and self-determination are virtually interchangeable. It is matter of personal dignity to decide the time and way of one's death. As a supportive argument, quality of life is used: if the person decides that the quality of his/her life is too low and not acceptable to him/her then he/she has the right to choose death while one's dignity is still (relatively) intact. Some argue that dignity, being complex and unique to each person, includes not only physical and physiological aspects, but also emotional, intellectual, spiritual and existential ones (Quill, 1993).

For the second group, dignity belongs to human nature: we posses it in the mode which is not limited and therefore dignity cannot be denied or damaged. They argue that the (rational) nature of humankind cannot be attacked as such, only some aspect can be hidden: an incurable disease affects one's life but not one's nature. Dignity to them consists of the intrinsic worth of human nature (Ramsey, 1997). So despite pain and heavy suffering, there is dignity in such a case; human dignity cannot be undermined. It is obvious that such a hermeneutic of dignity is based on certain metaphysical presumptions which can be taken as granted or refused as false.
From a clinical point of view, contemporary medicine can impose medical technology on a dying person to the extent to which it can be seen as incompatible with and contradictory to human dignity. This has been recently described by an Iranian neurosurgeon in the following way: "Rob a human being of his dignity and you have robbed him of the essence of being human. Confine him, immobilize him, make him dependant, deprive him of hope and then inflict pain upon him and you have all the ingredients of the highest form of torture." (Nayernouri, 2011, p. 55)

2.5.6 Evaluation

On one hand a patient's choices, limited by existing legal constrains which do not allow a physician to comply with the patient's request for euthanasia as a deliberately hastened death, result in a violation and/or loss of dignity. On the other hand a patient's choices in many countries are limited by insufficient palliative care; this results in a violation of human dignity because persons have to die in indignant conditions.

2.5.7 Conclusion

Any conclusion regarding human dignity depends on the meaning given to the term "human dignity".

2.6 Patient's best interest

The argument of the patient's best interest is related to the argument of dignity. In the later case it was human dignity which demanded a dignified death; in some situations the respect for human dignity could justify termination of the life of a person suffering in a way which violates human dignity (when understood as a changeable feature of human beings). Here it is on the grounds of the patient's best interest that euthanasia is justified. It is either the patient self who is interpreting his/her best interest or another person (physician, nurse, relative) who is assessing the patient's best interest and who acts in the patient's best interest. Some people think that euthanasia does not go against the goals of medicine, considering it to be possibly in the patient's best overall interest. Some authors relate *euthanasia* to *eudaimonia* (living well, flourishing) of the Aristotelian tradition, arguing that in virtue ethics, euthanasia can be regarded as a continuation of *eudaimonia* insofar as euthanasia facilitates good dying (dying is a part of life), avoiding bad dying which would be frustrating and not a vibrant way to finish life. (Begley, 2008). Therefore medical and other health care professionals have to balance their own *integrity* with professional concerns and patients' interests. In this way they will recognize good and be able to realize it. Finally, helping another will lead, from a teleological perspective, to human flourishing. (Begley, 2008). So if euthanasia is understood as the upholding of a patient's best interest, then it is a catalyst to human flourishing.

The counter-argument points out that if a patient's best interest is interpreted by another person such as a health care professional, then such an interpretation will be paternalistic. Another objection does not deny the legitimacy of the patient's best interest, however in scenarios involving killing, it is not given precedence.

2.7 Quality of life

The quality of life argument is related to the patient's best interest argument in the way that it is the patient's best interest to live a life which has certain qualitative features, which are valuable and worthwhile. Quality of life is therefore an indicator as to how these qualitative features can be assessed by the patient. In contrast to the patient's best interest, quality of life is purely subjective and can be measured by the patient only. There is an affinity with the suffering argument: once suffering becomes unbearable, quality of life is very low, possibly so low that the patient does not want to live a life of such poor quality, giving euthanasia a role and upon the patient's evaluation of his/her life, a good death can be administrated.

Insofar as death is a part of life, quality of life can be referred to the quality of dying. As there has been an enormous emphasis on the quality of life in all areas of medicine in the last decades, the same impetus should be given to death and dying. (Hoffmann, 2009; Nordenfelt, 1994; Walter & Shannon, 1990). Quality of life can become a secondary argument of autonomy (as the primary argument): Once the quality of life or dying is too low and no longer acceptable or intolerable, the patient can express his/her autonomy by requesting euthanasia.

The counter-argument to the quality of life argument is based on a critique of the concept of quality of life in health care. This critique emphasizes life as a gift which is valuable as such and which should not be measured by subjective criteria of quality. In a comparable way as the dignity of life cannot be measured, the value of life cannot be assessed. Although quality of life is very important both individually and for society as a whole, quality of life in itself cannot be the reason to terminate those suffering low quality of life or life which is not deemed worthy of being lived. And this line of counter-argument could continue with references to the Nazi period (the killing of people with low quality of life and with unworthy life).

2.8 Health care costs

It is a trivial statement that health care resources are limited. Since some treatments (e.g. intensive care or in oncology) are very expensive, they should be used with good justification in order to prevent that health care resources are not used in an unfair and irresponsible way but in the ways in which the criteria of social justice are satisfied.

From an economic standpoint, one package of morphine costs a few Euros while one day in an Intensive Care Unit can cost thousands of Euros. On top of that if the treatment is futile anyway and the patient's prospect is one mainly of pain, suffering and dying then not only principles such as autonomy or dignity apply but also principles like justice, solidarity (which would not justify futile treatment) and health care costs as distribution of limited resources criteria have to be taken into account.

There are various scenarios for the economical calculation in this context; from very liberal ones to those based more on social coherence and social solidarity (which has its limits as well). Then euthanasia could become a smooth solution for generally expensive health care and for health care systems suffering from financial deficiency. It should be mentioned that palliative care is much less expensive than many medically aggressive, technically advanced and economically costly treatments.

The counter-argument is based on the impropriety of a financial argument in the context of dying patients. The counter-objection stresses the fact of limited resources for health care and the validity of health care cost calculations. The middle-ground position argues that care for terminally ill and dying patient certainly cannot be limited to economic calculations however health care costs do have to be considered.

2.9 Regulation - legalization

The basic form of the regulation argument concerns the legalization of euthanasia. Proponents argue, while referring to autonomy, right to die, compassion and dignity, that euthanasia should be a legal right for everyone; the criminalization of euthanasia is contrary to the many arguments for which euthanasia should be decriminalized. The fear of decriminalization of euthanasia has the consequence that euthanasia will be practised "in the shadows", beyond any social control. The legalization argument is more policy oriented, focusing more on social and legislative strategies than on morality as such.

Opponents argue that the right to die cannot be legally acknowledged since such a right does not exist, moreover such a legal provision would violate human rights, in particular the right to life. Even opponents who would otherwise condone legal voluntary euthanasia under certain conditions argue that once legalized, euthanasia would be abused. Referring to the Dutch practice where not all performed cases of euthanasia have been reported, they argue that there is a slippery slope from active voluntary euthanasia to involuntary euthanasia which, again, can be proven empirically. (Keown, 1995, 2002).

A pragmatic view on regulation appreciates a legal provision on euthanasia under the argument "regulation is better as no regulation at all". Once regulated, obligatory rules have been established and they provide an enforceable framework. The alternative scenario of no regulation is much worse because euthanasia will be performed anyway but in the chaotic and confused setting of a grey zone.

Those who hold euthanasia as wrong in principle argue that an immoral practice cannot be transformed into a moral one by legalization: immorality cannot be legalized.

2.10 Transparency

The transparency argument is associated with the regulation argument. As is generally known, euthanasia is being practiced in many countries in which it is illegal. So the transparency argument states as follows: let us be transparent, let us continue doing what we are doing anyway in the open and honest way, let us terminate hypocrisy (criticising euthanasia in Benelux, not being able to address the issue in our home countries, behaving as if euthanasia is not presently being practised in our cities).

The argument to the contrary holds that if euthanasia is completely wrong, then transparency only serves to corrupt existing morality. A similar objection as above would apply.

3. Conclusion

In the analysis of this chapter, it became clear that for any argumentation on euthanasia, regardless of whether for or against, the first crucial step is clarity in terminology: what exactly do we mean by the term "euthanasia". So to avoid confusion, misunderstanding and frustration, it is crucial to start with clear semantics. Within this analytical study, euthanasia, having been distinguished from assisted suicide and from other instances of the end-of-life decisions such as withholding, withdrawing or terminal sedation, was defined as a deliberate act of termination of the life of *B* by *A* upon an explicit request of *B* for the sake of *B*. This means that the term euthanasia is understood to be so-called active voluntary euthanasia. Moreover, for a precise definition, some additional criteria apply such as terminal stage of the illness, unbearable suffering, enduring and voluntary wish to die (expressed repeatedly), and the act of euthanasia being performed by a physician.

In the discussions on euthanasia various numbers of arguments are listed. Similarly different types of argumentations can be identified which use different or the same arguments taken from different fields and contexts; so one and the same argument is used within diverse argumentations. In summary, philosophical, legal, religious and social types of argumentations on euthanasia should be distinguished. So if, for instance, an argument is made on the basis of a "right", while one argumentation uses the argument of "right" in the legal sense (e.g. human rights), another uses the argument of "right" in the sense of moral right (moral claim, not based on specific legislation). The next one uses the argument of "right" in a theological way (God's right over life) or in a psychological way (one's right to an authentic expression of his/her self).

It became evident that there are no unequivocal arguments for or against euthanasia. Any list of arguments *for* euthanasia is, to a large extent, at the same time also a list of the arguments *against* euthanasia in the sense that another list of objections to these *pro* arguments has to be considered. Some of the *pro* arguments are simultaneously *contra* arguments and vice versa (e.g. dignity). Despite this fact, some arguments are prevalently arguments *pro* (e.g. autonomy) while the other ones are arguments *against* (e.g. slippery slope). If the argumentation is not to be biased, it has also to deal with the argument's contra position in an intellectually honest way.

The analysis demonstrated that some arguments which at first glance seemed quite convincing were found to be not so if questioned and analyzed critically, and once their weak points are also brought to light. So for instance the autonomy argument (autonomy of the dying person asking for euthanasia) is not as convincing as its proponents argue, being replaced or invalidated by the argument of compassion - unless there is clear evidence that euthanasia was the genuine choice and authentic option of the person concerned. While the autonomy argument has its justifications and explanatory powers, it is however diminished by other arguments such as competence or social pressure which affect the authenticity of an autonomous choice.

As an auxiliary tool, a matrix of arguments (Fig. 1) demonstrating the interconnectedness of the individual arguments was provided. The matrix shows both the prevalent dichotomy *"pro et contra"* and complementariness. As the main arguments *for* euthanasia, autonomy, the right to die, unbearable suffering, compassion, dignity, the patient's best interest, quality of life, health care costs, policy arguments of legalization (regulation) and transparency have been identified. By contrast, as the arguments *against* euthanasia, the following ones have been listed: competence, inviolability of human life, prohibition of killing, abuse, slippery slope, quality palliative care, physician's role, vulnerability, and social pressure. All these arguments have to be placed into the operational framework of the proposed matrix whose purpose is to illustrate the correlation of individual arguments. Some arguments can be used simultaneously both ways, for or against euthanasia; each of them has its own different explanatory and justifying power; some of them remain mutually exclusive (e.g. autonomy, compassion).

There is an immense interrelation between the arguments which sometimes goes unnoticed but what can be described by comparative analysis based on the proposed matrix. Many arguments rely on specific meaning or interpretations, as derived by the semantics of a singular term, or by a specific philosophical approach upon which the argument is based (e.g. dignity); last but not least the arguments also rely on their use in a particular cultural and/or religious context.

Such an understanding of the backgrounds, mechanisms and strategies of the arguments on euthanasia contributes significantly to a meaningful and respectful discussion of the controversial issue of euthanasia, which will surely continue into the coming decades.

4. References

Achille, M.A. & Ogloff, J.R. (1997). When Is a Request for Assisted Suicide Legitimate? Factors Influencing Public Attitudes Toward Euthanasia, *Canadian Journal of Behavioral Science*, Vol. 29, No. 1 (January 1997), pp. 19-27, ISSN 0008400X

Battin, M.P. (2003). Euthanasia and Physician-Assisted Suicide. In: *LaFollette, H. (Ed.)*, pp. 673-704, *The Oxford Handbook of Practical Ethics*, Oxford University Press, ISBN 0198241054, Oxford, UK - New York, USA

Battin, M.P.; Leslie, F.P. & Landesman, B.M. (2007). *Death, Dying and the Ending of Life*, Ashgate Publishing, ISBN 075462174X, Burlington, USA

Bauer-Maglin, N. & Perry, D. (2010). *Final Acts. Death, Dying, and the Choices We Make*, Rutgers University Press, ISBN 0813546278, New Brunswick, USA

Beauchamp, T.L. & Childress, J.F. (2001). *Principles of Biomedical Ethics*, Oxford University Press, 5th edition, ISBN 0195143329, Oxford, UK - New York, USA

Beauchamp, T.L. (Ed.). (1996). *Intending Death: The Ethics of Assisted Suicide and Euthanasia*, Prentice Hall, ISBN 0131995553, Upper Saddle River, USA

Beech, I. (1995). Suicide and Voluntary Active Euthanasia. Why the Difference in Attitude? *Nursing Ethics*, Vol. 2, No. 2 (June 1995), pp. 161-170, ISSN 09697330

Begley, A.M. (1998). Beneficent Voluntary Active Euthanasia. A Challenge to Professionals Caring for Terminally Ill Patients, *Nursing Ethics*, Vol. 5, No. 4 (July 1998), pp. 294-306, ISSN 09697330

Begley, A.M. (2008). Guilty But Good. Defending Voluntary Active Euthanasia From a Virtue Perspective, *Nursing Ethics*, Vol. 15, No. 4 (July 2008), pp. 446-456, ISSN 09697330

Behnke, J.A. & Bok, S. (Eds.). (1975). *The Dilemmas of Euthanasia*, Anchor Press, ISBN 0385097301, Garden City, USA

Ben Mitchell, C. (2010). Killing Euthanasia, *Ethics & Medicine. An International Journal of Bioethics*, Vol. 26, No. 1 (Spring 2010), pp. 5-6, ISSN 0266688X

Berlin, I. (1969). *Four Essays on Liberty*, Oxford University Press, ISBN 0192810340, Oxford, UK - New York, USA

Bernards, N. (Ed.). (1989). *Euthanasia: Opposing Viewpoints*, Greenhaven Press, ISBN 0899084427, San Diego, USA

Biggar, N. (2004). *Aiming to Kill. The Ethics of Suicide and Euthanasia*, Pilgrim Press, ISBN 0829815031, Cleveland, USA

Biggs, H. (2001). *Euthanasia, Death With Dignity, and the Law,* Hart Publishers, ISBN 1841130915, Oxford, UK - Portland, USA

Blocher, M. (1999). *The Right to Die? Caring Alternatives to Euthanasia,* Moody Press, ISBN 0802477399, Chicago, USA

Brock, D.W. (1992). Voluntary Active Euthanasia, *The Hastings Center Report,* Vol. 22, No. 2 (March-April 1992), pp. 10-22, ISSN 00930334

Brody, B.A. (Ed.). (1989). *Suicide and Euthanasia: Historical and Contemporary Themes,* Kluwer Academic Publishers, ISBN 0792301064, Dordrecht, NL - Boston, USA

Callahan, D. (1984). Autonomy: A Moral Good, Not a Moral Obsession, *The Hastings Center Report,* Vol. 14, No. 5 (March-April 1984), pp. 40-42, ISSN 00930334

Campbell, N. (1999). A Problem for the Idea of Voluntary Euthanasia, *Journal of Medical Ethics,* Vol. 25, No. 3 (June 1999), pp. 242-244, ISSN 14734257

Cantor, N.L. (1993). *Advance Directives and the Pursuit of Death With Dignity,* Indiana University Press, ISBN 025331304X, Bloomington, USA

Cassell, E.J. (2004). *The Nature of Suffering and the Goals of Medicine,* Oxford University Press, ISBN 0195156164, Oxford, UK - New York USA

Cassell, E.J. (2004a). Pain and Suffering. In: *Post, S.G. (Ed.),* Vol IV, pp. 1961-1969, *Encyclopedia of Bioethics,* 3rd edition, Thomson, ISBN 0028657748, New York, USA

Cavan, S. (2000). *Euthanasia: The Debate Over the Right to Die,* Rosen Publishing Group, ISBN 082393215X, New York, USA

Cohen-Almagor, R. (2001). *The Right to Die With Dignity: An Argument in Ethics, Medicine, and Law,* Rutgers University Press, ISBN 0813529867, New Brunswick, USA

Cosic, M. (2003). *The Right to Die: An Examination of the Euthanasia Debate,* New Holland, ISBN 1864368098, Sydney, Australia

The Danish Council of Ethics (Det Etiske Råd). (2006). *End of Life - Ethical Challenges and Problems.* Available at http://etiskraad.dk/. Cited 20.03.2011.

Dorman, J. (Ed.). (2010). *The Right to Die,* Greenhaven Press, ISBN 0737746846, Detroit, USA

Downing, A.B. (Ed.). (1970). *Euthanasia and the Right to Death. The Case for Voluntary Euthanasia,* Humanities Press, ISBN 0391000225, New York, USA

Downing, A.B. & Smoker, B. (Eds.). (1986). *Voluntary Euthanasia. Experts Debate the Right to Die,* Owen, ISBN 0391033654, London, UK

Draper, H. (1998). Euthanasia. In: *Chadwick, R. (Ed.),* Vol II, pp. 175-187, *Encyclopedia of Applied Ethics,* Academic Press, ISBN 012227066, San Diego…, USA

Dworkin, G.; Frey, R.G. & Bok, S. (1998). *Euthanasia and Physician-Assisted Suicide,* Cambridge University Press, ISBN 0521582466, Cambridge, UK - New York, USA

Dworkin, R. (1993). *Life's Dominion: An Argument about Abortion, Euthanasia, and Individual Freedom,* Knopf, ISBN 0394589416, New York, USA

Ells, C. (2001). Shifting the Autonomy Debate to Theory as Ideology, *Journal of Medicine and Philosophy,* Vol. 26, No. 4, pp. 417-430, ISSN 0360-5310

Engdahl, S. (Ed.). (2007). *Euthanasia,* Greenhaven Press, ISBN 0737732512, Detroit, USA

Feinberg, J. (1992). In Defence of Moral Rights, *Oxford Journal of Legal Studies,* Vol. 12, No. 2 (Summer 1992), pp. 149-169, ISSN 0143-6503

Ferguson, J.E. (2007). *The Right to Die,* Chelsea House Publishers, ISBN 0791092873, New York, USA

Finkel, N.J.; Hurabiell, M.L. & Hughes, K.C. (1993). Right to Die, Euthanasia, and Community Sentiment: Crossing the Public/Private Boundary, *Law and Human Behavior*, Vol. 17, No. 5 (October 1993), pp. 487-506, ISSN 01477307

Gaylin, W. & Jennings, B. (2003). *The Perversion of Autonomy: Coercion and Constraints in a Liberal Society*, Georgetown University Press, ISBN 0878409068, Washigton DC, USA

Gentles, I. (1995). *Euthanasia and Assisted Suicide: The Current Debate*, Stoddart, ISBN 0773757317, Toronto, Canada

Gill, R. (Ed.). (1998). *Euthanasia and the Churches*, Cassell, ISBN 0304703524, London, UK – New York, USA

Gomez, C.F. (1991). *Regulating Death: Euthanasia and the Case of the Netherlands*, Free Press, ISBN 0029124409, New York, USA

Grisez, G. & Boyle, J.M. (1979). *Life and Death with Liberty and Justice: A Contribution to the Euthanasia Debate.* University of Notre Dame Press, ISBN 0268012628, Notre Dame, USA

Gunning, K.F. et al. (1991). Euthanasia, *Lancet*, Vol. 338, No. 8773 (October 1991), pp. 1010-1011, ISSN 01406736

Haley, J. (2003). *Death and Dying: Opposing Viewpoints*, Greenhaven Press, Thomson/Gale, ISBN 0737712244, Farmington Hills - San Diego, USA

Harris, N. (Ed.). (2005). *The Ethics of Euthanasia*, Thomson, ISBN 0737721847, San Diego, USA

Hillyard, D. & Dombrink, J. (2001). *Dying Right: The Death With Dignity Movement*, Routledge, ISBN 0415927986, New York, USA

Hoffmann, E.C. (Ed.). (2009). *Health-Related Quality of Life*, Nova Biomedical Books, ISBN 1607417231, New York, USA

Holm, S. (1998). Autonomy. In: *Chadwick, R. (Ed.)*, Vol I, pp. 267-274, *Encyclopedia of Applied Ethics*, Academic Press, ISBN 012227066, San Diego…, USA

Humphry, D. (1992). *Dying With Dignity: Understanding Euthanasia*, Carol Publishing Group, ISBN 1559721057, New Brunswick, USA

Humphry, D. & Wickett, A. (1986). *The Right to Die: Understanding Euthanasia*, Harper & Row, ISBN 0060155787, New York, USA

Chervenak, F.A.; McCullough, L.B. & Arabin, B. (2006). Why the Groningen Protocol Should Be Rejected, *The Hastings Center Report*, Vol. 36, No. 5 (September - October 2006), pp. 30-33, ISSN 00930334

Childress, J. (2000). Autonomy. In: *Veatch, R.M. (Ed.)*, pp. 148-156, *Cross-Cultural Perspectives in Medical Ethics*, Jones and Bartlett Publishers, ISBN 0763713325, London, UK

Christman, J. & Anderson, J. (Eds.). (2009). *Autonomy and the Challenges of Liberalism*, Cambridge University Press, ISBN 0521839513, Cambridge, UK - New York, USA

Jennings, B. (2007). Autonomy. In: *Steinbock, B. (Ed.)*, pp. 72-89, *The Oxford Handbook of Bioethics*, Oxford University Press, ISBN 0199273355, Oxford, UK - New York, USA

Jussim, D. (1993). *Euthanasia: The "Right to Die" Issue*, Enslow Publishers, ISBN 0894904299, Hillside, USA

Kay, R.S. (2006). Causing Death for Compassionate Reasons in American Law, *The American Journal of Comparative Law*, Vol. 54 (American National Report, Fall 2006), pp. 693-716, ISSN 0002919x

Keown, J. (Ed.). (1995). *Euthanasia Examined. Ethical, Clinical, and Legal Perspectives*, Cambridge University Press, ISBN 0521451418, Cambridge UK - New York, USA

Keown, J. (2002). *Euthanasia, Ethics, and Public Policy: An Argument Against Legalisation,* Cambridge University Press, ISBN 0521804167, Cambridge, UK - New York, USA

Kinzbrunner, B.M. & Policzer, J.S. (2010). *End of Life Care: A Practical Guide,* McGraw-Hill Professional Publishing, ISBN 0071545271, New York, USA

Kohl, M. (1975). *Beneficent Euthanasia,* Prometheus Books, ISBN 0879750472, Buffalo, USA

Larson, E.J. & Amundsen, D.W. (1998). *A Different Death: Euthanasia & the Christian Tradition,* InterVarsity Press, ISBN 083081518X, Downers Grove, USA

Leone, D.A. (Ed.). (1999). *The Ethics of Euthanasia,* Greenhaven Press, ISBN 0737700041, San Diego, USA

Lesley, M. (2006). *To Cry Inside: Love, Death and Prison - the Hidden Face of the Euthanasia Debate,* Penguin Group, ISBN 0143020382, Auckland, New Zealand

Lewis, P. (2007). *Assisted Dying and Legal Change,* Oxford University Press, ISBN 0199212872, Oxford, UK - New York, USA

Lewy, G. (2011). *Assisted Death in Europa and America,* Oxford University Press, ISBN 0199746415 Oxford, UK, New York, USA

Lindemann, H. & Verkerk, M. (2008). Ending the Life of A Newborn: The Groningen Protocol, *The Hastings Center Report,* Vol. 38, No. 1 (January-February 2008), pp. 42-51, ISSN 00930334

Maas, van der P.J. et al. (1991). Euthanasia and Other Medical Decisions Concerning the End of Life, *Lancet,* Vol. 335, No. 8767 (September 1991), pp. 669-773, ISSN 0140-6736

Mak, Y.Y. & Elwyn G. (2005). Voices of the Terminally Ill. Uncovering the Meaning of Desire for Euthanasia, *Palliative Medicine,* Vol. 19, No. 4 (June 2005), pp. 343-350, ISSN 1477030X

Manning, M. (1998). *Euthanasia and Physician-Assisted Suicide: Killing or Caring?* Paulist Press, ISBN 0809138042, New York, USA

Mattews, M.A. (1987). Suicidal Competence and the Patient's Right to Refuse Lifesaving Treatment, *California Law Review,* Vol. 75, No. 2 (March 1987), pp. 707-758, ISSN 00081221

Mayer, M.J. (1995). Dignity, Death and Modern Virtue, *American Philosophical Quarterly,* Vol. 32, No. 1 (January 1995), pp. 43-54, ISSN 21521123

Medina, L.M. (Ed.). (2005). *Euthanasia,* Greenhaven Press, ISBN 0737720050, Detroit, USA

Misbin, R.I. (Ed.). (1992). *Euthanasia: The Good of the Patient, the Good of Society,* University Publishing Group, ISBN 155572017X, Frederick, USA

Moreno Villares, J.M. & Villa Elízaga, I. (2005). Eutanasia en niños: Una reflexión sobre el protocolo de Groningen, *Acta Pediátrica Española,* Vol. 63, No. 8 (July 2005), pp. 307-313, ISSN 00016640

Moreno, J.D. (Ed.). (1995). *Arguing Euthanasia: The Controversy Over Mercy Killing, Assisted Suicide, and the "Right to Die",* Simon & Schuster, ISBN 0684807602, New York, USA

Morgan, J. (Ed.). (1996). *An Easeful Death? Perspectives on Death, Dying and Euthanasia,* Federation Press, ISBN 1862872228, Sydney, Australia

Muller, M.T.; Van der Wal, G. & van Eijk, J.T. (1994). Voluntary Active Euthanasia and Physician-Assisted Suicide in Dutch Nursing Homes. Are the Requirements For Prudent Practice Properly Met? *The Journal of the American Geriatrics Society,* Vol. 42, No. 6 (June 1994), pp. 624-629, ISSN 15325415

Nayernouri, T. (2011). Euthanasia, Terminall Illness and Quality of Life, *Archives of Iranian Medicine*, Vol. 14, No. 1 (January 2011), pp. 54-55, ISSN 10292977

Nordenfelt, L. (1994). *Concepts and Measurement of Quality of Life in Health Care*, Kluwer Academic Publishers, ISBN 0792328248, Dordrecht, NL - Boston, USA

Ogden, R. (1994). The Right to Die: A Policy Proposal for Euthanasia and Aid in Dying, *Canadian Public Policy / Analyse de Politiques*, Vol. 20, No. 1 (March 1994), pp. 1-25, ISSN 03170861

Onwuteaka-Philipsen, B.D. et al. (2003), Euthanasia and Other End-of-Life Decisions in the Netherlands in 1990, 1995, and 2001, *Lancet*, Vol. 362, No. 9381 (August 2003), pp. 395-399, ISSN 01406736

Oosthuizen, G.C.; Shapiro, H.A. & Strauss, S.A. (Eds.). (1978). *Euthanasia,* Oxford University Press, ISBN 0195701437, New York, USA

Paust, J.J. (1995). The Human Right to Die with Dignity: A Policy-Oriented Essay, *Human Rights Quarterly,* Vol. 17, No. 3 (August 1995), pp. 463-487, ISSN 1085794X

Peck, S.M. (1997). *Denial of the Soul: Spiritual and Medical Perspectives On Euthanasia,* Random House Large Print, ISBN 0679774246, New York, USA

Quill, T.E. (1993). *Death and Dignity: Making Choices and Taking Charge,* W.W. Norton, ISBN 0393034488, New York, USA

Quill, T.E. & Battin, M.P. (2004). *Physician-Assisted Dying: The Case for Palliative Care and Patient Choice,* Johns Hopkins University Press, ISBN 0801880696, Baltimore, USA

Quill, T.E.; Lo, B. & Brock, D.W. (1997). Palliative Options of Last Resort. A Comparison of Voluntarily Stopping Eating and Drining, Terminal Sedation, Physician-Assisted Suicide, and Voluntary Active Euthanasia, *The Journal of the American Medical Association,* Vol. 278, No. 23 (December 1997), pp. 2099-2104, ISSN 00987484

Rachels, J. (1986). *The End of Life: Euthanasia and Morality,* Oxford University Press, ISBN 019217746X, Oxford, UK - New York, USA

Ramsey, H. (1997). Euthanasia: Compassion, Dignity and Respect, *Sophia*, Vol. 36, No. 2 (September-October 1997), pp. 43-54, ISSN 00381527

Rebman, R.C. (2002). *Euthanasia and the "Right to Die": A Pro/Con Issue*, Enslow, ISBN 0766018164, Berkeley Heights/N.J., USA

Roberts, C.S. & Gorman, M. (1996). *Euthanasia: A Reference Handbook*, ABC-CLIO, ISBN 0874368316, Santa Barbara, USA

Rosenblatt, S.M. (1992). *Murder of Mercy: Euthanasia on Trial*, Prometheus Books, ISBN 0879757728, Buffalo, USA

Russell, O.R. (1975). *Freedom to Die: Moral and Legal Aspects of Euthanasia,* Human Sciences Press, ISBN 0877052166, New York, USA

Sheldon, T. (1994). Dutch Argue that Mental Torment Justifies Euthanasia, *The British Medical Journal,* Vol. 308, No. 6926 (February 12, 1994), p. 431, ISSN 09598146

Sheldon, T. (2003). Being "Tired of Life" Is Not Grounds For Euthanasia, *The British Medical Journal*, Vol. 326, No. 7380 (January 11, 2003), p. 71, ISSN 09598146

Schachter, O. (1983). Human Dignity as a Normative Concept, *American Journal of International Law,* Vol. 77, No. 4 (October 1983), pp. 848-854, ISSN 00029300

Scherer, J.M. & Simon, J.R. (1999). *Euthanasia and the Right to Die. A Comparative View*, Rowman & Littlefield Publishers, ISBN 0847691667, Lanham, USA

Schneewind, J.B. (1998). *The Invention of Autonomy: A History of Modern Moral Philosophy,* Cambridge University Press, ISBN 052147938X, Cambridge, UK

Schneider, C.E. (1988). Rights Discourse and Neonatal Euthanasia, *California Law Review,* Vol. 76, No. 1 (January 1988), pp. 151-176, ISSN 00081221

Schotsmans, P. & Gastmans, C. (2009). How to Deal with Euthanasia Requests: A Palliative Filter Procedure, *Cambridge Quarterly of Healthcare Ethics,* Vol. 18, No. 4 (Fall 2009), pp. 420–428, ISSN 09631801

Skevington, S. (2002). Pain. In: *Howarth, G. & Leaman, I. (Eds.),* pp. 341-342, *Encyclopedia of Death and Dying,* Routledge, ISBN 0415188253, London, UK - New York, USA

Smith, G.P. (1989). *Final Choices: Autonomy in Health Care Decisions,* Thomas, ISBN 0398055912, Springfield, USA

Smith, W.J. (2006). *Forced Exit: Euthanasia, Assisted Suicide, and the New Duty to Die,* Encounter Books, ISBN 1594031193, New York, USA

Smook, A.O. & de Vos-Schippers, B. (Eds.). (1990). Right to Self-Determination, *Proceedings of the 8th World Conference of the International Federation of Right to Die Societies.* Organized by the Nederlandse Vereniging voor Vrijwillige Euthanasie (NVVE) in Maastricht on June 7-10, 1990, VU University Press, ISBN 9062569307, Amsterdam, NL

Snyder, C.L. (Ed.). (2006). *Euthanasia,* Greenhaven Press, ISBN 0737729333, Detroit, USA

Stefoff, R. (2009). *The Right to Die,* Marshall Cavendish Benchmark, ISBN 0761429487, New York, USA

Sullivan, W.F. (2005). *Eye of the Heart: Knowing the Human Good in the Euthanasia Debate,* University of Toronto Press, ISBN 0802039235, Toronto, Canada

Sunstein, C.R. (1997). The Right to Die, *The Yale Law Journal,* Vol. 106, No. 4 (January 1997), pp. 1123-1163, ISSN 00440094

Swarup, H. (2009). *Who Owns Your Life? The Right to Die and Die With Dignity,* Macmillan, ISBN 0230636699, New Delhi, India

Tada, J.E. (1992). *When Is It Right to Die? Suicide, Euthanasia, Suffering, Mercy,* Zondervan, ISBN 0310585708, Grand Rapids, USA

ten Have, H. (2001). Euthanasia. In: *ten Have, H. & Gordijn, B. (Eds.),* pp. 469-486, *Bioethics in a European Perspective,* Kluwer Academic Publishers, ISBN 1402001266, Dordrecht, NL - Boston, USA - London, UK

ten Have, H. & Welie, J.V.M. (1992). Euthanasia: Normal Medical Practice? *The Hastings Center Report,* Vol. 22, No. 2 (March-April 1992), pp. 34-38, ISSN 00930334

Thomasma, D.C. (Ed.). (1998). *Asking to Die: Inside the Dutch Debate about Euthanasia,* Kluwer Academic Publishers, ISBN 0792351851, Dordrecht, NL - Boston, USA

Torr, J. (Ed.). (2000). *Euthanasia: Opposing Viewpoints,* Greenhaven Press, ISBN 0737701269, San Diego, USA

Tulloch, G. (2008). *Euthanasia – Choice and Death,* Edinburgh University Press, ISBN 0748618813, Edinburgh, Ireland

Uhlmann, M.M. (Ed.). (1998). *Last Rights? Assisted Suicide and Euthanasia,* William B. Eerdmans Publishing Company, ISBN 0802841996, Grand Rapids, USA

Van Zyl, L. (2000). *Death and Compassion: A Virtue-Based Approach to Euthanasia,* Ashgate, ISBN 0754612317, Aldershot, UK

Velleman, J.D. (1999). A Right of Self-Termination? *Ethics,* Vol. 109, No. 3 (April 1999), pp. 606-628, ISSN 00141704

Verhagen, E. & Sauer, P.J.J. (2005). The Groningen Protocol: Euthanasia in Severely Ill Newborns, *The New England Journal of Medicine,* Vol. 352, No. 10 (March 10, 2005), pp. 959-962, ISSN 00284793

Vries, de M.C. & Verhagen, A.A. (2008). A Case Against Something That Is Not the Case: Groningen Protocol and the Moral Principle of Non-maleficence, *The American Journal of Bioethics,* Vol. 8, No. 11, pp. 29-31, ISSN 15360075

Walter, J.J. & Shannon, T.A. (Eds.). (1990). *Quality of Life: The New Medical Dilemma,* Paulist Press, ISBN 08909131919, New York, USA

Wanzer, S.H. & Glenmullen, J. (2007). *To Die Well. Your Right to Comfort, Calm, and Choice in the Last Days of Life,* Da Capo Press, ISBN 0738210838, Cambridge, USA

Watts, D.T. & Howell T. (1992). Assisted Suicide Is Not Voluntary Active Euthanasia, *The Journal of the American Geriatrics Society,* Vol. 40, No. 10 (October 1992), pp. 1043-1046, ISSN 15325415

Wekesser, C. (Ed.). (1995). *Euthanasia: Opposing Viewpoints,* Greenhaven Press, ISBN 1565102444, San Diego, USA

Wennberg, R.N. (1989). *Terminal Choices: Euthanasia, Suicide, and the Right to Die,* W.B. Eerdmans Publishing Company, ISBN 0802804543, Grand Rapids, USA

Williams, P.C. (1977). Rights and the Alleged Right of Innocents to be Killed, *Ethics,* Vol. 87, No. 4 (July 1977), pp. 383-394, ISSN 00141704

Wilshaw, C. (1974). *The Right to Die: A Rational Approach to Voluntary Euthanasia,* British Humanist Association, ISBN 0901825085, London, UK

Woodward, J. (Ed.). (2006). *The Right to Die,* Greenhaven Press, ISBN 0737734396, Detroit, USA

Young, M. (Ed.). (2007a). *Euthanasia,* Greenhaven Press, ISBN 0737727890, Detroit, USA

Young, R. (2007). *Medically Assisted Death,* Cambridge University Press, ISBN 0521880246, Cambridge, UK

Yount, L. (2007). *Right to Die and Euthanasia, Facts on File,* ISBN 0816062751, New York, USA

Part 3

Policy and Attitude

8

The Impact of the Dutch Euthanasia Act on the Number of Requests for Euthanasia and Physician Assisted Suicide - A Cohort Study in General Practice Between 1977 and 2007

G.A. Donker and J.E. van Alphen
NIVEL - Netherlands Institute for Health Services Research
Utrecht
The Netherlands

1. Introduction

In 2002 Euthanasia (E) and Physician assisted suicide (PAS) were legalised by passing of the Euthanasia Act in the Netherlands. In this law E was defined as the administration of drugs with death of the patient as the ultimate result, at the explicit request of a patient. PAS was defined as the prescription of drugs by a physician for the purpose of self-administration by the patient. Recent studies showed that the number of deaths in the Netherlands due to E/PAS has decreased after the implementation of the Euthanasia Act in 2002. E decreased from 2.6% of all deaths reported in 2001 to 1.7% in 2005.[1,2] PAS decreased from 0.2% of all deaths in 2001 to 0.1% in 2005.[1] Improved palliative care, including the use of deep continuous sedation at the end of life, and an increase of the average life expectancy are some of the possible explanations for this decrease.[1,2] In addition, the general misperception that morphine shortens life is more and more condemned.[1] This could also explain a decrease, as fewer palliative treatments are registered as E. Our main research question is, whether the number of requests for E or PAS has changed after the implementation of the Euthanasia Act in 2002.

Few publications have reported on requests for E/PAS and the rate of these which is actually granted in the Netherlands.[4-6] Van der Maas et al described an increase in the number of requests between 1990 and 1995 of 37% in terminally ill patients.[4] Trend analysis by Marquet et al, on the incidence of requests for E/PAS with Dutch GPs in the period 1977 to 2001 showed an increase which stabilised during the nineties.[5] Other studies reported that about 44% of the requests actually results in E or PAS.[6] The 56% of requests not resulting in an actual E/PAS was also evaluated. In 13% of the cases the patient passed before E, 13% of patients died even before completion of the preparation process.[6] In 13% of the cases the patient withdrew the request and in 12% of the cases the physician considered the request not eligible.[6]

Several studies examined patients' reasons for requesting E/PAS, in the last decades.[5,7,8] Marquet et al found that hopelessness and deterioration are frequent reasons for a request

and that pain and dyspnoea are declining in frequency as a reason.[5] Emanuel et al considered pain, depressive symptoms and dependence as the most frequent reasons to consider E/PAS.[7] Especially patients with depressive symptoms and pain are changing their minds over time.[7]
This study examines the impact of the Euthanasia Act (2002) on the incidence and reasons for E/PAS in Dutch general practice during the period 1977 to 2007.

2. Methods

Data were collected annually by a standardized questionnaire on requests for E/PAS in Dutch general practice in the period from 1977 to 2007. The GPs included participate in the Dutch Sentinel Practice Network. This network of 45 general practices represents 0.8% of the Dutch population and is representative at a national level for age, gender, geographic distribution and population density. Annually the GPs were requested to report the number of and reasons for requests of E/PAS, they were consulted for in the past year. Definition for E and PAS were applied as formulated in the Dutch Euthanasia Act (2002). Only serious requests of terminally ill patients were noted. Therefore, requests for possible E/PAS in the future, not related to an existing disease, were excluded. Age, gender, underlying disease, reason for the request and presence of a living will were recorded on the questionnaire. GPs reported a maximum of three reasons per request by open question. No age group was excluded. Stemming from the period when euthanasia was not legalized in the Netherlands purposely there is no registration whether the requests were executed or not.
Incidence was calculated as the number of requests per 10,000 patients on GP's lists. Diseases were classified using the International Classification of Primary Care (ICPC) system. Incidence analyses were stratified by patient and practice characteristics. Linear regression trend analysis was performed on the incidence of requests for E/PAS and presented in graphs. Data for the period 1997 to 2000 were adapted to fit in the regression analysis.
The reasons for requesting E/PAS were classified into 22 different subcategories, e.g. pain, dyspnoea, deterioration, and hopelessness. For the most frequently claimed reasons the data were calculated into proportions per category and entered into graphs using linear regression analysis.

3. Results

In the period from 1977 to 2007 the GPs of the Dutch Sentinel Network were consulted for 1011 requests for E/PAS; 54% (546) male and 46% (465) female. In 74.8% the patient was diagnosed with cancer and in 6.4% with a cardiovascular disease. The age distribution showed a peak between 70 and 79 years (28.8%); 26.6% of patients between 60 and 69 years, and 17.3% between 80 and 89 years of age. A rather large group (23.7%) is younger than 60 years of age including 12.7% between 50 and 59, 6.5% between 40 and 49 and 3.3% between 30 and 39 years of age.

Requests for E/PAS, 1977-2007

The number of requests per 10,000 patients (figure 1) shows an increase in the period until 1990. After 1991 trends are slightly decreasing until 2004. After 2004 the incidence stabilised around 2.2 per 10,000 patients ($P<0.05$). No increase after the implementation of the Euthanasia Act in 2002 was observed.

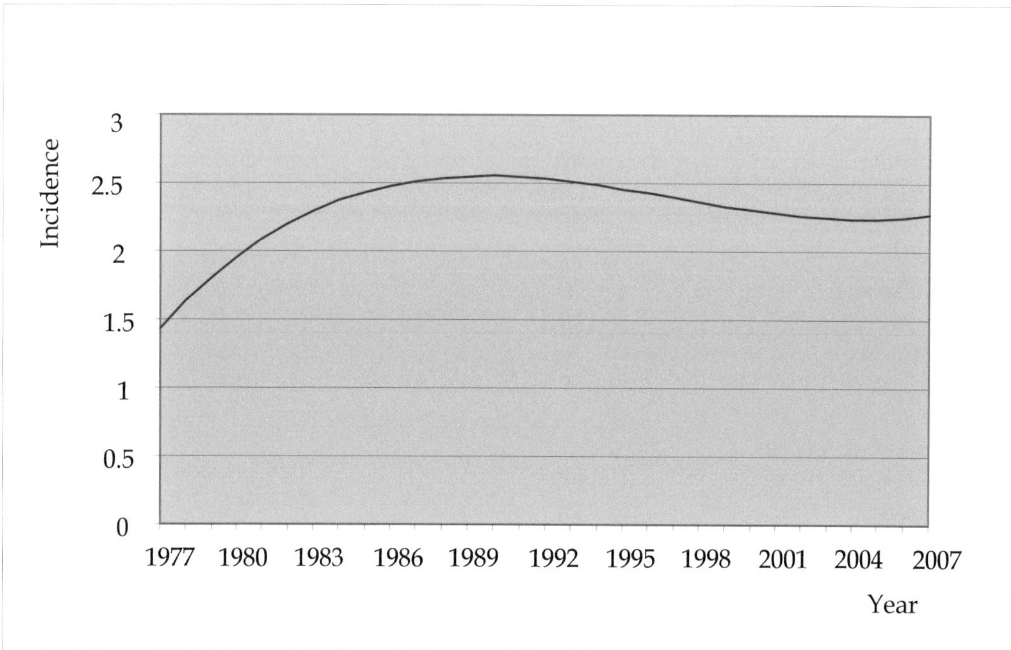

Fig. 1. Annual requests for E/PAS to GPs in the Netherlands, per 10,000 patients (1977-2007).

	B (SE)	95% CI	P-value
Intercept	1.434412 (0.152603)	---	---
1977-1990	0.208166 (0.04684)	0.11127 - 0.305061	0.000186
1991-2004	-0.012 (0.003834)	-0.01993 - (-0.00407)	0.004693
2005-2007	0.0002 (8.56E-05)	2.28E-05 - 0.000377	0.028625

Table 1. Annual requests for E/PAS to GPs in the Netherlands, per 10,000 patients (1977-2007). Results from linear regression analysis.

Reasons to request E/PAS

The most frequently mentioned reason for requesting E/PAS was pain in 31.4% (table 2). Deterioration (26.1%), hopelessness (19.0%) and dyspnoea (12.6%) were also frequent reasons for patients to ask for E/PAS. Fear in general was in 9.7% a reason for the request; fear without a specific reason 4.0%, fear of pain 2.1%, fear of losing dignity 2.2%, fear of deterioration 1.8%, and fear of dependency in 0.7% of the requests. Loss of dignity was one of the reasons for requesting E/PAS in 7.9% of the cases and dependency in 5.1%. Metastatic disease, vomiting and depression were less frequently reported, respectively 3.9%, 3.0%, and 2.8% of all requests in general practice in the Netherlands in the period of 1977 to 2007.

Reason request	N	Percentage of requests
Somatic reasons		
Pain	317	31.4%
Deterioration	264	26.1%
Dyspnoea	127	12.6%
Metastatic disease	36	3.9%
Vomiting	27	3.0%
Bowel disorder	20	2.2%
Swallowing disorder	19	2.1%
Dementia	4	0.4%
Pressure ulcers	3	0.3%
Psychosomatic reasons		
Hopelessness	192	19.0%
Humiliation	80	7.9%
Dependency	47	5.1%
Fear not specified	37	4.0%
Depression	26	2.8%
Fear of humiliation	20	2.2%
Fear of pain	19	2.1%
Fear of deterioration	16	1.8%
Loneliness	11	1.2%
Fear of dependability	6	0.7%
Other medical disorders	112	12.3%
Other reasons	72	7.9%

* Combined group of Fear not specified, Fear of losing dignity, Fear of pain, Fear of deterioration and Fear of dependability.

Table 2. Percentage of reasons for request E/PAS representing different subgroups.

Through the years *pain* is declining in frequency as (one of) the reason(s) for a patient to request E/PAS ($p<0.001$) (Figure 2 and Table 3). In 1977 in almost half of the cases listed by the GPs *(fear of) pain* was mentioned as one of the reasons for the request; in 2007 in one fifth of the cases. Despite this decrease *(fear of) pain* is still the most frequent reason to request in 2007. *(Fear of) deterioration* was increasingly one of the reasons until 1991, but during the last 16 years this trend has decreased ($p<0.01$). *Dyspnoea* shows a declining frequency during the period 1977 to 2007 ($p>0.05$). *Hopelessness* as the reason for a request initially increased and later decreased during the years ($p>0.05$).

4. Discussion

The number of requests per 10,000 patients showed an increase in the first phase of the study 1977-1990, then slightly decreased and stabilised during the past three years. The number of requests remained low since the implementation of the Euthanasia Act in 2002 and through the years concerned a small proportion of all deaths in general practice. Three quarter of the patients that requested E/PAS were suffering from malignant diseases. Reasons for requesting E/PAS were changing over time. *Pain* was declining in frequency as the reason for a request over the years, but remained the most frequent reason for requesting E/PAS throughout the study period. *Deterioration* and other *non somatic reasons* for requesting E/PAS were increasing until the beginning of the nineties, whereafter these reasons declined again.

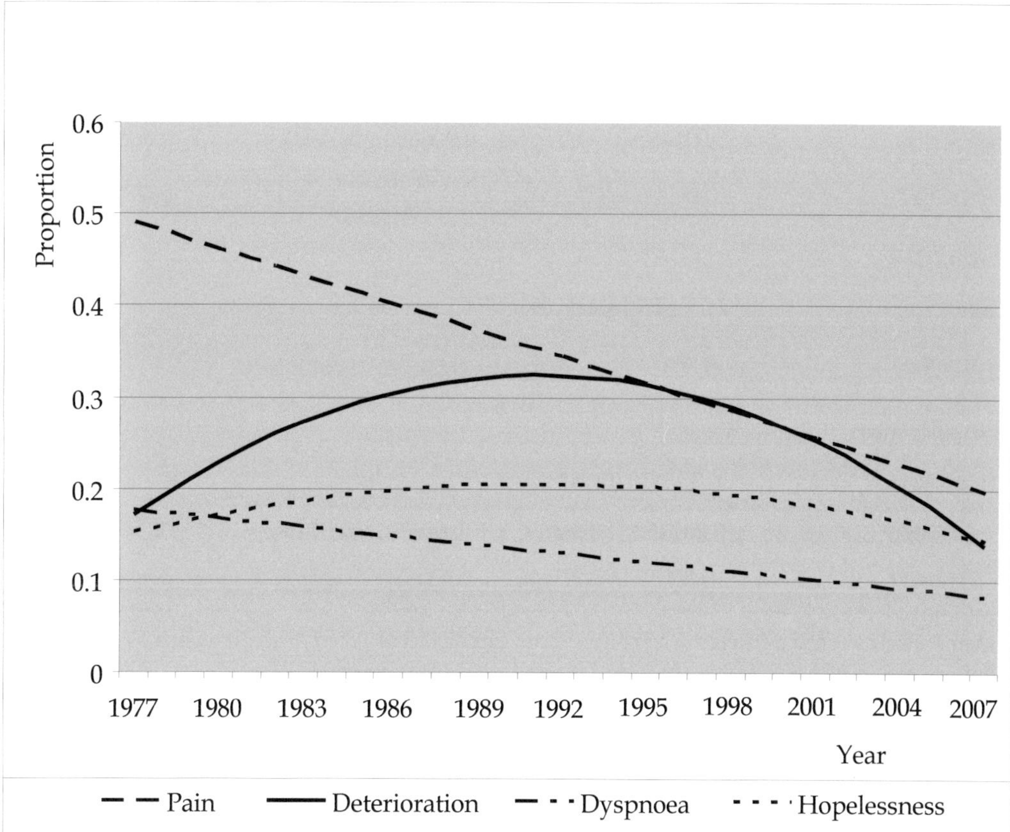

Fig. 2. Reasons for requesting Euthanasia or physician assisted suicide with GPs in the Netherlandsin proportion per category (1977-2007)

This study presents data collected over a 31 year period, partly before any regulation or law had passed. Some limitations need to be mentioned. First, the retrospective design of the study could have induced recall bias among the GPs and, therefore, could have influenced the results. However, we assumed serious consultations about E/PAS would be the consultations least subjective to such bias due to the impact of such consultations on the GP. In addition, the GPs know in advance they will be requested to report their cases of E/PAS each year which enhances correct registration.

Secondly, the definition of E changed over the period 1977 to 2007. In the first years, before the discussion about E in The Netherlands started, the term 'passive euthanasia' was used for various conditions, now called palliative treatment. E as included in our study is formulated as deliberate use of a treatment that was assumed to be life shortening. This definition has not changed during the study period of more than 30 years.

Pain	B (SE)	95% CI	P-value
Intercept	0,491129 (0,038781)	---	---
1977-2007	-0,00977 (0,002221)	-0,01432 – (-0,00523)	0,000133
Deterioration			
Intercept	0,171239 (0,046684)	---	---
1977-1991	0,021448 (0,007203)	0,006693 - 0,036203	0,005938
1992-2007	-0,00075 (0,000232)	-0,00123 – (-0,00028)	0,003063
Dyspnoea			
Intercept	0,177379 (0,027109)	---	---
1977-2007	-0,00314 (0,001552)	-0,00631 - 3,76E-05	0,052598
Hopelessness			
Intercept	0,152416 (0,04465)	---	---
1977-1991	0,007352 (0,006889)	-0,00676 - 0,021464	0,295027
1992-2007	-0,00025 (0,000222)	-0,00071 - 0,0002	0,261701

Table 3. Reasons for requesting Euthanasia or Physician assisted suicide with GPs in the Netherlands (1977-2007). Results from linear regression analysis.

Furthermore, there are no data on the amount of granted requests for E/PAS. This variable was not included in the past due to the illegal condition of E/PAS before the implementation of the Euthanasia Act in The Netherlands in 2002. Onwuteaka-Philipsen et al described 44% of the requests for E/PAS is granted by GPs in The Netherlands.[6] In 12% of requests it was considered not eligible by the physician and in 13% it was withdrawn by the patient.[6] The patient died before the E/PAS was actually carried out in the rest of the cases (31%).[6]

Our study is unique in collecting data about E/PAS in general practice over a long time period, even before these practices were legalized. The major contribution of this study is the finding that requests for E/PAS in general practice did not increase after implementation of the Euthanasia Act in 2002. As The Netherlands was the first country worldwide to do so, a cohort study embracing a period of over 30 years assessing the impact of the implementation of a Euthanasia Act has not been performed elsewhere.

For the interpretation of the results the representativeness of the network is important. The network is designed to be nationally representative for geographical distribution and distribution in population density.[9] As far as type of practice is concerned, solo practices are slightly overrepresented.[9] There is no indication, however, that this would bias the results.

This network is well-suited for reporting in retrospect, prospectively-collected data through a continuous morbidity registration (CMR) process. Results are typically used for monitoring and harmonising health information.[9-12] In the Netherlands, registration with a GP is compulsory for access to health care.[9,12] The Dutch primary care system is equally accessible to all socio-demographic subgroups.[12] However, it is important to realize that in The Netherlands in general nursing home residents are not under the care of a GP. Therefore, we consider our data representative for euthanasia requests in general practice, but not for nursing homes and other institutions not cared for by GPs, such as prisons and mental health institutions.
Earlier research showed that comparing the five years before and after the implementation of the Euthanasia Act did not show an increased demand for euthanasia after implementation of the new guidelines as well.[13] However, some gender differences in the reasons for requesting euthanasia were revealed in that study. Loss of dignity as a reason declined especially in females. Excellent communication skills including gender sensitivity are important in exploring end of life wishes and underlying reasons for requesting for euthanasia with patients.[13]

5. Conclusions

The incidence of requests for E/PAS in Dutch General Practice increased considerably in the years between 1977-1990 after which it slightly decreased and stabilised in the period 2005-2007. No increase during the first five years after the implementation of the Dutch Euthanasia Act in 2002 was observed. Pain has declined, but remained the most frequent reason for requesting E/PAS in Dutch General Practice despite improved palliative care.

6. Acknowledgement

The study was funded by the Ministry of Health. We would like to thank all GPs from the Dutch Sentinel Network for their contributions to the study. We thank Mrs. M. Heshusius-Valen for her crucial role in the data collection process.

7. References

[1] Van der Heide A, Onwuteaka-Philipsen BD, Rurup ML, Buiting HM, van Delden JJM, Hanssen-de Wolf JE, Janssen AGJM, Pasman HRW, Rietjens JAC, Prins CJM, Deerenberg IM, Gevers JKM, van der Maas PJ, van der Wal G. End-of-life practices in the Netherlands under the Euthanasia Act. N Engl J Med 2007;356:1957-65.

[2] Onwuteaka-Philipsen BD, van der Heide A, Koper D, Keij-Deerenberg I, Rietjens JAC, Rurup ML, Vrakking AM, Georges JJ, Muller MT, van der Wal G, van der Maas PJ. Euthanasia and other end-of-life decisions in the Netherlands in 1990, 1995 and 2001. The Lancet 2003;362:395-9.

[3] Georges JJ, Onwuteaka-Philipsen BD, van der Wal G, van der Heide A, van der Maas PJ. Differences between terminally ill cancer patients who died after euthanasia had been performed and terminally ill cancer patients who did not request euthanasia. J Palliat Med 2005;19:578-586.

[4] Van der Maas PJ, van der Wal G, Haverkate I, de Graaff CLM, Kester JGC, Onwuteaka-Philipsen BD, van der Heide A, Bosma JM, Willems DL. Euthanasia, physician-

assisted suicide, and other medical practices involving the end of life in the Netherlands, 1990-1995. N Engl J Med 1996;335:1699-1705.
[5] Marquet RL, Bartelds A, Visser GJ, Spreeuwenberg P, Peters L. Twenty five years of requests for euthanasia and physician assisted suicide in Dutch general practice: trend analysis. BMJ 2003;327:201-202.
[6] Onwuteaka-Philipsen BD, Jansen-van der Weide MC, van der Wal G. Granted, undecided, withdrawn, and refused requests for euthanasia and physician-assisted suicide. Arch Int Med 2005;165:1698-704.
[7] Emanuel EJ, Fairclough DL, Emanuel LL. Attitudes and desires related to euthanasia and physician-assisted suicide among terminally ill patients and their caregivers. JAMA 2000;284:2460-68.
[8] Rurup ML, Onwuteaka-Philipsen BD, Jansen-van der Weide MC, van der Wal G. When being 'tired of living' plays an important role in a request for euthanasia or physician-assisted suicide: patient characteristics and the physician's decision. Health policy 2005;74:157-66.
[9] Donker GA. Continuous Morbidity Registration Sentinel Stations The Netherlands 2007. Annual Report. Utrecht, NIVEL, 2008.
[10] Van den Block L, van Casteren V, Deschepper R, Bossuyt N, Drieskens K, Bauwens S et al. Nationwide monitoring of end-of-life care via the Sentinel Network of General Practitioners in Belgium: the research protocol of the SENTI-MELC study. BMC Palliat Care 2007; 6:6.
[11] Busse R, Wagner HP, Krauth C, Klein-Lange M, Schwartz FW. Sentinel practices in evaluating longer periods of care: quality of life and drug therapy of terminally ill persons in Lower Saxony (Germany). J Epidemiol Community Health. 1998 Apr;52 Suppl 1:56S-60S.
[12] Van der Zee S, Saskia C, Hoek G, Brunekreef B. Incidence of Influenza-like Illness, Measured by a General Practitioner Sentinel System, Is Associated with Day-to-day Variations in Respiratory Health in Panel Studies. American Journal of Epidemiology 2000; 152(4):389-392.
[13] Alphen JJ van, Donker GA, Marquet RL. Requests for euthanasia in general practice before and after implementation of the Dutch Euthanasia Act. Brit J Gen Pract 2010;60:263-7.

9

Turkish Health Professional's Attitudes Towards Euthanasia

Gulten Kaptan[1], Lecturer Ozden Dedeli[2] and Levent Önen
[1]*Maltepe University, Istanbul*
[2]*Celal Bayar University, Manisa*
Turkey

1. Introduction

Death, the end of life, is one of the most real things in life. Therefore it has always been the major concern of people to meet with it. It is not the death but the process of dying worries people. Although the moment of death may be at any time, for some reason, it has been perceived as identical with the old age. Much research has indicated that almost in every country, particularly in the developed countries, aged population increases, which brings extra burden to the health care systems and social services. The diseases encountered in old age are mostly chronic and long lasting, which necessitate the provision of health care services in long and costly manner. This, inevitably, brings the problem of the distribution of limited sources into discussion (Aksoy, 1998). Every country has its own priorities in health services. Although most attention in the West has focused on the elderly as terminal patients, in some countries the major focus might be on younger adult AIDS patients or on children dying from malnutrition or infectious diseases. Another important category, although much smaller in number, are critically ill or extremely low birth weight babies. In each of these categories, the issues might be similar but the solutions differ significantly from country to country.

Before getting into detail on end of life decision-making, it is of benefit to give some basic information about the country. Turkey is a nation state with almost 68 million population comprising people from different ethnic backgrounds. The male and female populations are almost equal to each other. It has a young population with 55% under the age of 20 (Republic of Turkey, Prime Ministry State Institute of Statistics, 2002). The major faith tradition in Turkey is Islam (95%). There are some Jews, Christians and others. Although Turkey is a secular state by its governmental system, since there is such a great majority of Muslims with a long tradition, religion plays a significant role in ethical reasoning in public mind, though not in official level. The rate of population over 65 is 8%, and the life expectancy at birth is 70.2. (Republic of Turkey, Prime Ministry State Institute of Statistics, 2002) Turkey is a unique country in its region as a Muslim State officially committed to adapt western life style and tradition.

Decision-making is an important process, especially in terminal stages of the illnesses. The moral quality of a clinical decision is dependent on the process of that decision and not only on the outcome. We are accountable and responsible for the way in which our decisions are reached. Since our understanding of the patient's perspective will always be limited, good communication and acceptance of the patient's view is essential in reaching the desired goal of a consensus decision. (Randall and Downie, 1996) It is pretty easy to make the 'right decision' if the patient can involve to the decision making process. Autonomous patients can choose the extent to which they wish to participate in decisions about these treatments; if they wish to be fully involved they are adequately informed. However, non-autonomous patients are unable to participate in deriving the balance of benefits to burdens and risk in the particular situation. Advance statements are offered as a solution in case of non-autonomous patients.

There is not a proper advance statement in Turkey. Even it is not legal to put Do-Not-Resuscitate (DNR) orders. However this does not mean that it is not practiced in clinics. Many doctors and nurses in anaesthesiology and reanimation departments reported to us that there are many voluntary and involuntary DNR orders are practiced in ICUs and the wards. Therefore there is no point to talk about the legal binding of advance statements and DNR orders. In recent years some Turkish bioethicists strongly suggested the necessity of advance statements and DNR orders. (Oguz, 2001) Oguz argues that a good application of DNR order, under the light of the concept of 'futility of treatment', the number of euthanasia requests will decrease.

2. Information

Euthanasia is a terribly troubling word, meaning literally, according to some, “a good death,” but according to others a morally outrageous death. According to some researchers euthanasia is the act of taking the life, for reasons of mercy, of a person who is hopelessly ill. A basic distinction is made between two kinds of euthanasia, namely passive and active.

Active euthanasia is identical with mercy killing and involves taking direct action to end a life, for example, intentionally giving a person a lethal dose of a drug to end a painful and prolonged period of dying. Passive euthanasia is allowing a patient to die when he or she could have been kept alive by the appropriate medical procedures. Active euthanasia can be defined as any treatment initiated by a physician with the intent of hastening the death of another human being who is terminally ill and in severe pain or distress with the motive of relieving that person from great suffering.

Passive euthanasia can be defined or considered as discontinuing or not starting a treatment at the request of the patient. Further distinction is made between voluntary, involuntary, and non-voluntary euthanasia. According to this distinction, voluntary euthanasia occurs when the decision to terminate life by the physicians corresponds with the patient’s desire to do so and the patient willfully gives consent of its implementation. Involuntary euthanasia occurs when the decision to end life is implemented against the patient’s wishes. Non-voluntary euthanasia refers to cases where patients are unable to make their wishes known, for example a person who is brain dead and in a permanent or irreversible coma. According to another researchers active voluntary euthanasia and physician-assisted suicide are often combined and mentioned in one breath. They defined active voluntary euthanasia as the deliberate termination of life, by someone other than the patient, at the patient’s request and physician-assisted suicide as intentionally helping a patient to end his or her life at his or her request. Euthanasia means ending a patient's life according to certain principles and under certain circumstances, where medicine can not cure or provide a life of acceptable quality. In two different ways based on physicians' action and patients' consent. It can be active or passive according to physicians' actions, and it is important to separate DNR orders and physician-assisted suicide from them; especially in countries like Turkey that are debating the level of technological development and their values. According to patients' consent, it is necessary to emphasize voluntary, non-voluntary and involuntary types of euthanasia (Aksoy 2000,Aksoy 1998, Ozkara et al 2001).

3. Attitudes towards euthanasia in Turkey

Euthanasia has deep historical roots. Before Hippocrates, euthanasia was a routine procedure and physicians assumed that they had the authority to kill patients for whom they gave up the hope of recovery, without asking for their permission (Ney 1997). They accepted this as a part of their medical practice. Hippocrates regarded this procedure as a hindrance to the establishment of confidentiality between physicians and patients. Probably this is the reason for the words in The Hippocratic Oath, "I will give no deadly medicine to anyone if asked, nor suggest any such counsel." This guarantee which Hippocrates provided by his oath, established the basis of the confidence between physicians and patients for 2500 years.

The effects of the Hippocratic Oath were noticed in Anatolia in the 19th century after modern medical schools had been established. Written sources (Lequenne 1991) show that euthanasia continued to be widely used after Hippocrates and was a socially exalted procedure among Galatians who settled in Anatolia in 287 BC and some other civilizations followed them. During this period suicide was also exalted by the society, and had some similarities with the harakiri tradition in Japan. Islamic domination put an end to both the euthanasia practice and its high regard in society in Anatolia. Euthanasia was wiped out of the society's living conscience during the period when Anatolia used to be a part of Islamic civilization. But it has continued to be a part of the social subconscience. The contemporary situation of the concepts of death and euthanasia in Anatolia, which entered a new period after the establishment of modern Turkey, was determined by its culture which was considerably affected by this social subconscience and Islamic belief.

Euthanasia is another ethical issue related to end of life decision making. The concept of euthanasia entered the agenda in Turkey in 1975. At the beginning, it was thought to be the problem of the countries where medicine was highly developed. The medical technology in Turkey was not very well-developed to make the euthanasia debate necessary at that time. Life sustaining systems rarely existed, intensive care and health care facilities were in poor conditions and hardly accessible. It has become an important problem in Turkey in the last decade, as the result of technological and medical developments. There are still some problems about the attainment and purchasing of health care facilities, and also about the level of medical care. But especially the developments in life sustaining systems and their efficient usage in daily practice made euthanasia an important subject for society. As physicians, patients, patients' relatives, insurance companies and jurists met the dilemma routinely, and as the mass media began to put it on the agenda more, a lot of discussions have taken place. This is an important pressure which forces the State to form some attitude about euthanasia.

The first euthanasia discussions had started in 1990s in Turkey. Official religious authorities and medical associations declared euthanasia as unacceptable. In those days there were very few people who have supported euthanasia in Turkey (Oguz, 1996). However, during the course of the time the research conducted in different centers have indicated that health care professionals, especially nurses support the assisted suicide and euthanasia (Bahcecik et al, 1998; Akcil et al, 1998; Ersoy and Altun, 2001). Despite these findings both passive and active euthanasia remain unlawful in Turkish Criminal Law. While passive euthanasia is considered as unintentional killing by law (Turkish Criminal Law. Article: 455), active euthanasia is punishable as intentional killing (Turkish Criminal Law. Article: 448) (Artuk, 2001) Like in all divinely revealed religions euthanasia is absolutely forbidden in Islamic understanding. (Rispler-Chaim, 1993)

In Turkey there is a great difference between the level of medical technology and the physician-patient relationship regarding the contemporary norms. Paternalistic attitudes are common and this also suits the expectations of society. Physicians rarely inform their patients about their diagnosis and treatment, even when it is not a fatal or hopeless situation. The primary reasons which physicians put forward about this fact are that they had to attend to too many patients and patients' educational level was not adequate (Hayran, 1994). Undoubtedly these are important factors, but there are evidences which indicate that they can not be the main ones. Even in private clinics where the number of patients per physician is very low, physicians' preferences regarding the relationship are quite similar to those of their colleagues in general hospitals. I think the main reason is the physicians' identity which is determined by medical education and social status. The physician-patient relationship in Turkey totally leans on the belief that a physician always does the best for their patient and always protects life. This belief established the myth of the "little god" physician. This view began to change and be corrupted dramatically in the last few years. The most appropriate word which describes the contemporary situation is chaos.

Today, many social institutions especially the mass media severely criticize physicians' attitudes in Turkey. Sometimes these criticisms turn out to be unfair attacks on medicine. This is the result of corruption in the myth of "little god" physician, and social disappointment about that. The associations of medical professionals try very hard to avoid any harm to medicine as a social institution while passing through this chaotic period. They try to re-establish confidentiality in physician-patient relationships on a stronger basis like the "informed consent doctrine". The foundation of the associations for specialized doctors of medicine is one of the main positive steps in realizing this purpose.

One of the most important factors which determines society's attitude towards euthanasia is religion. 90% of the Turkish population are Muslims. As there are various sects and tariqas that cause significant differences, it is important to begin with an overall review of Islamic approach to euthanasia. There are important differences between Islamic countries. The first group contains the countries which are governed by Islamic rules. These countries accept sheria as their legal and administrative code, like Iran and Saudi Arabia. In Iran Shia Muslims and in Saudi Arabia Sunni Muslims as sects of Islam, rule the State. The second group consists of countries which have secularly governed states, but their laws are based on sheria, like Egypt and Algeria. Actually this is the largest group. Turkey differs from these countries. Although the majority of the population is Muslim, the State is totally secular. Secularism in Turkey includes both the administrative, legislative and all other social systems. Despite a radical Islamic movement, which takes Turkey as its main target, cultural characteristics and historical background in 20th century led to a strong resistance in the society. Islam's approach to death is quite clear. Allah is the master of life and death. A Muslim is expected to know and accept that there are divine purposes in life's turning to be a painful one and in the delay of desired death. Ending life personally or asking somebody to do it instead, is regarded as an attempt to share Allah's power, so this is assumed to be an unforgivable sin. According to the Koran the wish for death is forbidden (Sahih-i Buhari, 1982; Nisâ sura of Koran). Suicide is the biggest sin (Sahih-i Buhari, 1982). No funeral prayer is made for such people, this means they can never be recipients of Allah's forgiveness. This situation affects the family as well, and causes isolation in society. Murder is a lighter sin. Even if there is no adequate reason found for tolerance, there is a chance for Allah's final forgiveness, because there is no rule which hinders his last prayer. When Islam's approach to death is examined with regards to the results of euthanasia, it is clear that in countries where sheria is in operation either totally or only legally, practicing euthanasia is impossible. Since Imam-i Gazali, an Islamic commentator (Karaman, 1971), Islamic rules have been assumed to have reached perfection, so there could be no additional rules except the interpretation of the existing ones. In Islam, rules about death are very clear that there is no place for interpretation. Islamic rules put every aspect of life in an order and health care issues are one of these aspects. Because of this, medicine in Islamic countries has developed according to these rules. This development has not reached the level of modern medicine yet, so euthanasia is not considered a real problem yet.

4. Turkish heath professionals' attitudes towards euthanasia

The concept of euthanasia and heath professional's attitudes towards euthanasia have been discussed in many research in Turkey. Mayda et al (2005) in their study reported that 43.8% of the oncologists did not object to euthanasia. Some 33.7% had been asked to perform euthanasia and 41.5% believed that euthanasia was performed secretly although it is against the law in Turkey. Forty-two doctors (50.6%) noted that they had withdrawn treatment in patients. The most frequently cited reasons for objecting to euthanasia were its unethical nature and the possibility of abuse. Although the overwhelming majority of the population in Turkey is Muslim, religious rules are not seen as the leading cause of objection to euthanasia. In fact, secularism and education may have influenced people's attitudes toward euthanasia. This is clearly ref lected in the questionnaire completed by doctors, who have a high level of education. Doctors who encounter terminally ill patients with cancer should update their knowledge about patients' rights and euthanasia. Doctors, who are often asked to perform euthanasia, especially in the cancer setting, can help to illuminate the debates about euthanasia.

In Turkey several studies have shown the following to be the most frequently given reasons for objecting to euthanasia: the possibility of its abuse (41.6%-72.8%) and conf lict with ethical values (24.9% and %32.9) or with religious beliefs (18.7% and %21.7) (Ozkara et al 2001,2002,2003,2004a,2004b). In another study from Turkey have been administrated by

Turla et al (2006). The study paticipants 43.5 % were medical doctor and 45.5% auxiliary health professionals. Of all participants, 33.6% did not object to euthanasia and 7.9% were asked to perform euthanasia. Eighty point seven percent of the participants noted that euthanasia could be abused even if a euthanasia law were passed. Only 7.9% of the health professionals were requested to perform euthanasia. This can be explained by that fact that the study included not only physicians but also other health professionals. It can be concluded that the health professionals should have a chance to discuss euthanasia and that their attitude toward and their expectations and worries about euthanasia should be taken into account when a euthanasia law is drafted.

The one of cross-sectional study was evaluated health professional's attitudes towards euthanasia in Manisa and Erciyes in Turkey (Karadeniz et al. 2008). Participants were doctors, nurses, and midwives in this study. Whereas 38.4% of the health personnel utterly agree to the definition of euthanasia as an act or practice of painlessly putting to death a person suffering from an incurable disease at his or her will, 11.2% of them express their absolute objection to the definition. While 46.7% of them fully support the idea that religious beliefs affect the decision to undergo euthanasia, 28% support the idea simply, and 4.3% of them don't support the idea at all. The idea that life support to a patient should be decreased if he or she expresses his wish to undergo euthanasia is rejected by 35.4% of them, but welcomed by 28.2%. However, 18.7% of them were undecided; 40.7% of them completely disagreed to the idea that a patient should not be fed if he or she expresses his wish to undergo euthanasia; 33.9% simply disagreed the idea; and 15% were undecided. The patient's wish to undergo euthanasia if he or she cannot live without a life support is rejected by 27.9% of them, whereas 25% of them are undecided. The view that euthanasia should be a legal procedure in all countries is supported by 16.5% and rejected by 29.3%. However, 24.4% of them are undecided. Those who say they will not perform euthanasia at all even if it becomes a legal procedure comprise 43.4% of them; while 5.7% say they can; and 23.9% of them are undecided. That the decision to undergo euthanasia should be given by the patient himself or herself is completely rejected by 21.7%; supported by 24.8%; and 19.9% are undecided. The percentages of health personnel who utterly disagree and who simply disagree to the opinion that the life of a patient should be terminated if he or she is in the vegetative state are the same: 26.6%. Those who are undecided are 28.2%; 42.4% of them say that they themselves would undergo euthanasia, while 17.9% of them say they would not; 5.7% of them were undecided. In Turkey, the approach of the health professional groups related closely with the subject and patients is being researched in many studies.

Another research investigates thoroughly the psychologists' approach to euthanasia practices in Turkey which is considered illegal in Turkey. The research participants were psychologists (n=100) who were working in Izmir (West Anatolia) and Ankara (Middle Anatolia). The participants were found to believe that euthanasia is being secretly practiced in Turkey despite being illegal and 85% view euthanasia as a legal right for patients with certain diseases (Ozkara 2004c).

Other study has been carried out to determine the opinions of nurses working in intensive care units (ICU) of the several hospitals in Adana (South Anatolia). This descriptive study was performed on 186 nurses working in the ICUs. The mean age of the nurses who 26.9 ±3.9, 73.7% of them had graduated from vocationals schools, and themean duration of professional experience was 6.6 ±5.1. Of all the nurses, 50.0% were married, 44.6% working at the ICU of internal medicine; 55.9% thought that euthanasia was the right of a patient as a human being, and 24.8% of them would ask for euthanasia if they were bedridden. Legal euthanasia in Turkey was not supported by 39.8% of the nurses, and there were more nurses supporting the legality of euthanasia (both active and passive). In case it becomes legal, 63.4% of the nurses think that euthanasia should be practiced by a team that determined by law, 81.7% would not want to take part in an euthanasia practice, 81.2% think that it could be exploited by people.of all the nurses 44.1% believe that euthanasia is being practiced in some conditions in our country. It was seen that nurses working in at ICU's support passive euthanasia rather than active euthanasia (Kumas 2005).

Tepehan, et al (2009) have evaluated doctors' and nurses' attitudes to euthanasia in intensive care units and surgical, internal medicine and paediatric units in Turkey. A total of 205 doctors and 206 nurses working in several hospitals in Istanbul participated. Significantly higher percentages of doctors (35.3%) and nurses (26.6%) working in intensive care units encountered euthanasia requests than those working in other units. Doctors and nurses caring for terminally ill patients in intensive care units differed considerably in their attitudes to euthanasia and patient rights from other health care staff. Recently, physician assisted suicide has been the topic of much controversy. Some nurses may see assisted suicide as an ethical dilemma; other nurses assisted suicide is still illegal.

A descriptive study investigated the current status of ethics instruction in Turkish nursing education programs. The sample for this study comprised 39 nursing schools, which represented 51% of all nursing schools in Turkey. The results revealed that 18 of these nursing schools incorporated an ethics course into undergraduate and three into graduate level programs. Most of the educators focused on the basic concepts of ethics, deontological theory, ethical principles, ethical problems in health care, patient rights and codes of ethics for nurses. More than half of the educators believed that students' theoretical knowledge of ethics is applied to their clinical experiences. The teaching methods used included discussion in class, lectures, case studies, small group discussion, dramatization and demonstration. Assessment was carried out by means of written essays and written examinations (Gorgulu & Dinc 2007).

Another study were to give Turkish university students on attitudes to euthanasia, and to assess the impact of type of education on attitudes towards euthanasia and to determine the influence of socio-demographics on attitudes of the students towards euthanasia. In total, 878 volunteered undergraduate registered students with the mean age of 21.13±1.92 year from six universities were surveyed. The students were divided into two groups according to education program as follows: Health Science students (HS) and Liberal Arts and Business students (LAB).Two students major groups-Health Science (n = 421) and Liberal Arts and Business (n = 457), were compared. 48.4% of the students were positive to euthanasia. The socio-demographic factors, including mother`s education level, family`s socio-economic background, religious belief and religiosity were seen to be influenced on attitudes towards euthanasia among the overall students. No significant difference regarding the acceptance of euthanasia between the Health Science majors and the Liberal Arts and Business majors. Mainly, 40% of the Muslim students are opposed to euthanasia, whereas 86.7% of the atheist students are the most in favour of euthanasia. The religion was selected as the most important reason for being negative to euthanasia. The results showed that resistance to euthanasia is apparently associated with demographics and non-scientific reasoning among Turkish undergraduate students (Bas Aslan & Cavlak 2007).

While a topic long debated in Western nations at a public level, euthanasia (Physician-assisted suicide) in Turkey has been a subject relegated to debate among a small group of subject experts. For the first time, as a component of Turkey's First Gerontology Atlas (GeroAtlas) research project, euthanasia has been investigated from the perspective of the elderly. Based on the analysis of gender specific data acquired in the project, a number of observations have been presented. The purpose of this research is not solely to present the perspectives of the elderly concerning euthanasia, but to call attention to the need to bring deliberation on this topic into the realm of public opinion, to go deeper and bring new perspectives to light, and emphasize the need for people from all segments of society to enter this debate (Tufan 2009).

In other interventional study was undertaken to assess the impact of physiotherapy education on the knowledge and attitudes of physiotherapists (PTs) and physiotherapy students (PSs) toward euthanasia. The study, which included a total of 494 participants (311 PTs; 183 PSs) aged 18 to 52 y from the western and central portions of Turkey. Results indicated that PTs (48.9%) were more likely to approve of euthanasia than PSs (38.3%) ($P<.05$). The legalization of euthanasia was favored by 43.7% of PTs, compared with 29.5% of PSs ($P<.05$). On the other hand, PTs and PSs expressed similar views regarding euthanasia, including reasons for accepting or opposing euthanasia and acceptable conditions for its use ($P>.05$). Overall results showed that sex and age had no effect on whether euthanasia was accepted ($P>.05$); religiousness was found to have the greatest effect on attitudes toward euthanasia ($P<.05$). The findings of the current study suggest that (1) the attitudes of PTs are different from those of PSs, and (2) the Islamic point of view has a negative impact on the attitudes of PTs and PSs toward euthanasia (Cavlak, et al 2007).

Kok, et al (2003) in their study to determine the approach and expectation of physicians at Erzurum (East Anatolia) on the subject of euthanasia. In this cross-sectional study, a questionnaire was applied to 69 physicians working at Erzurum. Out of 69 physicians that replied the questionnaire 55% was male, 63% of physicians declared that theyare against euthanasia practice to be legalised. 68 % of participants said that euthanasia discussion in our country is beneficial. In other study 87 physicians working at Duzce, an important city of Black Sea region. 72% of participants were male and the mean age is 33.14±7.29 years, and 54% of participants were specialist. 48% of physicians declared that they are against euthanasia practice to be legalised. While only 12% of the doctors attending our study declared that they had come across formal request of euthanasia 42% said that they believed that euthanasia in our country has been practiced secretly although it is forbidden. 84 % of participants said that euthanasia discussion in our country is beneficial (Ozkara, et al 2004d).

Bilgen, et al (2009) in their study was to assess the attitudes and practices of doctors and nurses about end-of-life decisions and compare our results with those observed in different European countries. The data was collected from nurses and doctors, using a standardized questionnaire adapted from the EURONIC study. A total of 250 structured questionnaires were delivered, and 135 (77%) of them were accepted for analysis. The end-of-life decision was taken in 39.4% of the hospitals and personal involvement was 40%. Although an ethical committee was present in the hospitals of 61.5% of responders, a written policy was present in only 3.1% of the units. The mean attitude score was 6.5. Seventy-five percent of the contributors agreed that everything possible should be done to ensure a neonate's survival regardless of the prognosis and 65.2% of responders believed that costs of health care should not affect nontreatment decisions. Most of the responders (65.2%) agreed that severe mental disability as an outcome was equal to or worse than death. In patients in whom medical intervention would be futile, or would not offer sufficient benefit to justify the burdens imposed, hospitals should set up a functional ethical committee in order to decide in matters of withholding or withdrawing intervention.

Another study was to reveal what pneumologists who worked in oncology clinics thought about euthanasia. The mean age of the pneumologists included in the study (n=110) was 32.90±7.01 years. Of the pneumologists, 40.8% were against euthanasia and 46.7% believed that euthanasia was performed in Turkey although it was illegal. Thirty-one point five percent of the pneumologists working in oncology clinics and 14.3% of the pneumologists working in clinics other than oncology clinics faced euthanasia requests. The opinions of health professionals taking care of terminally ill patients on euthanasia and patient rights are very important. Frequent requests for euthanasia and the health professionals' belief that euthanasia is performed secretly in Turkey demonstrate that euthanasia should be discussed openly and attitude and approach towards euthanasia should be investigated (Yalniz, et al 2010).

In many European countries, the last decade has been marked by an increasing debate about the acceptability and regulation of euthanasia and other end-of-life decisions in medical practice. Growing public sensibility to a 'right to die' for terminally ill patients has been one of the main constituents of these debates. Cohen, et al (2006) have described and compared acceptance of euthanasia among the general public in 33 European countries. Results showed that the acceptance of euthanasia tended to be high in some countries (e.g. the Netherlands, Denmark, France, Sweden), while a markedly low acceptance was found in others (e.g. Romania, Malta and Turkey). A multivariate ordinal regression showed that weaker religious belief was the most important factor associated with a higher acceptance; however, there were also socio-demographic differences: younger cohorts, people from non-manual social classes, and people with a higher educational level tended to have a higher acceptance of euthanasia. While religious belief, socio-demographic factors, and also moral values (i.e. the belief in the right to self-determination) could largely explain the differences between countries, our findings suggest that perceptions regarding euthanasia are probably also influenced by national traditions and history (e.g. Germany).

5. Factors of affecting attitudes towards euthanasia

According to several study of result have described various factors which have a great influence on most individuals' view of euthanasia. These factors include cultural and religious beliefs, age, gender and socio-demographic factors.

5.1 Age

Age has a very strong impact on people's attitudes towards euthanasia. An elderly person with a terminal illness is vulnerable. They may lack the knowledge and skills to alleviate their symptoms, and may well suffer from fear about the future and anxiety about the effect of the illness on others. The elderly person's decision making about euthanasia may be affected by confusion, dementia, depression or other related symptoms, which could be relieved with appropriate treatment and social support. Great pressure is experienced by elderly people to request euthanasia because many of them already feel a burden to their families and caregivers. Another study in India to determine the elderly's attitude towards death, the majority were not afraid of death, due to their strong faith in God. About 61.5% of the elderly supported euthanasia, but expressed concern that euthanasia might be misused as a means of getting rid of invalid elderly persons and avoiding the responsibility of caring for them. In the study conducted by one researcher a significant association between age and the choice for euthanasia was found. It was also reported another study that support for voluntary euthanasia is even stronger among the elderly.

5.2 Race

Life-prolonging techniques became increasingly available and there were possibly generational and cultural changes in patients' attitudes. According to several researchers attitudes towards the dying patient and the appropriate treatment approach are based on cultural and emotional factors. A cross-cultural perspective on any aspect of the attitude process could enrich our understanding in that it could provide insights that reach to the very core of societal stability. The first process is the way we express our attitudes toward other people and secondly is attitude change.

5.3 Religion

It is simply assumed that most Christians are united in their opposition to assisted suicide and voluntary euthanasia. Although many regular churchgoers apparently agree with legalizing some forms of active euthanasia, most theologians and church leaders remained opposed. Some church leaders suggest that to accept that one is not going to get well and therefore to request help to die is an act of faithless misery, a decree of hopelessness, and as such an offence against two of the central theological qualities, faith and hope. In the study conducted by another researcher, it was reported that Buddhists ideas in relation to euthanasia converge with Christian views.

In South Africa Muslims made a declaration that active euthanasia where patients may end their lives by lethal injection is impermissible under any circumstances and that passive euthanasia where patients may withhold treatment or artificial life-support is only permissible if a trustworthy, reliable opinion and specialist feels that there is no hope of survival. In the study to determine American attitudes toward the physician's role were found that various religious groups have strong effects on attitudes toward many social, political and moral issues.

Protestants have been found to hold different attitudes concerning active euthanasia than Catholics. Among Protestant clergy, 73.2% accepted active euthanasia as a viable option, as opposed to 63.1% of the Catholic clergy. Protestants tended to favour active euthanasia more often than Catholics.

5.4 Gender

Patients' choices for care in the event of terminal illness relate to a complicated set of demographic, educational and cultural factors. One of study found that women wanted life-sustaining treatments less often than did men. In a study that was conducted by another researcher about euthanasia and women, when mercy killings occur they are usually administered by men for women, with two-thirds of those being female. She also reported that women are over represented in assisted suicide and euthanasia reports. In addition, women will be affected most by euthanasia simply because they live longer and have fewer resources than men.

5.5 Socio-demographic factors

Researchers found that social changes, such as circumstantial changes, have an effect on people's attitudes towards euthanasia in South Africa. Another study was shown that economic factors play a role in the individuals' request for euthanasia. They mentioned that as medical treatment at the end of life becomes more than ever expensive, health insurance above all in the USA are beginning to question the economic soundness of providing long-term treatment to terminally ill patients. According to many researchers highly educated, politically liberal people with a less religious self-perception are most likely to accept active euthanasia in the case of a terminally ill patient (Ramabele 2004).

Many countries display their approach towards euthanasia according to their own conditions. Euthanasia is legal only in Holland and Belgium. Legal status of euthanasia varies from country to country. In contrast, euthanasia is stil illegal in many countrys. It was defined as "murder on request" in criminal laws of some countries such as Germany and Austria and it was not clearly defined but prohibited in some other countries such as Japan and Turkey.

In Japan, people who perform euthanasia are sentenced to six months to seven years imprisonment. In Turkey, active euthanasia is not clearly defined in the criminal law, but it is considered "murder." There is not an agreement about passive euthanasia, but it is not thought to deserve strict punishment. Assisted suicide is considered a kind of help to commit suicide.

6. Conclusions

In this book chapter we want to discuss Turkish health professional's attitudes towards euthanasia. Under these conditions, it is important to keep the discussion healthy and alive. Any effort which tends to reach a consensus on this subject will help us in finding a way towards a rational solution for the euthanasia debate in Turkey.

7. References

[1] Aksoy, S (1998). 'Saglik Kaynaklarinin Dagitiminda ve Tedavi Kararinin Verilmesinde Kullanilan Kriterlerin Etik Tartismasi' (Ethical Discussion of Criteria Used in the Distribution of Health Care Resources), (eds.) Pelin, S., Arda, B., Ozcelikay, G., Ozgur, A. ve Senler, F. 3. Tibbi Etik Sempozyumu Bildirileri, Ankara, pp 419-24. (in Turkish)

[2] Republic of Turkey, Prime Ministry State Institute of Statistics. http://www.die.gov.tr/ENGLISH/index.html

[3] Randall, F. & Downie, R.S (1996). Palliative Care Ethics. Oxford University Press, Oxford.

[4] Oguz, Y (2001). 'Tip etigi acisindan yasamin son doneminde karar verme surecleri.' (End of life decision making processes from medical ethics perspective.) Medikal Etik, 3: 61-67. (in Turkish)

[5] Aksoy, S (2000). 'Can Euthanasia be Part of a 'Good-doctoring'?' Eubios Journal of Asian and International Bioethics, 10(5): 152-54.

[6] Ney, PG (1994). The universal ethic of mutual benefit. T.Klin.TibbiEtik 2:53-56.

[7] Lequenne F (1991). *Galatlar. (Les Galates)*. 2nd. edition. Ankara. TTK Pub. 16-27 (in Turkish).

[8] Oguz, Y (1996). 'Euthanasia In Turkey: Cultural and Religious perspectives' Eubios Journal of Asian and International Bioethics 6:170-1.

[9] Bahcecik, N., Alpar, S.E., Yildirim, Y., Temiz, G., Ozen, C. and Keles, S (1998). 'Hemsirelerin Otanazi Konusundaki Gorusleri'. (Nurses' View on Euthanasia) Proceedings of 3rd National Bioethics Symposium. Ankara, pp 339-348. (In Turkish)

[10] Akcil, M., Bilgili, N., Turkan, S.K., Yardim, M. and Yildiz, A.N (1998). 'Universite Son Sinif Ogrencilerinin Otanazi Konusundaki Gorusleri' (Views of Final Year University Students on Euthanasia). Proceedings of 3rd National Bioethics Symposium. Ankara, pp 149-158. (In Turkish)

[11] Ersoy, N. & Altun, I (2001). 'Hemsirelerin Yardimli Intihar Hakkinda Gorusleri ile Ilgili Bir Calisma' (A Study on Nurses' Views on Assisted Suicide). Turkiye Klinikleri Journal of Medical Ethics. 9:49-55. (In Turkish)

[12] Artuk, M.E (2001). 'Hukukcu Gozuyle Otanazi' (Euthanasia from Lawyer's Perspective). In Ed. Hatemi, H. and Dogan, H. Medikal Etik. Yuce Publication, Istanbul, pp:42-60

[13] Rispler-Chaim (1993). V. Islamic Medical Ethics in the Twentieth Century. E.J. Brill, Leiden, pp 94-99.

[14] Hayran, O., Gürsoy, A., Akçay F., Savas, H (1994). Turkish physicians' attitudes to ethical issues. BME. 102:16-21.

[15] *Sahih-i Buhari*. (trans. Miras K.) (1982) 7th edition. Ankara. Turkish Religious Affairs Publication. Vol. 12. pp.70-1.(in Turkish)

[16] Nisâ sura of *Koran*. Verse no.29.(in Turkish)

[17] *Sahih-i Buhari*. (trans. Miras K.) (1982) 7th edition. Ankara. Turkish Religious Affairs Publication. Vol.4. pp.559-65.(in Turkish)

[18] Karaman, H (1971). Islam Hukukunda Içtihat. (Conviction in Islamic Legislation) 1st edition. Ankara. Turkish Religious Affairs Publication, pp.187-88. (in Turkish)

[19] Mayda, SA., Ozkara, E., Corapcioglu, F (2005). Attitudes of oncologists toward euthanasia in Turkey Pallative and Supportive Care. 3:221-25.

[20] Ozkara, E., Yemiscigil, A., & Dalgic, M (2001). The opinions of law school students on the issue of euthanasia. Journal of Forensic Medicine. 15:46–52 (in Turkish).

[21] Ozkara, E., Ozdemir, C., Hanci, IH., et al (2002). Attitudes of doctors working in Ankara towards euthanasia. Journal of Faculty of Law, University of Ankara, 51:207–214 (in Turkish)

[22] Ozkara, E., Sen, H., Tok, M., et al (2003). Attitudes of Istanbul physicians toward euthanasia. Forensic Science International. *136* (Suppl. 1) 330–1.

[23] Ozkara, E., Civaner, M., Oglak, S., et al (2004a). Euthanasia education for health professionals in Turkey: Students change their opinions. Nursing Ethics. 11:290–97.

[24] Ozkara, E., Hancı, H., Civaner, M., et al (2004b). Turkey's physicians' attitude towards euthanasia: A brief research report. Omega (Westport). 49(2):109–115.

[25] Turla, A., Ozkara, E., Ozkanli, C., Alkan, N (2006-2007). Health professional's attitudes toward euthanasia:A cross sectional study in Turkey.Omega. 54(2):135-145.

[26] Karadeniz, G., Yanikkerem, E., Pirinci, E., Erdem, R., Esen, A., Kitapcioglu, G (2008).Turkish health professional's attitude toward euthanasia.Omega. 57(1):93-112.

[27] Ozkara, E., Inceer, B., Hanci, IH., Ozan, G., Oral, G (2004c). Psikiyatristlerin otenaziye yaklasimi. Adli Tip Psikiyatri Dergisi. 1(1):35-42 (in Turkish).

[28] Kumas, G (2005). Adana ilindeki cesitli hastanelerin yogun bakim unitelerinde calisan hemsirelerin otanazi hakkindaki dusunceleri. (Master Thesis) Adana: Cukurova Universitesi Saglik Bilimleri Enstitusu Hemsirelik Anabilim Dali (in Turkish).

[29] Tepehan, S, Ozkara, E, Yavuz, FM (2009). Attitudes to euthanasia in icus and other hospital departments. Nurs Ethics 16(3):319-27.

[30] Gorgulu, RS, Dinc, L (2007). Ethics in Turkish nursing education programs. Nurs Ethics 14(6):741-52.

[31] Bas Aslan, U, Cavlak, U (2007). Attitudes towards euthanasia among university students: A sample based on Turkish population. J. Medical Sci., 7: 396-401.

[32] Tufan, I (2009). The View of Turkish Elderly on Euthanasia: Results from First Turkish Gerontology Atlas Study. Geriatri ve Geriatrik Nöropsikiyatri Dergisi 1(2):23-27 (In Turkish).

[33] Cavlak, U, Bas Aslan, U, Gurso, S, Yagci, N, Yeldan, I (2007). Attitudes of physiotherapists and physiotherapy students toward euthanasia: A comparative study. Advances in Therapy 24(1):135-45.

[34] Kok, NA, Ozkara, E, Dakgic, M, Sener, M (2003). The opinions of physicians working at Erzurum about euthanasia. Turk J Emerg Med. 3(2): 41-46 (In Turkish).

[35] Ozkara, E, Bukan, B, Dalgic, M, Mayda, S,A (2004d). Opinions of physicians working at düzce about euthanasia. Adli Psikiyatri Dergisi 1(1):9-13 (In Turkish).

[36] Bilgen, H, Topuzoglu, A, Kuscu, K, et al (2009). End-of-life decisions in the newborn period: attitudes and practices of doctors and nurses The Turkish Journal of Pediatrics 51:248-56.

[37] Yalniz, E, Ozkara, E, Komurcuoglu, B, et al (2010). Pneumologısts' approach towards euthanasıa Turkish Journal Geriatrics 13(4):219-24.

[38] Cohen, J, Marcoux, I, Bilsen, J, et al (2006). European public acceptance of euthanasia: Socio-demographic and cultural factors associated with the acceptance of euthanasia in 33 European countries Social Science & Medicine 63(3):743-56.

[39] Ramabele T (2004). Attitudes of the elderly towards euthanasia:A cross cultural study. (Master Thesis). Faculty of Humanities Departmant of Psychology University of Free State.

Part 4

Euthanasia of Animals

10

Medical and Bioethical Issues in Laboratory Animal

Matilde Jiménez-Coello, Karla Y. Acosta-Viana,
Antonio Ortega-Pacheco and Eugenia Guzmán-Marín
Universidad Autónoma de Yucatán
México

1. Introduction

Euthanasia in laboratory animals is a routinely procedure to properly complete the tests and experiments in which these models have a key role for the precise evaluation of various issues during the development of a scientific activity (Van Zutphen, 2001). The term euthanasia is derived from the Greek terms *eu* meaning good and *thanatos* meaning death (Webster, 1990). It is a necessary and accepted procedure in all aspects of veterinary medicine and many aspects of scientific procedures involving animals (Reilly, 2001). A "good death" would be one that occurs with minimal pain and distress.

It has been estimated that 75 to 100 million vertebrates are used per year worldwide in research, teaching and testing activities for a wide range of purposes. Only in Europe 10.7 million vertebrates are used annually for research purposes (Van Zutphen, 2001). Drug research, testing of vaccines and other biologicals, and cancer research account for about 70% of the animals used, while the remaining 30% are used for purposes such as fundamental research, for diagnostic purposes, for teaching, etc. (Fig. 1) (Baumans, 2005) therefore, animals need to be killed for various reasons, including the collection of blood and tissues, culling of breeding stock, disposal at the end of an experiment and in those circumstances where animals are experiencing pain and distress which cannot be alleviated (Reilly, 2001).

Euthanasia techniques should result in rapid loss of consciousness followed by cardiac or respiratory arrest and the ultimate loss of brain function. In addition, the technique should minimize distress and anxiety experienced by the animal prior to loss of consciousness (AVMA, 2007). For these reason, if an animal has to be killed, death must occur with the least fear, anxiety, pain and distress. The method used for euthanasia must either kill the animal very rapidly or instantaneously render the animal unconscious so that death ensues before consciousness is regained (Reilly, 2001).

Selection of the most appropriate method of euthanasia in any given situation depends on the species of animal involved, adequate methods of animal restraint, skill of personnel, number of animals, and other considerations. Available information focuses primarily on domestic animals, but the same general considerations should be applied to all species. For the best method of euthanasia, the following criteria must be considered: (1) ability to induce loss of consciousness and death without causing pain, distress, anxiety, or apprehension; (2) time required to induce loss of consciousness; (3) reliability; (4) safety of personnel; (5) irreversibility; (6) compatibility with requirement and purpose; (7) emotional effect on observers or operators; (8) compatibility with subsequent evaluation, examination, or use of tissue; (9) drug availability and human abuse potential; (10) compatibility with species, age, and health status; (11) ability to maintain equipment in proper working order; and (12) safety for predators/scavengers should the carcass be consumed (AVMA, 2007).

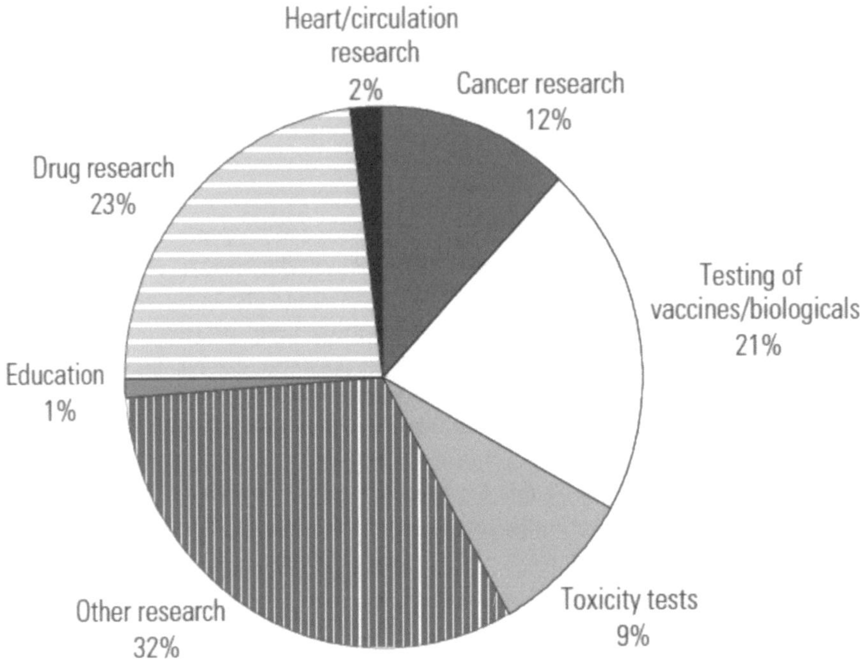

Fig. 1. Distribution of the purposes of animal use in research (Baumans, 2005)

In this chapter, attention is paid to provide investigators and technicians details of the current state of information relevant to the euthanasia of animals used for scientific purposes, so they can choose the better decision about the suitability of methods for euthanasia considering the welfare of animals.

2. Objectives of the euthanasia

The primary criteria for euthanasia in terms of animal welfare is that the method used should be painless, achieve rapid unconsciousness and death, require minimum restraint, avoid excitement, is appropriate for the age, species, and health of the animal, must minimize fear and psychological stress in the animal, be reliable, reproducible, irreversible, simple to administer (in small doses if possible) and safe for the operator, and, so far as possible, be aesthetically acceptable for the operator (Close et al., 1996).

Animals are killed in laboratories or breeding establishments for various reasons:	**Statements to consider when is necessary to kill an animal,**
At the end of an experiment or when there might be continuing adverse effects;	Humane procedures must be used (avoiding distress, reliable, producing rapid loss of consciousness without pain until death occurs and procedures should also be compatible with the scientific or educational aims
To provide blood and · other tissues for a scientific purpose;	Procedures must be performed only by persons competent in the method to be used, or under direct supervision of a competent person.
When levels of pain, distress and suffering are likely to exceed the designated level;	The appropriate means must be readily at hand
Where the health or welfare of the animals are grounds for concern;	Animals should be killed in a quiet, clean environment and normally away from other animals. There should be no disposal of the carcass until death is established.
When they are no longer suitable for breeding;	Dependent neonates of animals being killed must also be killed or provision made for their care
Unwanted stock or those with unsuitable characteristics, for example, type or sex, are not needed.	When fertilized eggs are used, the method of disposal must ensure the death of the embryo.

Table 1. Reasons to explain why the laboratory animals must be euthanatized and statements to consider for do it.

2.1 Signs of pain or distress in animals

When animals are killed, both the method of euthanasia, particularly the time taken to produce unconciseness, and how the technique is performed can result in animals experiencing pain, distress, fear and anxiety. Furthermore, the animal's psychological response to the environment in which it is killed, including interactions with other animals and humans and how it is handled, can result in emotional distress.

Pain may be defined as "an aversive sensory experience that elicits protective motor actions, results in learned avoidance and may modify species-specific traits of behaviour, including social behaviour" The use of the word pain implies a conscious awareness of the stimulus and not an unconscious reflex response (Close et al., 1996).

Physiologically, pain is that sensation (perception) that results from nerve impulses reaching the cerebral cortex via ascending neural pathways. Under normal circumstances, these pathways are relatively specific, but the nervous system is sufficiently plastic that activation of nociceptive pathways does not always result in pain and stimulation of other (non-nociceptive) peripheral and central neurons can give rise to pain. The term nociceptive is derived from the word *noci* meaning to injure and *ceptive* meaning to receive, and is used to describe neuronal input caused by noxious stimuli, which threaten to, or actually do, destroy tissue. These noxious stimuli initiate nerve impulses by acting at primary nociceptors and other sensory nerve endings that respond to noxious and non-noxious stimuli from mechanical, thermal, or chemical activity. Endogenous chemical substances such as hydrogen ions, potassium ions, ATP, serotonin, histamine, bradykinin, and prostaglandins, as well as electrical currents, are capable of generating nerve impulses in nociceptor nerve fibers. Activity in nociceptive pathways can also be triggered in normally silent receptors that become sensitized by chronic pain condition (Vierck et al., 1989; Wall, 1992).

Nerve impulse activity generated by nociceptors is conducted via nociceptor primary afferent fibers to the spinal cord or the brainstem where it is transmitted to two general sets of neural networks. One set is related to nociceptive reflexes (eg, withdrawal and flexion reflexes) that are mediated at the spinal level, and the second set consists of ascending pathways to the reticular formation, hypothalamus, thalamus, and cerebral cortex (somatosensory cortex and limbic system) for sensory processing. It is important to understand that ascending nociceptive pathways are numerous, often redundant, and are capable of considerable plasticity under chronic conditions (pathology or injury). Moreover, even the transmission of nociceptive neural activity in a given pathway is highly variable. Under certain conditions, both the nociceptive reflexes and the ascending pathways may be suppressed, as, for example, in epidural anesthesia. Under another set of conditions, nociceptive reflex actions may occur, but activity in the ascending pathways is suppressed; thus, noxious stimuli are not perceived as pain. It is incorrect to use the term pain for stimuli, receptors, reflexes, or pathways because the term implies perception, whereas all the above may be active without consequential pain perception (Breazile & Kitchel, 1969; Zinnerman, 1984).

Pain is divided into two broad categories: (1) sensory-discriminative, which indicates the site of origin and the stimulus giving rise to the pain; and (2) motivational-affective in which the severity of the stimulus is perceived and the animal's response is determined. Sensory-discriminative processing of nociceptive impulses is most likely to be accomplished by subcortical and cortical mechanisms similar to those used for processing other sensory-discriminative input that provides provides the individual with information about the intensity, duration, location, and quality of the stimulus. Motivational-affective processing involves the ascending reticular formation for behavioral and cortical arousal. It also involves thalamic input to the forebrain and the limbic system for perceptions such as discomfort, fear, anxiety, and depression. The motivational-affective neural networks also have strong inputs to the limbic system, hypothalamus and the autonomic nervous system for reflex activation of the cardiovascular, pulmonary, and pituitary-adrenal systems. Responses activated by these systems feed back to the forebrain and enhance perceptions derived via motivational-affective inputs. On the basis of neurosurgical experience in humans, it is possible to separate the sensory-discriminative components from the motivational-affective components of pain (Kitchel et al., 1993).

For pain to be experienced, the cerebral cortex and subcortical structures must be functional. If the cerebral cortex is nonfunctional because of hypoxia, depression by drugs, electric shock, or concussion, pain is not experienced. Therefore, the choice of the euthanasia agent or method is less critical if it is to be used on an animal that is anesthetized or unconscious, provided that the animal does not regain consciousness prior to death.

An understanding of the continuum that represents stress and distress is essential for evaluating techniques that minimize any distress experienced by an animal being euthanatized. Stress has been defined as the effect of physical, physiologic, or emotional factors (stressors) that induce an alteration in an animal's homeostasis or adaptive state

(Kitchen et al., 1989). The response of an animal to stress represents the adaptive process that is necessary to restore the baseline mental and physiologic state. These responses may involve changes in an animal's neuroendocrinologic system, autonomic nervous system, and mental status that may result in overt behavioral changes. An animal's response varies according to its experience, age, species, breed, and current physiologic and psychologic state (NRC, 1992).

2.2 Identification and recognition of death

It is essential that all personnel are trained to recognize and confirm death in the species they are working. The most important aspects in recognition of death include cessation of heartbeat and respiration, absence of reflexes, and in small laboratory animals, the lowering of the body temperature to below 25°C. The method chosen will depend on the species being handled. If there is any doubt about confirmation of death, a second method should be used to kill the animal (Close et al., 1996).

2.3 Personal training

All methods of euthanasia can be badly performed and therefore personnel carrying out euthanasia on animals must be suitably trained to carry out euthanasia in the most effective and humane manner. Professional advice should be sought (Close et al., 1996). Personnel who perform euthanasia must have appropriate certification and training, experience with the techniques to be used, and experience in the humane restraint of the species of animal to be euthanatized, to ensure that animal pain and distress are minimized during euthanasia. Training and experience should include familiarity with the normal behaviour of the species being euthanatized, an appreciation of how handling and restraint affects that behaviour, and an understanding of the mechanism by which the selected technique induces loss of consciousness and death. Prior to being assigned full responsibility for performing euthanasia, all personnel must have demonstrated proficiency in the use of the technique in a closely supervised environment (AVMA, 2007). Training programmes should include courses on the biology of the species to be used, suitable methods of euthanasia for each species and national and animal welfare regulations. Training must include aspects such as recognition of pain, fear, distress, anxiety, insensibility and death for all species to be used.
Experienced personnel who have developed a trusting relationship with the particular animals should be used for euthanasia of these animals as this will minimize stress and anxiety in the animals.
All people performing euthanasia should demonstrate professionalism and sensitivity for the value of animal life. The degree of distress experienced by those people observing or performing euthanasia in any form is dependent on their backgrounds and on their personal philosophies and ethical concerns about using animals in research. The stress of performing euthanasia is magnified when there are strong emotional bonds between personnel and individual animals or when large numbers of animals are killed on a regular basis (Close et al., 1996).

2.4 Equipment and Instrumentation required

Equipment, instruments and installations used for stunning or killing animals should be designed, constructed and maintained so as to achieve rapid stunning and death. They should be regularly inspected and cleaned to (Close et al., 1996).

2.5 Disposal of carcasses

After death has been verified, the carcase must be disposed of appropriately (Reilly, 2001). The possible hazards to humans when animals are known to be carrying a zoonotic agent or were treated with radioisotopes or toxic chemicals must be evaluated and personnel handling such carcasses should take the necessary precautions to protect themselves and others (Close et al., 1996). This is particularly important for animal such as sheep, cattle, pigs and horses which may be used for human or pet food (Reilly, 2001). Care should be taken when disposing of carcasses and other waste, for example water in which agents have been dissolved that it does not provide any danger to others or the environment (Close et al., 1996).

2.6 Modes of action of euthanatizing agents

Euthanatizing agents cause death by three basic mechanisms: (1) hypoxia, direct or indirect; (2) direct depression of neurons necessary for life function; and (3) physical disruption of brain activity and destruction of neurons necessary for life.
Agents that induce death by direct or indirect hypoxia can act at various sites and can cause loss of consciousness at different rates. For death to be painless and distress-free, loss of consciousness should precede loss of motor activity (muscle movement). Loss of motor activity, however, cannot be equated with loss of consciousness and absence of distress. Thus, agents that induce muscle paralysis without loss of consciousness are not acceptable as sole agents for euthanasia (eg, depolarizing and nondepolarizing muscle relaxants, strychnine, nicotine, and magnesium salts). With other techniques that induce hypoxia, some animals may have motor activity following loss of consciousness, but this is reflex activity and is not perceived by the animal.
A second group of euthanatizing agents depress nerve cells of the brain, inducing loss of consciousness followed by death. Some of these agents release inhibition of motor activity during the first stage of anesthesia, resulting in a so-called excitement or delirium phase, during which there may be vocalization and some muscle contraction. These responses do not appear to be purposeful. Death follows loss of consciousness, and is attributable to cardiac arrest and/or hypoxemia following direct depression of respiratory centers.
Physical disruption of brain activity, caused by concussion, direct destruction of the brain, or electrical depolarization of neurons, induces rapid loss of consciousness. Death occurs because of destruction of midbrain centers controlling cardiac and respiratory activity or as a result of adjunctive methods (eg, exsanguination) used to kill the animal. Exaggerated muscular activity can follow loss of consciousness and, although this may disturb some observers, the animal is not experiencing pain or distress (AVMA, 2007).

2.7 Acceptable methods of euthanasia in laboratory animals

2.7.1 Physical methods

These methods must cause immediate loss of consciousness through physical trauma to the brain. They are most useful when pharmacological methods would interfere with the purpose of the experiment. While physical methods may be aesthetically less pleasant for observers and those killing animals, in skilled hands they are quick and certain and possibly the least distressing for the animal.
Specialist training is essential for all of these methods. These methods require restraint which may cause extra stress for some animals. If possible the animal should not be killed in the sight or smell of other animals (Close et al., 1996).

2.7.1.1 Shooting

Shooting in the head to ensure immediate destruction of the brain is an effective and humane way of killing large reptiles and mammals. This may be divided into two types: captive bolt or free bullet. The type of weapon used must be selected according to the species to be killed and the environment.

Captive bolt: A penetrating captive bolt is used for euthanasia of ruminants, horses, swine, laboratory rabbits, and dogs. Its mode of action is concussion and trauma to the cerebral hemisphere and brainstem (Blackmore, 1985; Dennis et al., 1988; Daly and Whittington, 1989). Captive bolt guns are powered by gunpowder or compressed air and must provide sufficient energy to penetrate the skull of the species on which they are being used (Blackmore, 1985). Adequate restraint is important to ensure proper placement of the captive bolt. A cerebral hemisphere and the brainstem must be sufficiently disrupted by the projectile to induce sudden loss of consciousness and subsequent death. Accurate placement of captive bolts for various species has been described (Clifford, 1984; Blackmore, 1985; Daly and Whittington, 1989). A multiple projectile has been suggested as a more effective technique, especially for large cattle (Blackmore, 1985). A nonpenetrating captive bolt only stuns animals and should not be used as a sole means of euthanasia (must be stunning under adjunctive methods). An advantage of the penetrating captive bolt is that could be an effective method of euthanasia for use in research facilities, in slaughterhouses, and on the farm when use of drugs is inappropriate or unavailable, but the disadvantages of this method is that is aesthetically displeasing and the death may not occur if equipment is not maintained and used properly. The use of the penetrating captive bolt is an acceptable and practical method of euthanasia in horses, ruminants, and swine, and it is conditionally acceptable in other appropriate species. However the non-penetrating captive bolt must not be used as a sole method of euthanasia.

Free bullet: Special care must be taken to avoid danger to the operator using this method. All personnel must be trained in these techniques to ensure the correct positioning of the weapon to ensure a direct hit into the brain (Longair et al., 1991). Shooting using a free bullet must not be used inside a building because of danger to personnel from ricocheting bullets, but it may be used effectively in the field by skilled marksmen. When the animal can be appropriately restrained, the captive bolt method is preferable as there is less danger to personnel. A free bullet humane killer is preferred for example, on horses (Oliver, 1979; Blackmore, 1985; Dodd, 1985).

2.7.1.2 Concussion

This may be carried out by several means depending on the size of the animal. In smaller animals such as small rabbits, newborn kittens and newborn puppies, rats, mice, young guinea pigs, hamsters, birds, small reptiles, amphibians and fish (Clifford, 1984), a blow on the head may be sufficient to render the animal insensible (Green, 1987). Experience and training are essential for the correct choice of method to be used.

In larger animals specialized equipment such as the non-penetrating captive bolt must be used. **The use of the hammer or poleaxe is condemned as a method of stunning.** These methods must always be followed immediately by exsanguination, removal of the heart or destruction of the brain to ensure death. Training is essential for all operators. If not performed correctly, various degrees of consciousness with concomitant pain can ensue.

It is difficult to ensure consistency in performance by operators and therefore only a few animals should be killed using this method at any time. Death must be confirmed in each animal before the next animal is stunned.

High pressure water jet has been successfully used for the stunning of pigs and is an accepted method in Switzerland (Schatzmann et al., 1991, 1994).

2.7.1.3 Electrical stunning

Electrical current has been used for stunning species such as dogs, cattle, sheep, goats, hogs, fish and chickens (Warrington, 1974; Gregory & Wotton, 1986; Eikelenboom, 1986; Lambooy & Voorst, 1986; Anil & McKinstry, 1991).

Experiments with dogs have identified a need to direct the electrical current through the brain to induce rapid loss of consciousness. In dogs, when electricity passes only between fore-and hind limbs or neck and feet, it causes the heart to fibrillate but does not induce sudden loss of consciousness (Roberts, 1954). For electrical stunning of any animal, an apparatus that applies electrodes to opposite sides of the head, or in another way directs electrical current immediately through the brain, is necessary to induce rapid loss of consciousness. Attachment of electrodes and animal restraint can pose problems with this form of stunning. Signs of effective electrical stunning are extension of the limbs, opisthotonos, downward rotation of the eyeballs, and tonic spasm changing to clonic spasm, with eventual muscle flaccidity.

Electrical stunning should be followed promptly by electrically induced cardiac fibrillation, exsanguination, or other appropriate methods to ensure death (AVMA, 2007).

2.7.1.4 Cervical dislocation

Cervical dislocation is a technique that has been used for many years and, when performed by well-trained individuals, appears to be humane. However, there are few scientific studies to confirm this observation.

This technique is used to euthanatize poultry, other small birds, mice, and immature rats and rabbits. For mice and rats, the thumb and index finger are placed on either side of the neck at the base of the skull or, alternatively, a rod is pressed at the base of the skull. With the other hand, the base of the tail or the hind limbs is quickly pulled, causing separation of the cervical vertebrae from the skull. For immature rabbits, the head is held in one hand and the hind limbs in the other. The animal is stretched and the neck is hyperextended and dorsally twisted to separate the first cervical vertebra from the skull (Clifford, 1984). For poultry, cervical dislocation by stretching is a common method for mass euthanasia, but loss of consciousness may not be instantaneous (Lambooy, 1986).

Data suggest that electrical activity in the brain persists for 13 seconds following cervical dislocation (Vanderwolf, 1988), and unlike decapitation, rapid exsanguination does not contribute to loss of consciousness (Derr, 1991; Holson, 1992).

2.7.1.5 Decapitation

Decapitation can be used to euthanatize rodents and small rabbits in research settings. It provides a means to recover tissues and body fluids that are chemically uncontaminated. It also provides a means of obtaining anatomically undamaged brain tissue for study (Feldman & Gupta, 1976). Also, this procedure has been used for killing fish, amphibians and birds. Decapitation involves the severing of the neck of the animal, close to the head by using a sharp instrument. The use of scissors is discouraged unless they are suited to the species of animal (i.e. have sufficiently long blades) and the pressure is strong enough to sever the neck in one go with ease. Decapitation should be carried out using guillotines designed especially for that purpose to ensure rapid and quick severance in the correct position (Clifford, 1984). Guillotines that are designed to accomplish decapitation in adult rodents and small rabbits in a uniformly instantaneous manner are commercially available. Guillotines are not commercially available for neonatal rodents, but sharp blades can be used for this purpose.

Although it has been demonstrated that electrical activity in the brain persists for 13 to 14 seconds following decapitation (Mikeska & Klemm, 1975), more recent studies and reports indicate that this activity does not infer the ability to perceive pain, and in fact conclude that loss of consciousness develops rapidly (Vanderwolf et al., 1988; Derr, 1991; Holson, 1992). The immediate lack of circulation of blood to the brain and subsequent anoxia is thought to render the head rapidly insensible (Derr, 1991) making prior stunning or sedation unnecessary. Use of the puntilla is not acceptable (Commission of the European Communities, 1993). Use of other methods is preferred where possible until further research can show rapid loss of consciousness (Close et al., 1996).

The advantages described for this procedure, is that decapitation is a technique that appears to induce rapid loss of consciousness (Vanderwolf et al., 1988; Derr, 1991; Holson, 1992). It does not chemically contaminate tissues and it is rapidly accomplished. On the other hand, the disadvantages are that is a technique requiring handling and restraint to perform it, and could be distressful to animals. Also, it has been widely discussed about the presence of electrical activity in the brain following decapitation, creating controversy and for that reason its importance may still be open to debate (Mikeska & Klemm, 1975; Vanderwolf et al., 1988; Derr, 1991; Holson, 1992). Decapitation must be done by trained personnel to perform this technique, which should recognize the inherent danger of the guillotine and take adequate precautions to prevent personal injury. And finally, decapitation may be aesthetically displeasing to personnel performing or observing the technique.

The recommendations when decapitation has been chosen, is to consider that this technique is conditionally acceptable if performed correctly, and it should be used in research settings when its use is required by the experimental design and approved by a Bioethical Committee. The equipment used to perform decapitation should be maintained in good working order and serviced on a regular basis to ensure sharpness of blades. The use of plastic cones to restrain animals appears to reduce distress from handling, minimizes the chance of injury to personnel, and improves positioning of the animal in the guillotine.

2.7.1.6 Maceration

This method is acceptable for the destruction of chicks up to 72 hours old which often have to be killed in large numbers (Bandow, 1987; Commission of the European Communities, 1993). Only macerators designed specifically for this purpose must be used and under no conditions should domestic appliances be used (Close et al., 1996). The designed mechanical apparatus have rotating blades or projections, which causes immediate fragmentation and death of day-old poultry and embryonated eggs. A review (American Association of Avian Pathologists Animal Welfare and Management Practices Committee, 2005) about the use of commercially available macerators for euthanasia of chicks, poults, and pipped eggs indicates that death by maceration in day-old poultry occurs immediately with minimal pain and distress. Maceration is an alternative to the use of carbon dioxide for euthanasia of day-old poultry. Maceration is believed to be equivalent to cervical dislocation and cranial compression as to time element, and is considered to be an acceptable means of euthanasia for newly hatched poultry by the Federation of Agriculture Canada (1989), World Organization for Animal Health (OIE, 2006) and European Council (1993).

The advantage of this procedure is that death is almost instantaneous, the method is safe for workers and large numbers of animals can be killed quickly. But the disadvantages described for maceration are that special equipment is required and the macerated tissues may present bio-security risks. It is recommended to consider than maceration requires special equipment that must be kept in excellent working order. Chicks must be delivered to the macerator in a way and at a rate that prevents a backlog of chicks at the point of entry into the macerator and without causing injury, suffocation, or avoidable distress to the chicks before maceration.

2.7.1.7 Microwave irradiation

Heating by microwave irradiation is used primarily by neurobiologists to fix brain metabolites in vivo while maintaining the anatomic integrity of the brain (Stavinoha, 1983). Only specialist equipment (this does not include domestic microwave ovens) designed for this purpose is to be used (Close et al., 1996). Microwave instruments have been specifically designed for use in euthanasia of laboratory mice and rats. The instruments differ in design from kitchen units and may vary in maximal power output from 1.3 to 10 kw. All units direct their microwave energy to the head of the animal. The power required to rapidly halt brain enzyme activity depends on the efficiency of the unit, the ability to tune the resonant cavity and the size of the rodent head (Stavinoha et al., 1978). There is considerable variation among instruments in the time required for loss of consciousness and euthanasia. A 10 kw, 2,450 MHz instrument operated at a power of 9 kw will increase the brain temperature of 18 to 28 g mice to 79° C in 330 ms, and the brain temperature of 250 to 420 g rats to 94 C in 800 ms. (lkarashi et al., 1984). It is only to be carried out on small animals such as amphibians, birds, mice, rats and small rabbits (less than 300 g) (Zeller et al., 1989). This method requires specialist expertise, but when carried out correctly is humane as death occurs in milliseconds (Andrews et al., 1993, Bermann et al., 1985, Olfert et al., 1993). Care must be taken to ensure correct positioning of the microwave beam but time taken to restrain the animal should be kept to a minimum to reduce stress prior to euthanasia.

The advantages for this procedure are that it cause loss of consciousness achieved in less than 100 ms, and death in less than 1 second. Besides, this is the most effective method to fix brain tissue *in vivo* for subsequent assay of enzymatically labile chemicals. The disadvantages mentioned for this technique are that the specific instruments are expensive and only small animals (with the size of mice and rats) can be euthanatized with commercial instruments that are currently available.

2.7.2 Chemical methods

Many anaesthetics are used in overdose as euthanasia agents. An anaesthetic is an agent that produces, in a controllable manner, a drug-induced absence of perception of all sensation. It produces unconsciousness, analgesia, and muscle relaxation sufficient to perform procedures painlessly (Close et al., 1996).

2.7.3 Inhalational agents

Any gas that is inhaled must reach a certain concentration in the alveoli before it can be effective; therefore, euthanasia with any of these agents may take some time. The suitability of a particular agent depends on whether an animal experiences distress between the time it begins to inhale the agent and the time it loses consciousness. Some agents may induce convulsions, but these generally follow loss of consciousness. Agents inducing convulsions prior to loss of consciousness are unacceptable for euthanasia. Certain considerations are common to all inhalant agents:

- In most cases, onset of loss of consciousness is more rapid, and euthanasia more humane, if the animal is rapidly exposed to a high concentration of the agent.
- The equipment used to deliver and maintain this high concentration must be in good working order and in compliance with state and federal regulations. Leaky or faulty equipment may lead to slow, distressful death and be hazardous to other animals and to personnel.
- Most of these agents are hazardous to personnel because of the risk of explosions (eg, ether), narcosis (eg, halothane), hypoxemia (eg, nitrogen and carbon monoxide), addiction (eg, nitrous oxide), or health effects resulting from chronic exposure (eg, nitrous oxide and carbon monoxide).
- Alveolar concentrations rise slowly in an animal with decreased ventilation, making agitation more likely during induction. Other noninhalant methods of euthanasia should be considered for such animals.
- Neonatal animals appear to be resistant to hypoxia, and because all inhalant agents ultimately cause hypoxia, neonatal animals take longer to die than adults. Glass et al, (1944) reported that newborn dogs, rabbits, and guinea pigs survived a nitrogen atmosphere much longer than did adults. Dogs, at 1 week old, survived for 14 minutes compared with a 3-minute survival time after a few weeks of age. Guinea pigs survived for 4.5 minutes at 1 day old, compared with 3 minutes at 8 days or older. Rabbits survived for 13 minutes at 6 days old, 4 minutes at 14 days, and 1.5 minutes at 19 days and older. The panel recommended that inhalant agents not be used alone in animals less than 16 weeks old except to induce loss of consciousness, followed by the use of some other method to kill the animal.
- Rapid gas flows can produce a noise that frightens animals. If high flows are required, the equipment should be designed to minimize noise.
- Animals placed together in chambers should be of the same species, and, if needed, should be restrained so that they will not hurt themselves or others. Chambers should not be overloaded and need to be kept clean to minimize odours that might distress animals subsequently euthanatized
- Reptiles, amphibians, and diving birds and mammals have a great capacity for holding their breath and anaerobic metabolism (AMMVA, 2007).

2.7.3.1 Carbon dioxide

At concentrations above 60%, carbon dioxide acts as an anaesthetic agent and causes rapid loss of consciousness (Green, 1987). It is effective and humane for euthanasia of most small animals above 70%. Carbon dioxide stimulates the respiratory centre which may cause anxiety and stress in the animal as well as being aesthetically unpleasant for the observer. Carbon dioxide may form carbonic acid when in contact with the nasal mucous membranes which could produce a fizzy or tingling effect which may be mildly irritating to some species when applied at lower concentrations (Lucke, 1979). In most animals it is recommended to place them immediately into > 70% CO_2 where the animals lose consciousness very quickly due to the narcotic effect of the high intake of CO_2 on the brain without causing hypoxia (Forslid et a1., 1986; Blackshaw et a1., 1988). One hundred per cent CO_2 may cause severe dyspnoea and distress in conscious animals (van Zutphen et a1., 1993).

The advantages described for this procedure include: the rapid depressant, analgesic, and anesthetic effects of CO_2 are well established. Also, carbon dioxide is readily available and can be purchased in compressed gas cylinders. Carbon dioxide is inexpensive, nonflammable, nonexplosive, and poses minimal hazard to personnel when used with properly designed equipment. The euthanasia with carbon dioxide does not result in accumulation of tissue residues in food-producing animals and finally, carbon dioxide does not distort murine cholinergic markers (Bereger-Sweeney et al., 1994) or corticosterone concentrations (Urbanski & Kelly, 1991).

On the other hand, the disadvantages for using this euthanasia procedure are that CO_2 is heavier than air, and incomplete filling of a chamber may permit animals to climb or raise their heads above the higher concentrations and avoid exposure; some species, such as fish and burrowing and diving mammals, may have extraordinary tolerance for CO_2. Reptiles and amphibians may breathe too slowly for the use of CO2. Euthanasia by exposure to CO_2 may take longer than euthanasia by other means (Coenen et al., 1995). Also, induction of loss of consciousness at lower concentrations (< 80%) may produce pulmonary and upper respiratory tract lesions (Iwarsson & Rehbinder, 1993; Danneman et al., 1997) and must be considered that high concentrations of CO_2 may be distressful to some animals.

Room air contains 0.04% carbon dioxide (CO_2), which is heavier than air and nearly odourless. Inhalation of CO_2 at a concentration of 7.5% increases the pain threshold, and higher concentrations of CO_2 have a rapid anesthesic effect (Leake & Waters, 1929; Woodbury, 1958; Simonsen et al., 1981; Lecky, 1983; Matson et al., 1992; Klemm, 1994).

Several investigators have suggested that inhalation of high concentrations of CO_2 may be distressing to animals (Carding, 1968; Hoenderken, 1983; Gregory et al., 1987, Britt, 1987), because the gas dissolves in moisture on the nasal mucosa. The resulting product, carbonic acid, may stimulate nociceptors in the nasal mucosa. Some humans exposed to concentrations of around 50% CO_2 report that inhaling the gas is unpleasant and that higher concentrations are noxious (Anton et al., 1992; Danneman et al., 1997). Carbon dioxide has been used to euthanatize groups of small laboratory animals, including mice, rats, guinea pigs, chickens, and rabbits (Kline et al., 1963; Breazile & Kitchell, 1969; Kocula et al., 1971; Jaksch, 1981; Raj & Gregory, 1990), and to render swine unconscious before humane slaughter (Hoenderken, 1983; Gregory et al., 1987).

2.7.3.2 Carbon monoxide

This causes rapid death as it combines with the red blood cells in preference to oxygen, thus causing hypoxia (Chalifoux & Dallaire 1983).There is little or no distress as there is no smell (Breazile & Kitchell, 1969; Smith et a1., 1986; Green, 1987; Blackmore, 1993). It is not acceptable for use in reptiles because of their low metabolic rate and hypoxic tolerance. It is acceptable for small animals, but in dogs and cats vocalizations and convulsions may occur after unconsciousness making it aesthetically unpleasant. Death should be confirmed by physical means.

In the past, mass euthanasia has been accomplished by use of 3 methods for generating CO: (1) chemical interaction of sodium formate and sulfuric acid, (2) exhaust fumes from idling gasoline internal combustion engines, and (3) commercially compressed CO in cylinders. The first 2 techniques are associated with problems such as production of other gases, achieving inadequate concentrations of carbon monoxide, inadequate cooling of the gas, and maintenance of equipment. Therefore, the only acceptable source is compressed CO in cylinders.

The advantages for this procedure are: carbon monoxide induces loss of consciousness without pain and with minimal discernible discomfort; hypoxemia induced by CO is insidious, so that the animal appears to be unaware and death occurs rapidly if concentrations of 4 to 6% are used.
The disadvantages are that safeguards must be taken to prevent exposure of personnel and any electrical equipment exposed to CO (eg, lights and fans) must be explosion proof.
As recommendations, must be considered that carbon monoxide used for individual animal or mass euthanasia is acceptable for dogs, cats, and other small mammals, provided that commercially compressed CO is used and the following precautions are taken: (1) personnel using CO must be instructed thoroughly in its use and must understand its hazards and limitations; (2) the CO chamber must be of the highest quality construction and should allow for separation of individual animals; (3) the CO source and chamber must be located in a well-ventilated environment, preferably out of doors; (4) the chamber must be well lit and have view ports that allow personnel direct observation of animals; (5) the CO flow rate should be adequate to rapidly achieve a uniform CO concentration of at least 6% after animals are placed in the chamber, although some species (eg, neonatal pigs) are less likely to become agitated with a gradual rise in CO concentration (Lambooy & Spanjaard, 1980); and (6) if the chamber is inside a room, CO monitors must be placed in the room to warn personnel of hazardous concentrations.

2.7.3.3 Volatile inhalational anaesthetics

When using any liquid anaesthetic care must be taken to ensure that it is not allowed to come in contact with the animal. Sufficient air or oxygen should be provided during the induction period to prevent hypoxia (Andrews et al., 1993). Exposure to trace concentrations of anaesthetic gases is a recognized human health hazard and requires gas scavenging apparatus to be used in the work environment. Volatile inhalational anaesthetics are neither flammable nor explosive.
Halothane is a commonly used anaesthetic agent for small laboratory animals and is quick acting and stress free in overdose for euthanasia. It has a depressant effect on the cardiovascular and respiratory systems (Green, 1987).
Enflurane is a commonly used anaesthetic agent for small laboratory animals and is quick acting and stress free in overdose for euthanasia (Green, 1987). It has a depressant effect on the cardiovascular and respiratory systems. It may be preferred to halothane in situations where drug metabolism or toxicological work is being conducted as very little drug is metabolized in the liver.
Isoflurane is a commonly used anaesthetic agent which is quick acting and stress free in overdose for euthanasia. Isoflurane causes respiratory and cardiovascular depression. However, it has a pungent odour and must therefore not be used on animals which may be able to hold their breath. It is particularly useful where tissues such as liver are to be used for toxicological or microsomal studies as it undergoes no hepatic metabolism.
Nitrous oxide (N_2O) may be used with other inhalants to speed the onset of anesthesia, but alone it does not induce anesthesia in animals, even at 100% concentration. When used by itself, N_2O produces hypoxemia before respiratory or cardiac arrest. As a result, animals may become distressed prior to loss of consciousness.
The advantages of choose euthanasia with someone of these options are: Inhalant anesthetics are particularly valuable for euthanasia of smaller animals (< 7 kg) or for animals in which venipuncture may be difficult, and Halothane, enflurane, isoflurane, sevoflurane,

desflurane, methoxyflurane, and N_2O are nonflammable and nonexplosive under ordinary environmental conditions.
As disadvantages, animals may struggle and become anxious during induction of anesthesia because anesthetic vapors may be irritating and can induce excitement. Ether is flammable and explosive. Explosions have occurred when animals, euthanatized with ether, were placed in an ordinary (not explosion proof) refrigerator or freezer and when bagged animals were placed in an incinerator. Another disadvantage to consider is that the induction with methoxyflurane is unacceptably slow in some species. Nitrous oxide will support combustion, and as well personnel as animals can be injured by exposure to these agents, with a potential for human abuse of some of these drugs, especially N_2O.
As final recommendations, in order of preference, halothane, enflurane, isoflurane, sevoflurane, methoxyflurane, and desflurane, with or without nitrous oxide, are acceptable for euthanasia of small animals (< 7 kg). Ether should only be used in carefully controlled situations in compliance with state and federal occupational health and safety regulations. It is conditionally acceptable. Nitrous oxide should not be used alone, pending further scientific studies on its suitability for animal euthanasia. Although acceptable, these agents are generally not used in larger animals because of their cost and difficulty of administration.

Agents	Classifi-cation	Mode of action	Rapidity	Ease of perfor-mance	Safety	Species suita-bility	Efficacy and comments
Blow to head	Physical damage to brain	Direct concussion of brain tissue	Rapid	Requires skill, adequate restraint, and appropriate force	Safe	Young pigs < 3 weeks old	Must be properly applied to be humane and effective
Carbon dioxide (bottled gas only)	Hypoxia due to depression of vital centers	Direct depression of cerebral cortex, subcor-tical structures and vital centers; direct depression of heart muscle	Mode-rately rapid	Used in closed container	Minimal hazard	Non-human primates, free ranging wildlife	Effective, but time required may be prolonged in immature and neonatal animals
Carbon monoxide (bottled gas only)	Hypoxia	Combines with hemoglobin, preventing its combination with oxygen	Moderate onset time, but insidious so animal is unaware of onset	Requires appropriately maintained equipment	Extre-mely hazardous, toxic and difficult to detect	Non-human primates, free ranging wildlife	Effective, acceptable only when equipment is properly designed and operated

Agents	Classification	Mode of action	Rapidity	Ease of performance	Safety	Species suitability	Efficacy and comments
Cervical dislocation	Hypoxia due to disruption of vital centers	Direct depression of brain	Moderately rapid	Requires training and skill	Safe	Poultry, birds, lab mice, and rats (< 200 g) or rabbits (<1 kg)	Irreversible. Violent muscle contractions can occur after cervical dislocation
Chloral hydrate	Hypoxia from depression of respiratory center	Direct depre-ssion of brain	Rapid	Personnel must be skilled perform IV injection	Safe	Horses, ruminants and swine	Animals should be sedated prior to administration
Decapitation	Hypoxia due to disruption of vital centers	Direct depression of brain	Rapid	Requires training and skill	Guillotine pose potential employee injury hazard	Laboratory rodents, small rabbits, birds, some fish, amphibians, and reptiles (latter 3 with pithing)	Irreversible. Violent muscle contraction can occur after decapitation
Electrocution	Hypoxia	Direct depression of brain and cardiac fibrillation	Can be rapid	Not easily performed in all instances	Hazardous to personnel	Used primarily in foxes, sheep, swine, mink (with cervical dislocation), ruminants, animals <5 kg	Violent muscle contractions occur at same time as loss of unconsciousness
Gunshot	Hypoxia due to disruption of vital centers	Direct concussion of brain tissue	Rapid	Requires skill and appropriate firearm	May be dangerous	Large domestic and zoo animals, reptiles, amphibians, wildlife, cetaceans (<4 meters long)	Instant unconsciousness, but motor activity may continue

Agents	Classification	Mode of action	Rapidity	Ease of performance	Safety	Species suitability	Efficacy and comments
Inhalant anesthetics	Hypoxia due to depression of vital centers	Direct depression of cerebral cortex, subcortical structures, and vital centers	Moderately rapid onset of anesthesia; excitation may develop during induction	Easily performed with closed container; can be administered to large animals by means of a mask	Must be properly scavenged or vented to minimize exposure to personnel	Nonhuman primates, swine	Highly effective provided that subject is sufficiently exposed
Nitrogen, Argon	Hypoxia	Reduces partial pressure of oxygen available to blood	Rapid	Use closed chamber with rapid filling	Safe if used with ventilation	Cats, small dogs, birds, rodents, rabbits, other small species, mink, zoo animals, nonhuman primates, free ranging wildlife	Effective except in young and neonates; an effective agent, but other methods preferable
Penetrating captive bolt	Physical damage to brain	Direct concussion of brain tissue	Rapid	Requires skill, adequate restraint, and proper placement of captive bolt	Safe	Dogs, rabbits, zoo animals, reptiles, amphibians, free ranging wildlife	Instant loss of consciousness but motor activity may continue
Pithing	Hypoxia due to disruption of vital centers, physical damage to brain	Trauma of brain and spinal cord tissue	Rapid	Easily performed, but requires skill	Safe	Some ectotherms	Effective, but death not immediate unless brain and spinal cord are pithed
Thoracic compression	Hypoxia and cardiac arrest	Physical interference with cardiac and respiratory function	Moderately rapid	Requires training	Safe	Small to medium sized free ranging birds	Apparently effective

Table 2. Summary of Conditionally Acceptable Agents and Methods of Euthanasia - Characteristics and Modes of Action

2.8 Recommended methods of euthanasia in each species

Below are described the main methods of euthanasia suggested for the various species that can be used in the laboratory. A summary of these recommendations indicating characteristics of the euthanasia methods is presented on table 2.

2.8.1 Fish

There are over 20 000 species of fish with enormously varying lifestyles which makes it very difficult to generalize on methods of euthanasia. Although fish may not have the same spinothalamic pathways as mammals for pain perception, there is evidence that they do feel pain and should therefore be killed with the same care and consideration. All fish are sensitive to changes in the physical and chemical parameters of their water (especially temperature, dissolved gas levels, salinity, pH, etc.) but some species are much more tolerant of changes in anyone of these factors than are others. Therefore unless the species' response is known it is advisable to practise euthanasia in the fish's normal water. If drugs are used the water level should be lowered to ensure rapid sedation but not so much as to distress the fish before the addition of the agent. Dosing is always preferable to injection as the latter technique involves handling the fish and thus induces stress.

In general, larvae and adults can be euthanized by:

Physical methods: Concussion, Cervical dislocation (Clifford, 1984) and Maceration. Cervical dislocation it is feasible and effective in small fish, but should be confirmed by exsanguination or destruction of the brain. The stress caused by handling reduces the acceptability of this method. It is not possible or humane in larger fish. Maceration must be choose only for small fish of less than 2 cm in length may be humanely killed by placing down a waste disposal unit.

Chemical methods: Agents can be administered by dissolving the chemical in the tank water. Water temperatures often alter the efficacy of the drug and induction is often more rapid at higher temperatures. However, the temperature must not be raised so that it causes any stress to the fish. Drugs may also be administered by intramuscular or intraperitoneal injection. For euthanasia, anaesthetic drugs are generally used at double or triple the recommended anaesthetic dose.

The most common chemical agents used are: Tricaine methane sulphonate (buffered MS-222), Benzocaine (ethyl aminobenzoate), Etomidate, Metomidate, Quinaldine (2-methylquinoline), Halothane, injectable agents (barbiturates).

The methods considered as acceptable for unconscious fish are decapitation and exsanguinations. By other hand, the methods not acceptable for euthanasia of fish are : removal from water, whole body crushing, electrical stunning, hypothermia, hyperthermia, carbon dioxide, diethyl ether, Urethane, Chloral hydrate, tertiary amyl alcohol, tribromoethanol, chlorobutanol, Methyl pentynol, pyridines.

2.8.2 Amphibians

Because amphibians are ectothermic and thus accustomed to fluctuations in body temperature, their central nervous system (CNS) is less sensitive to hypoxia and anoxia. Even when the cranial nerves and brain are deprived of blood supply these animals are able to respond to stimuli for some time. Although decapitation, by itself, does not produce rapid unconsciousness in the severed heads of amphibians, rapid destruction of the brain does extinguish responses usually thought to indicate consciousness (AVMA, 2007).

There is, however, a remarkably intact set of somatic responses to stimuli long continued body movements, foot withdrawals in response to toe pinching, etc., as well as continued heartbeat in many cases for hours following brain destruction. This continued somatic activity is attributed to:

1. prolonged tolerance of the spinal cord, peripheral nerves and muscle (smooth, cardiac and skeletal) to hypoxic and hypotensive conditions, and
2. a far greater degree of integration of somatic responses at the level of the spinal cord instead of the brain (Close et al., 1996)

For those reasons, death may be recognized by cessation of heartbeat and respiration and in cases where this is not obvious; it may be confirmed by destruction of the brain. In larvae, Tadpoles and newts can be effectively killed by placing in a dish of water with MS-222 or benzocaine (dissolved in acetone). These produce rapid anesthesia, followed by death. For adults, it is important to obtain a firm hold, for example by wearing rough textured but non-abrasive gloves or by holding them in coarse material.

Cooling to 3-4°C will reduce metabolic and locomotory processes, thus facilitating handling prior to euthanasia. However, it must be remembered that cooling does not reduce the ability to feel pain. However, the physical methods for adult amphibians include: Concussion, microwave and electrical stunning. The procedures where chemical agents are considered, usually are used: Tricaine methane sulphonate (buffered MS-222), Benzocaine, sodium pentobarbitone, T-61. The methods considered as acceptable for unconscious amphibians are: Pithing and decapitation. Contrarily, the methods not acceptable for euthanasia of amphibians are: hypothermia, hyperthermia, exsanguinations, strangulation, carbon dioxide, ether, chloroform, volatile inhalational anesthetics, chloral hydrate, ketamine, hydrochloride, chlorbutanol, methylpentynol, 2-phenoxyethanol, tertiary amyl alcohol, tribromoethanol, and urethane (Close et al., 1996; Reilly, 2001).

2.8.3 Reptiles

Similarly to the amphibians, reptiles are also ectothermic and even when the cranial nerves and brain are deprived of blood supply following decapitation; they are able to respond to stimuli for some time. Although decapitation, by itself, does not produce rapid unconsciousness in the severed heads of reptiles (Warwick, 1990) rapid destruction of the brain does extinguish responses usually thought to indicate consciousness. For that reason, good methods of restraint are important to ensure minimal stress prior to carrying out euthanasia.

Particular care must be taken when handling venomous species, such as many types of snake, especially when they are not used to being handled (Close et al., 1996). Padded grasping implements are useful in handling lizards and snakes to ensure a firm but non-damaging restraint. Cooling of most reptiles to 3-4°C will reduce metabolic and locomotory processes (this temperature may kill some tropical species), thus facilitating handling prior to euthanasia. In tortoises, turtles and terrapins, retraction of the head and protection by the carapace can cause difficulty for euthanasia. To assist in exposing the head, land tortoises can be placed in shallow, tepid water large marine species may be put on a frame at 45° head up, inducing neck extension and soft-shelled species can be placed on their backs to induce neck extension. Rough textured but non-abrasive gloves may be worn when handling aquatic species to facilitate handling (Reilly, 2001).

Effective restraint of the jaws and tail is the key factor to' operator safety for restraining crocodilians and this should only be done by experts. As it is difficult to determine whether reptiles are unconscious or dead, it is recommended that death be confirmed by destruction of the brain. Usually, but by no means always, a lack of pupillary-blink-nictitating membrane responses, except in snakes which do not possess movable eyelids, implies a lack of consciousness. Rigor mortis is a reliable indicator of death as is the prolonged absence of a heartbeat and/or circulation (Close et al., 1996).
For eggs of reptiles, are recommended methods would include disruption of the egg and killing of the embryos by injection of sodium pentobarbitone, anaesthetic overdose or an appropriate physical method to destroy the brain or whole egg or early life form. For all practical purposes, all newly hatched reptiles can be treated inthe same way as adults. As the class Reptilia is varied, it is best to consider three main groups: the snakes and lizards (Squamata); tortoises, turtles and terrapins (Testudines); and crocodiles and alligators (Crocodilia). Larger reptiles may need to be sedated before being killed. Physical accepted methods include the captive bolt, concussion and shooting. The chemical method considered is to overdoses of pentobarbital by intraperitoneal route. The methods acceptable for unconscious reptiles are phithing and decapitation; contrarily between the methods not acceptable for euthanasia of reptiles are: spinal cord severance, hypothermia or hyperthermia, exsanguination, chloroform, and tricaine methane sulphonate (MS-222). Because reptiles are capable of holding their breath for a relatively long period of time and therefore inhalational methods cannot be considered as practicable or humane due to slow induction (Close et al., 1996; AVMA, 2007).

2.8.4 Birds

Birds have a complex respiratory system comprising the lungs and numerous air sacs with a one-way flow of air. This may influence the rate of absorption of inhalational agents and thus increase their efficiency. The dead of birds, Death may be recognized by the absence of signs of breathing, cardiac arrest and absence of reflexes in the head (Close et al., 1996). Reflexes to be checked would include pinching of wattles or blink reflexes. The most commonly used method of destroying eggs is cooling or freezing. The recommended temperature is<4°C for 4 h. In cases where the embryo has been exposed to experimental conditions for studies, decapitation is considered an acceptable method of euthanasia as is an overdose of anaesthetic (AVMA, 2007).
For adult birds, the physical methods considered are: cervical dislocation, maceration, concussion, microwave and electrical stunning (Reilly, 2001). The chemical methods for euthanasia in birds are inhalational agents (carbon dioxide, volatile inhalational anaesthetics, carbon monoxide) and injectable agents (Sodium pentobarbitone, T-61). The acceptable methods for unconscious in birds include decapitation, pithing and potassium chloride. And the methods not acceptable for euthanasia of birds are neck crushing, exsanguination, decompression creating a vacuum, nitrous oxide, ether/chloroform, cyclopropane, hydrogen cyanide gas and must be consideder that there are other agents which have not to be used (methoxyflurane, trichlorethylene, chloral hydrate, strychnine, nicotine, magnesiumsulphate, ketamine alone and neuromuscular blocking agents)(Close et al., 1996).

2.8.5 Rodents

Rodents are the most commonly used animals for experimental purposes and include mice, rats, hamsters, guinea pigs, gerbils, shrews, and dormice (Close et al., 1996; AVMA, 2007).

Physical methods for rodents include concussion, cervical dislocation (only animals under 150 g), decapitation, and rapid freezing (only for fetus and neonates) (Reilly, 2001). There are many chemical methods including: the use of Inhalational agents, as volatile inhalational anaesthetics (Halothane, enflurane, isoflurane), carbon dioxide. Also are used injectable agents like sodium pentobarbitone (diluted, because it can cause irritation of the peritoneum). The methods acceptable for unconscious rodents are: rapid freezing (only for rodents <4g), exsanguination, air embolism, potassium chloride and ethanol. The methods not acceptable for euthanasia of rodents are hypothermia, nitrogen, nitrous oxide, cyclopropane, ether, chloroform, decompression, asphyxia, drowning, trichlorethylene, methoxyflurane, hydrogen cyanide gas, carbon monoxide, strychnine, nicotine, chloral hydrate, magnesium sulphate, curariform drugs and other neuromuscular blocking agents (see table 3) (Close et al., 1996, Reilly, 2001).

Techniques	**Recommended**	**Acceptable with reservations**	**Not acceptable**
Chemical			
Inhalant	Carbon dioxide 💣	Halothane ☢	Either ☢👎 Hydrogen cyanide ☢☹ Carbon monoxide ☢ Nitrogen ☢ Chloroform
Injectable	Pentobarbitone sodium Ip (diluted)	Ethanol Ip	
Physical		Cervical dislocation	Microwave irradiation -not yet proven to be humane 💣
		Possibly👎 in animals heavier than 150 g (acceptable if stunned or anaesthesied first)	Decompression ☹💣
		Decapitation ☹🕮	Asphyxia ☹👎💣
		Stunning and exsanguinations ☹🕮	Rapid freezing (unconscious and <4 g) 👎💣

💣 Requires specialised equipment 🕮 Training required
☢ Occupational health and Safety Issues $ Expensive
☹ Aesthetically unpleasant 👎 Inhumane

Table 3. Recommended, acceptable with reservation and not accepted methods for euthanasia in rodents (Reilly, 2001).

2.8.6 Rabbits

Death must be recognized and confirm with the absence of reflexes. Must be confirm with exsanguinations, evisceration or decapitation. To euthanize embryos, they must be removed for decapitation, with a previous administration of increased amount of anaesthetic to the dam for longer to ensure that the anesthetic has crossed placenta. The foetuses that are not removed from the dam will die of anoxia when the dam is killed and no further method is necessary to ensure death of the foetus (Reilly, 2001).

The physical methods of killing adult rabbits include: concussion, cervical dislocation, captive bolt, decapitation, electrical stunning, and microwave. The chemical methods include inhalational methods with volatile agents (Halothane, isoflurane, enflurane, carbon dioxide, and carbon monoxide) or injectable agents.

The methods considered as acceptable for unconscious rabbits are: Exsanguination, nitrogen, potassium chloride and air embolism (5-50 mL/Kg) (AVMA, 2007). The non acceptable methods for euthanasia of rabbits are: nitrous oxide, methoxyflurane, clyclopropane, ether and chloroform and ketamine hydrochloride. Other agents not to be used for killing rabbits include decompression, asphyxia, drowning, trichlorethylene, hydrogen cyanide gas, hydrocyanic acid, strychnine, nicotine, chloral hydrate, magnesium sulphate and neuromuscular blocking agents (Close et al., 1996).

2.8.7 Carnivores (dogs, cats and ferrets)

Recognition and confirmation of death must be verified. Cessations of respiration and heartbeats, as well loss of reflexes are good indicators of death in carnivores. To euthanize embryos, must be considered similar indications as previously described for rabbits. Neonate carnivores should generally be treated as adults. Sodium pentobarbitone is the preferred method, but CO_2, cervical dislocation and concussion may be considered (Hall, 1972).

For adults, the physical procedures includes: Captive bolt, shooting and electrocution. The chemical methods used for carnivore adults are: Inhalational methods (with volatile inhalational anaesthetics), injectable agents (sodium pentobarbitone, secobarbital/dibucaine and T-61). The acceptable methods for unconscious carnivores includes: exsanguination, dislocation of neck, and potassium chloride; and the not acceptable methods for carnivores are stricking of chest of cats, decompression, carbon dioxide, carbon monoxide, nitrogen, ether and chloroform (AVMA, 2007). The following agents are also not to be used for killing carnivores: drowning, concussion (adults), decapitation, asphyxia, strangulation, nitrous oxide, hydrogen cyanide gas, cyclopropane, methoxyflurane, trichlorethylene, air embolism, hydrocyanic acid, chloral hydrate, strychnine, nicotine, magnesium sulphate, and neuromuscular blocking agents (Close et al., 1996).

Personnel using and having to kill any large mammal must receive special training in the handling, restraint and techniques of euthanasia of these animals. It is important to avoid actions which may increase the animals' awareness of the unusual situation. The animal is best killed in a familiar environment. It may be necessary to take the animals to approved slaughterhouses where specialized equipment is available for humane euthanasia of these animals. Euthanasia may have to be carried out by a person who has been trained and holds a certificate under national slaughter legislation or by a veterinarian with appropriate training (Close et al., 1996).

Cessation of respiration and heartbeat, and loss of reflexes are good indicators of irreversible death in these species. Death should be confirmed by exsanguination. The foetuses of these large mammals are well developed at birth and therefore considerable care must be taken to ensure that they are killed humanely if removed from the uterus (Reilly, 2001). Foetuses may also be large and in general any method used on an adult is considered acceptable. Because the neonates of large mammals are born in an advanced stage of development, they should be treated as adults.

Physical methods for adults must be considered: captive bolt, free bullet, shooting, concussion and electrical stunning (Blackmore, 1979). The chemical methods include: inhalational methods, with volatile inhalational anaesthesics (halothane, isoflurane, enflurane using a mask for kids and lambs) and carbon dioxide -only for pigs - (death must be confirmed by exsanguination) but other methods are considered preferable and carbon dioxide must not be used on any other large animal (AVMA, 2007). Other methods acceptable for unconscious large mammals are exsanguination, potassium chloride and the intravenously administration of chloral hydrate in conjunction with magnesium sulphate and sodium pentobarbitone. The methods not acceptable for euthanasia of large mammals are methoxyflurane, trichlorethylene, strychnine, nicotine, magnesium sulphate, thiopentone sodium, ketamine hydrochloride, curariform drugs and other neuromuscular blocking agents (Close et al., 1996).

2.8.8 Non-human primates

Personnel handling primates should be specially trained for these purposes. It is preferable that if primates have to be killed, that this be carried out by someone familiar to them in order to reduce stress and anxiety. For all larger primates, sedation (e.g. ketamine) should be administered prior to euthanasia (Reilly, 2001). Cessation of heartbeat and respiration, and absence of reflexes may be considered as indicators of death. The only recommended method for killing primates is by overdose of anaesthetic. Sodium pentobarbitone injected intravenously is the most acceptable agent. Exsanguination under inhalation anesthesia is also considered acceptable, but this must be followed by perfusion (Close et al., 1996; AVMA, 2007).

2.8.9 Other animals not commonly used for experiments

As vertebrate animals vary so much in size and physiology, the method chosen to kill any animal not included above should be chosen from those methods for animals that are most similar biologically. Advice should be obtained from a veterinarian. In general, an overdose of sodium pentobarbitone injected intravenously may be considered as a humane method of killing most animals. It is advisable in most cases to sedate the animal prior to euthanasia (Close et al., 1996).

3. Conclusion

The use of animals in the laboratory is very useful as these are excellence models for the evaluation and development of multiple scientific studies. It is for this reason that researchers need to consider that in the course of these animal experiments, assure that they have a good quality of life and likewise, must choose the right method to perform euthanasia in order to avoid stress, anxious or pain when it is done.

4. References

Agriculture Canada (1989) Recommended code of practice for the care and handling of poultry from hatchery to processing plant. Publication 1757/E. 1989. Ottawa: Agriculture Canada. 12.02.2011. Available from: http://www.agr.gc.ca/poultry/pub1757e.pdf

American Association of Avian Pathologists (2005) Animal Welfare and Management Practices Committee: Review of mechanical euthanasia of day-old poultry. Athens, Ga.

Andrews, E.J.; Bennett, T.; Clark, J.D.; Houpt, K.A.; Pascoe, P.J.; Robinson, G.W. & Boyce, J.R. (1993). Report of the AVMA panel on euthanasia. *Journal of the American Veterinary Medical Association*, Vol.202, No.2, (January 1993), pp. 229-249, ISSN 0003-1488

Anil, M.H. & McKinstry, J.L. (1991) Reflexes and loss of sensibility following head-to-back electrical stunning in sheep. *Veterinary Record* Vol. 128, No. 5 (February, 1991) pp. 106–107. ISSN 0042-4900

Anton, F.; Euchner, I. & Handwerker, H.O. (1992) Psycophysical examination of pain induced by defined CO2 pulses applied to nasal mucosa. *Pain* Vol. 49, No. 1 (April, 1992) pp.53–60 ISSN 0304-3959

Baumans, V. (2005) Science-based assessment of animal welfare: laboratory animals. *Revue Scientifique et Technique* Vol. 24, No. 2 (August, 2005) pp. 503-514 ISSN 0253-1933

Bereger-Sweeney, J.; Berger, U.V.; Sharma, M. & Paul, C.A. (1994). Effects of carbon dioxide-induced anesthesia on cholinergic parameters in rat brain. *Laboratory Animal Science*, Vol. 44, No. 4 (August, 1994) pp. 369–371. ISSN 0023-6764

Berman, E.; King, J.B.; All, J.; Carter, H.B.; Rehnberg, B. & Stead, A.G. (1985) Lethality ill mice and rats exposed to 2450 MHz circulatory polarized microwaves as a function of exposure duration and environmental factors. *Journal of Applied Toxicology* Vol. 5, No 1 (February, 1985) pp.23-31. ISSN 0260-437X

Blackmore, D.K. (1993) Euthanasia; not always eu. *Australian Veterinary Journal* Vol. 70, No. 11 (November, 1993) pp. 409-13 ISSN 0005-0423

Blackmore, D.K. (1985) Energy requirements for the penetration of heads of domestic stock and the development of a multiple projectile. *Veterinary Record* Vol. 116, No. 2 (January, 1985) pp. 36–40. ISSN 0042-4900

Blackshaw, J.K.; Fenwick, D.C.; Beattie, A.W. & Allan, D.J. (1988) The behaviour of chickens, mice and rats during euthanasia with chloroform, carbon dioxide and ether. *Laboratory Animals* Vol. 22, No. 1 (January, 1988) pp. 67-75 ISSN 0093-7355

Breazile, J.E. & Kitchell, R.L. (1969) Euthanasia for laboratory animals. Federal Proceedings Vol. 28, No. 4 (July, 1969) pp. 1577-1579 ISSN 0014-9446

Britt, D.P. (1987) The humaneness of carbon dioxide as an agent of euthanasia for laboratory rodents. In: Euthanasia of unwanted, injured or diseased animals for educational or scientific purposes. *University Federation for Animal Welfare* (UFAW) pp. 19-31 Potters Bar, UK

Carding, A.H. (1968) Mass euthanasia of dogs with carbon monoxide and/or carbon dioxide: preliminary trials. *Journal Small Animal Practice* Vol. 9, No. 5 (May, 1968) pp. 245–259. ISSN 0022-4510

Chalifoux, A. & Dallaire, A. (1983) Physiologic and behavioral evaluation of CO euthanasia of adult dogs. *American Journal of Veterinary Research.* Vol. 44, No. 12 (December, 1983) pp. 2412-2417. ISSN 0002-9645

Clifford, D.H. (1984) Preanesthesia, anaesthesia, analgesia, and euthanasia. In: Fox, J.G.; Cohen, B.J. & Loew, F.M. eds. *Laboratory Animal Medicine.* Academic Press Inc pp. 528–563. ISBN 0122639510 New York

Close, B.; Banister, K.; Baumans, V.; Bernoth, E.M.; Bromage, M.; Bunyan, J.; Erhardt, W.; Flecknell, P.; Gregory, N.; Hackbarth, H.; Morton, D. & Warwick, C. (1996). Recommendations for euthanasia of experimental animals: Part 1. DGXI of the European Commission. *Laboratory Animals* Vol. 30, No. 4 (October, 1996) pp. 293-316 ISSN 0093-7355

Coenen, A.M.; Drinkenburg, W.H.; Hoenderken, R. & van Luijtelaar, E.L. (1995) Carbon dioxide euthanasia in rats: oxygen supplementation minimizes signs of agitation and asphyxia. *Laboratory Animals* Vol. 29 No. 3 (July, 1995) pp. 262–268 ISSN 0093-7355

Commission of the European Communities (1993) *Council directive on the protection of animals at the time of slaughter or killing.* 93/119/EC. No L340/21. 03.05.2011. Available from: http://ec.europa.eu/food/animal/welfare/references_en.htm

Daly, C.C. & Whittington, P.E. (1989) Investigation into the principal determinants of effective captive bolt stunning of sheep. *Research Veterinary Science* Vol. 46, No. 3 (May, 1989) pp.406-408 ISSN 0034-5288

Danneman, P.J.; Stein, S. & Walshaw, S.O. (1997) Humane and practical implications of using carbon dioxide mixed with oxygen for anesthesia or euthanasia of rats. *Laboratory Animal Science* Vol. 47, No. 4 (August, 1997) pp. 376–385 ISSN 0023-6764

Dennis, M.B.Jr.; Dong, W.K.; Weisbrod, K.A. & Elchlepp, C.A. (1988). Use of captive bolt as a method of euthanasia in larger laboratory animal species. *Laboratory Animal Science* Vol. 38 No. 4 (August, 1988) pp.459–462 ISSN 0023-6764

Derr, R.F. (1991) Pain perception in decapitated rat brain. *Life Sciences* Vol. 49, No. 19 pp. 1399–1402. ISSN 0024-3205

Dodd, K. (1985) Humane euthanasia. I. Shooting a horse. *Irish Veterinary Journal* Vol. 39, No. 3 pp. 150-151. ISSN 0368-0762

Eikelenboom, G. (1983) *Stunning of Animals for Slaughter. Current Topics in Veterinary Medicine.* 1st ed. Martinus Nijhoff Publishers pp. 1–227. ISBN 0898385989. Boston Massachusetts.

European Council (1993) European Council Directive 93/119/EC of 22 December 1993 on the protection of animals at the time of slaughter or killing. Annex G: killing of surplus chicks and embryos in hatchery waste. Brussels: European Council. 05.03.2011, Available from: http://ec.europa.eu/food/fs/aw/aw_legislation/slaughter/93-119-ec_en.pdf

Feldman, D.B. & Gupta, B.N. (1976) Histopathologic changes in laboratory animals resulting from various methods of euthanasia. *Laboratory Animal Science* Vol. 26, No. 2 (April, 1976) pp. 218-221 ISSN 0023-6764

Forslid, A.; Ingvar, M.; Rosen, I. & Ingvar, D.H. (1986) Carbon dioxide narcosis: influence of short-term, high concentration carbon dioxide inhalation on EEG and cortical evoked responses in the rat. *Acta Physiologica Scandinavica* Vol. 127, No. 3 (July, 1986) pp. 281-287 ISSN 0001-6772

Green, C.J. (1987) Euthanasia. In: *Laboratory Animals: An Introduction for New Experiments.* (Tuffery, A.A. ed.). John Wiley &. Sons, pp. 171-177 ISNB 978-0471952572 Hoboken, NJ

Gregory, N.G.; Moss, B.W. & Leeson, R.H. (1987) An assessment of carbon dioxide stunning in pigs. *Veterinary Record* Vol. 121, No. 22 (November, 1987) pp.517–518 ISSN 0042-4900

Gregory, N.G. & Wotton, S.B. (1986) Effect of slaughter on spontaneous and evoked activity of the brain. *British Poultry Science* Vol. 27, No. 2 (June, 1986) pp.195–205. ISSN 0007-1668.

Ikarashi, Y.; Marvyama, Y. & Stavinoha, W.B. (1984) Study of the use of the microwave magnetic field for the rapid inactivation of brain enzymes. *Japanese Journal of Pharmacology* Vol. 35, No. 4 (August, 1984) pp. 371–387. ISSN 0021-5198.

Hoenderken, R. (1983) Electrical and carbondioxide stunning of pigs for slaughter. In: Eikelenboom, G. ed. *Stunning of Animals for Slaughter* Martinus Nijhoff Publishers, pp. 59-63 ISBN 978-0898385984, Boston Massachusetts.

Holson, R.R. (1992) Euthanasia by decapitation: evidence that this technique produces prompt, painless unconsciousness in laboratory rodents. *Neurotoxicology and Teratology* Vol. 14, No. 4 (July, 1992) pp.253–257. ISSN 0892-0362

Iwarsson, K. & Rehbinder, C. (1993) A study of different euthanasia techniques in guinea pigs, rats, and mice. Animal response and postmortem findings. *Scandinavian Journal Laboratory Animal Science* Vol. 20 pp.191–205. ISSN 09013393

Jaksch, W. (1981) Euthanasia of day-old male chicks in the poultry industry. *International Journal for the Study of Animal Problems* Vol. 2 pp.203–213. ISSN: 0195-7554

Kitchell, R.L.; Erickson, H.H.; Carstens, E. & Davis L.E. (1983). *Animal pain: perception and alleviation.* Bethesda: American Physiological Society. pp 221. ISBN 068304625X Baltimore, USA

Kitchen, N.; Aronson, A.L.; Bittle, J.L.; McPherson, C.W.; Morton, D.B.Pakes, S.P.; Rollin, B.; Rowan, A.N.; Sechzer, J.A.;Vanderlip, J.E.; Will, J.A.; Clark, A.S. & Gloyd J.S. (1987) Panel report on the colloquium on recognition and alleviation of animal pain and distress. *Journal American Veterinary Medical Association* Vol. 191, No. 10 (November, 1987) pp.1186–1191. ISSN 0003-1488

Klemm, W.R. (1964) Carbon dioxide anesthesia in cats. *American Journal Veterinary Research* Vol. 25 (July, 1964) pp.1201–1205 ISSN 0002-9645.

Kline, B.E.; Peckham, V. & Heist, H.E. (1963) Some aids in handling large numbers of mice. *Laboratory Animal Care* Vol. 13 (April, 1963) pp. 84–90 ISSN 094-5331

Kocula, A.W.; Drewniak, E.E- & Davis, L.L. (1961).Experimentation with in-line carbon dioxide immobilization of chickens prior to slaughter. *Poultry Science* Vol. 40 pp. 213–216. ISSN 1537-0437

Lambooy, E. & Spanjaard, W. (1980) Euthanasia of young pigs with carbon monoxide. *Veterinary Record* Vol. 107, No. 3 (July, 1980) pp. 59–61. ISSN 0042-4900

Lambooy, E. & van Voorst, N. (1986) Electrocution of pigs with notifiable diseases. *Veterinary Quarterly* Vol. 8, No. 1 (January, 1986) pp. 80–82 ISSN 0165-2176

Leake, C.D. & Waters, R.M. (1929) The anesthetic properties of carbon dioxide. *Current Researches in Anaesthesia and Analgesia* Vol. 8, No. 1 (December, 1929) pp. 7–19 ISSN 0003-2999

Lecky, J.H. (1983) Waste anesthetic gases in operating room air: a suggested program to reduce personnel exposure. *The American Society of Anesthesiologists*, Park Ridge Illinois USA.

Longair, J.A.; Finley, G.G.; Laniel, M.A.; Mackay, C.; Mould, K.; Olfert, E.D.; Rowsell, H. & Preston A. (1991) Guidelines for euthanasia of domestic animals by firearms. *Canadian Veterinary Journal* Vol. 32, No.12 (December, 1991) pp. 724-726.ISSN 0008-5286

Lucke, I.N. (1979) Euthanasia in small animals. *Veterinary Record* Vol. 104, No. 14 (April, 1979) pp. 316-18 ISSN 0042-4900

Mattsson, J.L.; Stinson, J.M. & Clark, C.S. (1972). Electroencephalographic power-spectral changes coincident with onset of carbon dioxide narcosis in rhesus monkey. *American Journal Veterinary Research* Vol. 33, No. 10 (October, 1972) pp.2043–2049. ISSN 0002-9645.

Mikeska, J.A. & Klemm, W.R. (1975) EEG evaluation of humaneness of asphyxia and decapitation euthanasia of the laboratory rat. *Laboratory Animal Science* Vol. 25, No. 2 (April, 1975) pp.175–179. ISSN 0023-6764

National Research Council (1992) Recognition and alleviation of pain and distress in laboratory animals. *Committee on Pain and Distress in Laboratory Animals Institute of Laboratory Animal Resources Commission on Life Sciences.* National Academy Press. ISBN 0-309-04275-5 Washington, DC.

Olfert, E.D.; Cross, B.M., & McWilliam, A.A. (1993) Guide to the care and use of experimental animals, Volume 1. *Canadian Council on Animal Care*, Ottawa, Canada. ISBN: 0-919087-18-3

Oliver, D.F. (1979) Euthanasia of horses. *Veterinary Record* Vol. 105, No. 10 (September, 1979) pp. 224-245. ISSN 0042-4900

Raj, A.B.M. & Gregory, N.G. (1990) Investigation into the batch stunning/killing of chickens using carbon dioxide or argon-induced hypoxia. *Research Veterinary Science* Vol. 49, No. 3 (November, 1990) pp. 364–366. ISSN 0034-5288

Reilly, J.S. (2001) Euthanasia of Animals Used for Scientific Purposes. *Australian and New Zealand Council for the Care of Animals in Research and Teaching* 2nd edition. Adelaide University ISBN 0 9586821 4 3 Adelaide Australia.

Roberts, T.D.M. (1954) Cortical activity in electrocuted dogs. *Veterinary Record* Vol. 66, No.5 pp.561–567. ISSN 0042-4900

Schatzmann, U.; Howard, J.; Pittino, J. & Fuchs, P. (1993) Jet injection for the stunning of slaughter pigs. *Fleischwirtschafst* Vol 73, No. 9 pp. 1027-1028 ISSN 0015-363X

Schatzmann, V.; Leuenberger, T.; Fuchs, P.; Howald, M. & Howard, J. (1991) Jet injection: the possibility of using a high pressure water jet for the stunning of slaughter pigs. *Fleischwirtschaft* Vol. 71, No. 8 pp 899-901 ISSN 0015-363X

Simonsen, H.B.; Thordal-Christensen, A.A. & Ockens, N. (1981) Carbon monoxide and carbon dioxide euthanasia of cats: duration and animal behavior. *British Veterinary Journal* Vol. 137, No. 3 (May, 1981) pp. 274-278. ISSN 0007-1935

Stavinoha, W.B.; Frazer, J. & Modak, A.T. (1978) Microwave fixation for the study of acetylcholine metabolism. In: Jenden, D.J. ed. Cholinergic mechanisms and psychopharmacology. *Proceedings of a Symposium on Cholinergic Mechanisms and Psychopharmacology,* held in La Jolla, California, March 28-31, 1977 Plenum Publishing Corp, 169–179. ISBN 0306379244 New York

Stavinoha, W.R. (1983) Study of brain neurochemistry utilizing rapid inactivation of brain enzyme activity by heating and mirowave irradiation. In: Black, C.L.; Stavinoha, W.B. & Marvyama, Y. eds. *Microwave irradiation as a tool to study labile metabolites in tissue* Pergamon Press; 1–12 Elmsford, NY

Urbanski, H.F. & Kelly, S.F. (1991) Sedation by exposure to gaseous carbon dioxide-oxygen mixture: application to studies involving small laboratory animal species. *Laboratory Animal Science* Vol. 41, No. 1 (January, 1991) pp. 80–82. ISSN 0023-6764

Van Zutphen, L.F.M. (2001). History of animal use. In: *Principles of Laboratory Animal Science* Van Zutphen, L.F.M.; Baumans, V. & Beynen A.C. eds. Elsevier, 2-5. ISBN 0444506128, Amsterdam

Vanderwolf, C.H.; Buzsaki, G.; Cain, D.P.; Cooley, R.K. & Robertson, B. (1988) Neocortical and hippocampal electrical activity following decapitation in the rat. *Brain Research* Vol. 451, No 1-2 (June, 1988) pp. 340–344. ISSN 0006-8993

Vierck, C.J.; Cooper, B.Y.; Ritz, L.A. & Greenspan, J.D. (1989). Inference of pain sensitivity from complex behaviors of laboratory animals. In: Chapman, C.R. & Loeser, J.D. eds. *Issues in Pain Measurement: Advances in Pain research and Therapy.* Raven Press, 93–115. ISBN 10 088167530X New York.

Wall, P.D. (1992) Defining pain in animals. In: Short, C.E. & Poznak, A.V. eds. *Animal pain.* Churchill-Livingstone Inc. 63-79. ISBN 978-0721659374, New York

Warrington, R. (1974) Electrical stunning, a review of the literature. *Veterinary Bulletin* Vol. 44, No.10 pp. 617–635. ISSN 0042-4854

Woodbury, D.M.; Rollins, L.T.; Gardner, M.D.; Hirschi, W.L; Hogan, J.R.; Rallison, M.L.; Tanner, G.S. & Brodie, D.A (1958) Effects of carbon dioxide on brain excitability and electrolytes. *American Journal of Physiology* Vol. 192, No. 1 (January, 1958) pp.79–90. ISSN 0002-9513

World Organization for Animal Health (OIE). (2006) Terrestrial animal health code, appendix 3.7.6: *Guidelines for the killing of animals for disease control purposes.* 15.03.2011. Available from http://www.oie.int/print.php?p=http://www.oie.int/eng/normes/mcode/en_chapitre_3.7.6.htm

Zeller von, W.; Mettler, D. & Schatzmann, U. (1989) Untersuchungen zm tierschutzgerechten Betiiubung des Schlachtgeflugels mit Mikrowellen 12550 MHzl. *Deutsche Tierdrtzliche Wochenschrift* Vol.96, pp. 285-332. ISSN: 0341-6593.

Zimmerman, M. (1984). Neurobiological concepts of pain, its assessment and therapy. In: Bromm B., ed. *Pain measurement in man. Neurophysiological correlates of pain*. Elsevier Publishing Co. 15–35. ISBN-10: 0444805710, Amsterdam.

11

Euthanasia for the Zoonosis Control Program

Márcia Dalastra Laurenti[1] and Marcio Antônio Batistela Moreira[2]
[1]*Laboratory of Pathology of Infectious Diseases, School of Medicine, University of São Paulo, São Paulo (SP),*
[2]*Laboratory of Clinical Pathology, School of Veterinary, Anhembi-Morumbi University, São Paulo (SP), Brazil*

1. Introduction

With regarding to public health, there are two major zoonoses in which is recommended euthanasia for dogs, rabies and visceral leishmaniasis. There are government agencies responsible for the control of these diseases as the Center for Zoonoses Control (CZC), which develops prophylactic programs such as: anti-rabies vaccination in urban and rural population of pets, public awareness, and monitoring and tracking of cases positive. According to the CZC of São Paulo, despite the human and canine rabies being virtually eradicated in the city, all infected animals should be euthanized after clinical signs such as paralysis. This decision comes by the fact of dog becomes a potential transmitter, there are no available treatment and the neurological disorders caused by the disease are progressive and irreversible, both in man and animals.

In relation to the visceral leishmaniasis, the treatment of canine disease is prohibited in Brazil, with drugs used for humans disease and are not registered in the Ministry of Agriculture, Livestock and Supply; on the grounds of risk of resistance developing for the causing agent of the disease, *Leishmania*, and increased risk of death to human patients suffering from disease. In spite of, the law is incisive with regarding to the requirement of euthanasia for seropositive dogs there is considerable discussion and controversy about the constitutionality and effectiveness of implementation.

2. Leishmaniasis

The leishmaniasis are represented by a group of diseases with zoonotic character that affects humans and several species of wild and domestic animals. Caused by a protozoan digenetic belonging to *Trypanosomatidae* family (DOFLEIN, 1991) *Leishmania* genus (ROSS,1903), have their biological cycle performed on two hosts, a vertebrate and invertebrate. Vertebrate hosts include wide variety of mammals, among them: rodents, edentulous, marsupials, primates, including canids and humans. The invertebrate hosts are small insects belonging to Psychodidae family, Phlebotominae subfamily, *Lutzomyia* genus in the New World and *Phlebotomus* in the Old World.

According to estimates by the World Health Organization, the global prevalence of the different clinical forms of the disease, cutaneous and visceral, exceeds 12 million cases with a population of 350 million individuals in areas at risk of contracting the infection (WHO, 2001). The leishmanioses are endemic on five continents, in 88 countries located in tropical and sub-tropical regions. The notification is mandatory only in 32 of 88 countries where the disease is prevalent. Thus, the two million new cases are estimated annually, only 600 thousand are officially notified, which shows a high rate of sub-notification (WHO, 2001). Socio-economic changes and behavioral arising from the globalization process hamper not only the control of the illness but also increase the number of victims. Good examples refer to the process of urbanization course of leishmanioses, a process closely related to rural exodus, unemployment, the expansion of slums, wars, among others.

Parasites belongs to the *Leishmania* genus present two main forms: the promastigote, found in the digestive tube of invertebrate hosts females, and amastigote, observed inside cells of the Phagocytic Mononuclear System in the tissues of vertebrate hosts (Genaro, 2002). The evolutionary cycle of these parasites includes a phase in invertebrate hosts where the promastigotes multiply by binary division in the digestive tube of sand fly female, and another stage in vertebrate hosts, reservoirs mammals, in which the amastigotes forms survive, live and multiply, also by binary division within the parasitophorous vacuoles of macrophages (Figure 1).

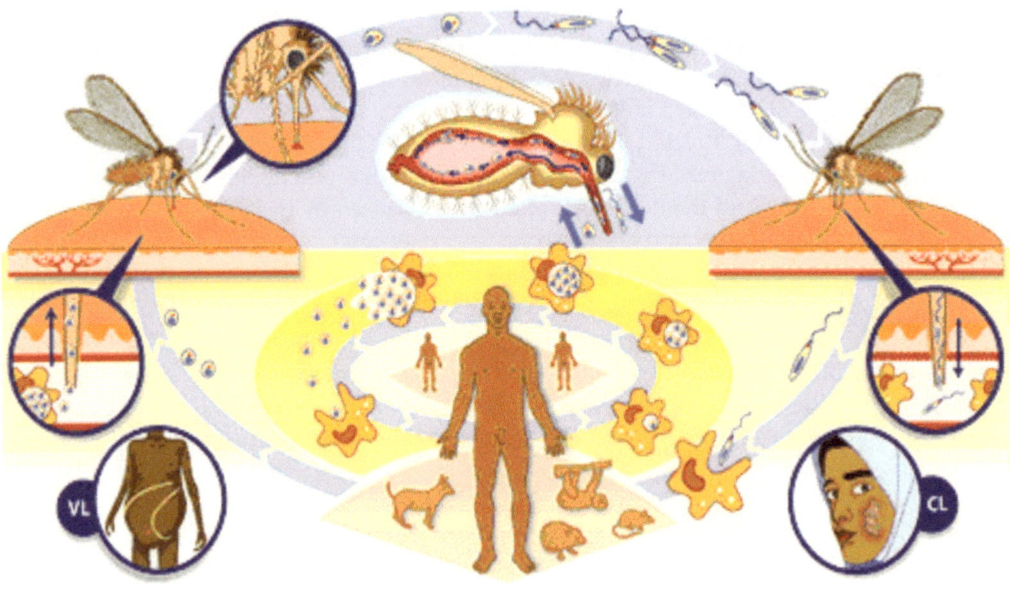

Source: TDR Welcome/Trust

Fig. 1. Biological cycle of *Leishmania* parasite.

Infection occurs when the sand fly female bite the vertebrate, blood feeding and ingests infected macrophages. In the gut of sand flies, these macrophages released de amastigotes, which are rapidly converted into promastigotes which multiply adhered to the peritrophic matrix secreted by cells of the stomach of the insect. After the blood digestion, the peritrophic matrix breaks releasing the promastigotes that colonize different parts of the digestive tube of the vector depending on the species of the parasite. The promastigotes remain anchored to the gut epithelium in the process of binary division. After that, biochemistry changes occur in the parasite surface, called metacyclogenesis. The parasites migrate to the anterior part of the vector alimentary tract. The vertebrate host infection is established when the sand fly female infected bite another vertebrate host and regurgitates the promastigotes in the mammalian skin. On that occasion, it is believed that most parasites are eliminated by lytic action of the complement system and by the action of neutrophils and eosinophils present in inflamed skin (Laurenti et al., 1996). However, some promastigotes that escape to nonspecific defense mechanisms of the host are phagocytized by macrophages in the skin, surviving and multiplying in the parasitophorous vacuoles. After successive binary divisions, the countless parasites cause increased on the pressure inside the macrophage lysing the host cell. The released amastigotes are phagocytized by other macrophages initiating an inflammatory reaction that is responsible for maintaining *Leishmania* in the skin or escape to viscera, depending on the species of the parasite (Genaro, 2002).

2.1 Cutaneous Leishmaniasis (CL)

The pathogenesis of cutaneous leishmaniasis is heavily influenced by two fundamental factors: first, related to the immunogenetic background of the vertebrate host and the second, related to virulence of *Leishmania* species, since there are several species *Leishmania* parasites causing cutaneous leishmaniasis. As a result of these interactions a spectrum of clinical histopathologic and immunological manifestation could be observed (Silveira et al., 2009) (Figure 2).

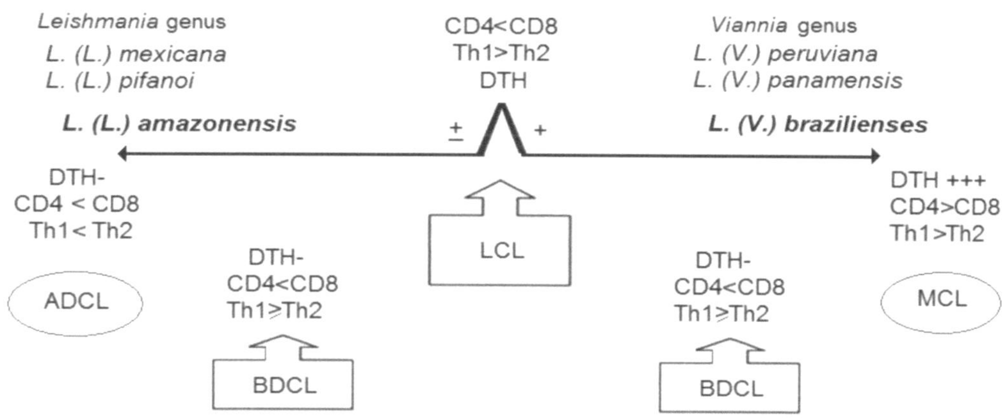

Fig. 2. New World cutaneous leishmaniasis: clinical and immunopathological classification according to Silveira et al., 2004.

The immunopathogenesis of American cutaneous leishmaniasis (ACL) has been regarded one of most interesting features concerning this parasitic protozoal disease in viewing of the complex interaction process between the variety of *Leishmania* species causing the disease and the human immune response. Actually, there are, at least, fourteen recognized *Leishmania* parasites within the subgenera *Viannia* and *Leishmania* which can give rise to clinical ACL (Lainson & Shaw, 1998; Lainson & Shaw, 2005). Recently, following new findings on the clinical and immunopathological spectrum of the disease caused by *Leishmania (V.) braziliensis* and *Leishmania (L.) amazonensis* there has been increased the interest on the immunopathogenic competences of these two *Leishmania* species; i.e. they are implicated not only with the localized cutaneous leishmaniasis (LCL), the most common ACL form placed at the centre of the clinical spectrum and supported by a moderate T-cell hypersensitivity, but also with the mucocutaneous leishmaniasis (MCL) and anergic diffuse cutaneous leishmaniasis (ADCL), the more severe ACL forms respectively. In this regard, while MCL represents the extreme expression of T-cell hypersensitivity pole, linked to a strong species-specific T-cell immune response against to *L. (V.) braziliensis*, ADCL means, in contrast, the extreme expression of T-cell hyposensitivity pole, associated to a high *Leishmania*-specific inhibition of T-cell response (Silveira et al., 2004). Moreover, these *Leishmania* parasites can also induce an intermediary form between the central LCL and the two polar MCL and ADCL, the borderline disseminated cutaneous leishmaniasis (BDCL), which is distinguished by a partial inhibition of T-cell response (Silveira et al., 2005). Furthermore, as BDCL can be caused by parasites belong to both subgenus of *Leishmania*, *Viannia* and *Leishmania*, as well as there are some clinical and immunological characteristics that differ between *Viannia* and *Leishmania* cases, then BDCL can occupy the two places between the centre (LCL) and the two polar forms (MCL and ADCL) in the clinical spectrum of disease (Silveira et al., 2009).

2.1.1 Control and prophylaxis of CL

The control of cutaneous leishmaniasis is difficult, since their cycle happens mainly in forests, often extensive, preventing the use of insecticides in large-scale. Deforestation for agriculture and livestock development reduces the endemic areas, but determines the appearance of large number of cases during the process. The use of repellents and musketeers of fine mesh, in some situations it becomes possible, as individual protection to avoid the bite of sand flies. Recent colonization areas near forests, can avoid transmitting intra-and peri-domestic with the construction of houses at a minimum distance of 500 m from the forest, due to the low flight capacity of these vectors. But the ideal solution for control of CL would produce an effective vaccine (Genaro, 2002).

3. Visceral Leishmaniasis (VL)

Visceral leishmaniasis is a widespread chronic infectious illness, characterized by irregular fever, hepatosplenomegaly, lymphadenopathy, anemia with leukopenia, hypergammaglobulinemia with hypoalbuminemia, lost weight, edema and progressive weakness leading to cachexia and, finally, to death if the patient is not subjected to special treatment. The human visceral leishmaniasis can assume a spectral character, which determines different clinical forms, ranging from a silent asymptomaatic or subclinical forms to oligosymptomatic, acute up to the classical form (Figure 3) of the disease (Badaró et al., 1986). American and European visceral leishmaniasis are considered zoonosis, while in India it is considered an anthropozoonosis.

3.1 Geographic distribution of VL

Visceral leishmaniasis occurs in several countries of the Old and New World and it is caused by *L. (L.) donovani*, *L. (L.) infantum* and *L. (L.) chagasi*. The *L. (L.) donovani* is found in regions of India, Bangladesh, Sudan, Pakistan, Nepal and parts of Eastern China. This species of the parasite can cause dermal leishmaniasis post-calazar, besides to classical visceral leishmaniasis, which is transmitted from man to man, characterizing an anthroponosis. It is possible that in Sudan the transmission occurs in a similar way to India, but other mammals were found parasitized; among them, three species of rodents (*Arvicanthis niloticus, Acomys albigena, Rattus rattus*) and two carnivorous (*Genetta genetta* and *Cat felis*). The vector of leishmaniasis in India is the *Phlebotomus argentipes* and in the region of China is the *Phlebotomus alexandri*. The *L. (L.) infantum* show extensive distribution by the Old World, occurring in Central Asia, North and Northeast China, West Asia (Iraq, Yemen, Saudi Arabia, Iran and Afghanistan), Africa (Algeria, Ethiopia, Tunisia, Libya, Egypt, Central African Republic, Congo, Chad, Gabon, Kenya, Nigeria, Malawi, Morocco, Niger, Senegal, Somalia, Sudan, Zaire and Zambia). In Europe, *L. (L.) infantum* is found in countries belonging to the Mediterranean basin, extending to Hungary and Romania. The main host is the domestic dog, *Canis familiaris,* considered the primary reservoir of infection for humans. Wild hosts are identified as the jackal, *Canis aureus*, wolf, *Canis lupus*, and the fox, *Vulpes vulpes*. In China was also mentioned the canid, *Nyctereutes procyonides,* as reservoir. In Georgia and Azerbaijan infection affects the badgers, *Meles meles,* and the fox, *Vulpes corsak*. The sand fly responsible for the transmission and spread of the disease, according to the region, are *Phlebotomus perniciosus, P. ariasi, P. major, P. alexandri, P. chinensis, P. perfiliewi, P. tobbi, P. longicuspis, P. mongolensis, P. kandelaki and P. caucasicus* (WHO, 2001). The *L. (L.) chagasi* shows wide distribution in the New World, occurring in Argentina, Bolivia, Brazil, Colombia, Paraguay, Venezuela, Guatemala, Guadeloupe, Martinique, Mexico, Honduras and El Salvador. The wild hosts in Brazil are the foxes, *Dusicyon vetulus* and *Lycalopex vetulus*, in the Northeast, *Cerdocyon thous*, Amazon, and skunks *Didelphis marsupialis*. The domestic dog is considered as the main source of infection for humans and the main vector is *Lutzomyia longipalpis* (Brazilian Health Ministry, 2006).

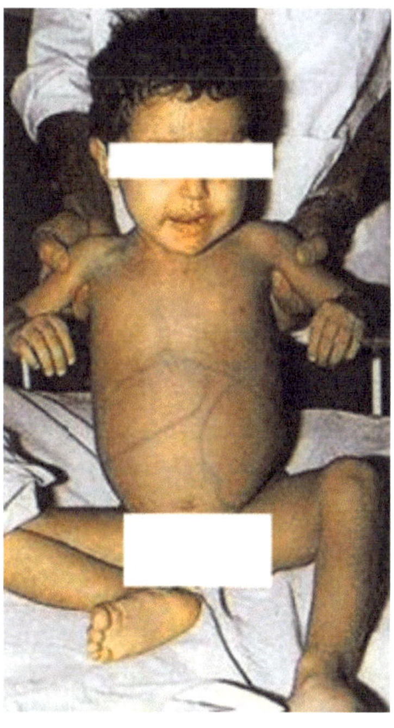

Fig. 3. Classical clinical form of visceral leishmaniasis characterized by hepatosplenomegaly. Photo kindly provided by Dra. Monica Elinor Alves Gama.

3.1.1 Ecology and epidemiology of VL

Visceral leishmaniasis is currently emerging and reemerging diseases, both in rural areas as in urban areas. The World Health Organization estimates a global annual incidence of 500 thousand cases. Although the VL is known even today as a disease typically rural, several urban epidemic outbreaks have been reported, due to the favorable epidemiological conditions, mainly in function of the expansion of slums with high population density that have poor sanitary conditions where individuals and infected dogs from endemic areas are your choice of housing in major cities.

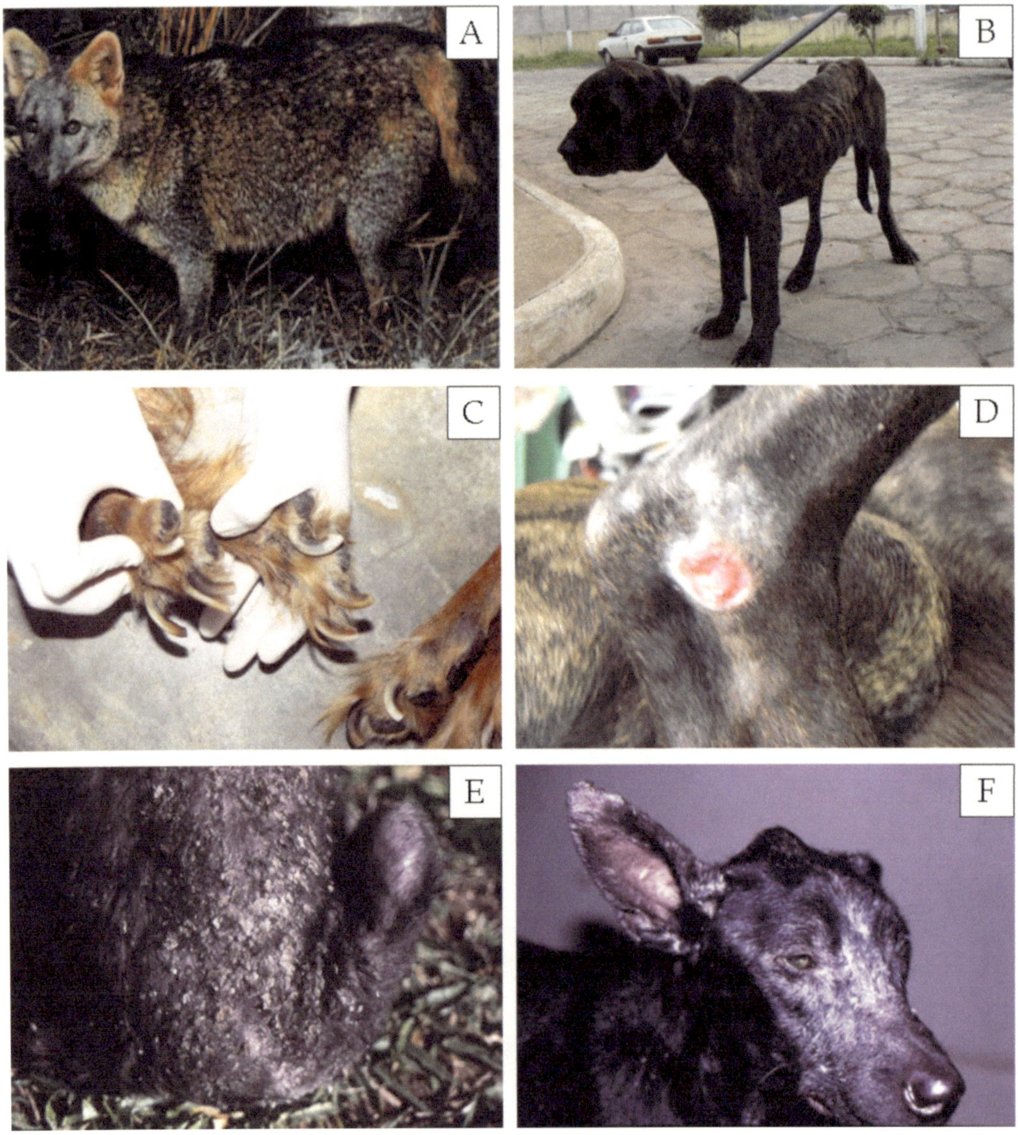

Fig. 4. *Leishmania (Leishmania) chagasi* wild reservoir (A) and domestic reservoir showing typical clinical features of the disease such as: weight loss (B), onychogryphosis (C), skin lesions: ulcer (D), hyperkeratosis (E) and alopecia (F).

Currently, what call attention is the increase in the number of cases of HIV co-infection, especially in southern Europe. This region of Europe HIV infection occurs in rural and suburban areas where visceral leishmaniasis is endemic. Many of these cases are associated with injection drug due to the habit of some groups of users to share disposable syringes and needles. This type of transmission has expanded to Europe's Nordic countries such as Germany, Finland, Norway, changing the classic epidemiological profile of transmission, without the presence of the insect vector and reservoir dogs.

Another aspect relevant in this context of expansion and urbanization of visceral leishmaniasis in the World and especially in Brazil is the possibility of contracting the disease through blood transfusion. This fact is aggravated since serological diagnosis for visceral leishmaniasis is not yet included in the screening of donors in all countries (Brazilian Health Ministry, 2006).

Two distinct epidemiological cycle of VL is observed, a wild cycle and domestic or per-domestic cycle. In the wild cycle are involved as vector, *Lutzomyia longipalpis*, and as a reservoir, the foxes (Figure 4A), which inhabit niches still undisturbed by man in forest or wilderness areas. Dogs are considered the domestic reservoir and have been found infected in all outbreaks of human disease; they are considered the main source of parasites in the chain of transmission of VL (Figure 4B). While the wild reservoir shows no clinical signs of the disease pointed to an adaptative relationship between parasite-host, the domestic reservoir shows important clinical manifestations of the disease with severe visceral involvement that causes the animal death. Among the main clinical features observed in canine visceral leishmaniasis, it is observed weight loss, lymphadenopathy, hepatosplenomegaly, onychogryphosis, skin lesions (ulcers, hyperkeratosis and alpecia), among others (Figure C-F) (Feitosa et al, 2000). The domestic cycle can occurs on rural or peri-urban environment, where *Lutzomyia longipalpis* is involved as the vector, which breeds and remains in the peri-domestic environment transmitting the infection to man and dog. The dog has an important role in maintaining of local infection, serving as a source of infection to the sand fly. The transmission occurs subsequently to the man, who is also able to serve as a source of infection for the vector. These two cycles can overlap, since man and the dog into wild environment may acquire the infection by the sand fly bite, and when return to domestic environment serves as a source of infection to local sand fly, starting the transmission in the domestic area. The reservoir presented intense cutaneous parasitism, so they are excellent source of infection to the sand fly, favoring the maintenance of the cycle of the disease (Genaro, 2002).

3.1.2 Prophylaxis of VL

If the control of visceral leishmaniasis is continuous and well conducted, can produce good results; however to the results obtained are durable, there is a requirement of permanent and effective epidemiological surveillance, otherwise gradually the outbreaks arise avoiding previous work. Since that the epidemiological role of dog is established as domestic reservoir and *Lutzomyia longipalpis* as vector, the control can be based on three fundamental points: treatment of human cases, elimination of infected dogs and combating vector.

The use of euthanasia to the control of canine visceral leishmaniasis began with Adler and Tchernomoretz, 1946 after failing to succeed with human treatment and concluded that the best form to disease control would be the elimination of dog. The program carried out in China (Leng, 1982) was based on a triad: the treatment of positive human cases, use of insecticides (DDT) and disposal of dogs in some locations. Using these methods for the control, the anthroponotic leishmaniasis almost finished and the zoonotic leishmaniasis continued and continues in China. They concluded that the removal of dogs helped in the control of leishmaniasis, but it was only one of the control measures.

The Brazilian program for control of VL advocates the canine serologic surveys, targeting to know canine epidemiological situation of the disease in areas with active transmission or with potential to transmission and at the same time, identify the positive dogs to later disposal. However, there are controversial data concerning to this subject. Some studies showed that there are no significant differences between regions where euthanasia was only used as a control measure, when compared to others in which the dog was not eliminated (Dietze et al., 1997), by the other side another study related the reduction of human VL incidence correlated to dog euthanasia but not exclude the possibility to consider other factors that may influence this relationship (Nunes et al., 2010). The difference is the use of the insecticide that presents good results in the control of leishmaniasis. Another point was emphasized by Braga et al. (1998), the importance of sensitivity and specificity parameters of the diagnostic assay, when evaluating the impact of the dog elimination in front of the employed methodology.

After two decades of attempts to control of VL in Brazil, the number of cases in the country increased sharply and broke into urban areas. The Brazilian program, started more than 40 years, is composed by integrating three measures of public health: the free distribution of specific treatment to human patients, the control of domestic reservoirs and the control of the vector. The control of reservoirs has been done by serological diagnosis of domestic dogs where transmission of *L. (L.) chagasi* for human occurs. For this, was structured a network of immunofluorescence assay (IFA) using eluate of filter paper; all dogs with positive result have been euthanized. However, dogs evaluate by IFA employing eluate when reevaluated by IFA using serum samples, 72% of the animals were negative (Silva et al., 2011). This result can be partially explained by the sample tested, serum and eluate, as previously reported by Figueiredo et al., (2010). Moreover, 59% of animals identified by IFA using eluate showed negative results for *L. (L.) chagasi* infection, characterizing a false positive result by IFA employing eluate. However, in areas where the circulation of other trypanosomatids occurs, parasitological confirmation of seropositive dogs is of great important in several aspects to avoid cross reaction. By the other side, according to Figueiredo et al. (2010), dogs infected by *Leishmania* could not be identified by IFA in dried blood on filter paper, possibly maintaining the transmission cycle in endemic area.

In respect of serologic methods employed in epidemiological investigations with the aim of knowing the prevalence of the disease in endemic areas or with potential for transmission of the VL, the parameters of sensitivity, specificity and predictive values of serological techniques employed are of the extreme importance to avoid erroneous interpretations, with false positive or negative. Although the serology is only an indirect method of measuring the infection, not defining the degree of parasitism, the presence of the disease, or even the potential for transmission that the dog may have to the vector. Decrease the number of false positive results would be very important for the efficiency and reliability of the program, avoiding the elimination of the dogs that do not provide risk in the transmission of infection.

The correlation between the clinical status of the dogs and its infectivity for the vector should also be considered in the discussions for the adoption of measures to the control of VL since Pinelli et al.(1994) observed that asymptomatic and symptomatic animals had severe immune response, quite distinct, favor or not the vector infection. Anyway, it is important to mention the report of Barata et al. (2005) showed infection in the laboratory reared vector which feeding in seropositive dogs from different clinical forms of the disease. Cutaneous parasitism in found in intact skin of dogs naturally infected by *L. (L.) chagasi*, irrespective of the presence or absence of clinical signs suggestive of visceral leishmaniasis (Madeira et al., 2004).

According to the technical report of the Ministry of Health of Brazil (Costa & Vieira, 2001), the program for the disposal of domestic dogs presents the lowest scientific-technical support between the three strategies of control program, and recommends that the systematic serological screening followed by dogs elimination should be suspended. Serological examination was recommended for dogs only from endemic areas who presents suspicious symptoms; however the serological test in eluate of blood on filter paper should be replaced by conventional serology; and that the elimination of dogs should be restricted only to the situations in which the diagnosis of visceral leishmaniasis was confirmed by parasitological exams. In addition, the treatment of dogs with drugs available for the human patients is not recommended, both for inefficiency as a measure of public health due to infectivity of treated dogs to the sand fly as for the risk of developing resistance to long-term medication.

Another point to be considered is that the elimination of the seropositive animals for the control of human VL provides the increase in the dog younger population, which is more susceptible to *Leishmania* infection (Nunes et al., 2008). Thus, it is necessary to investigate other methods for this zoonosis control in addition to the euthanasia of ill animals. The simple sacrifice itself proves to be ineffective and injure the owner and the life of the animals.

The increase in the number of VL cases and transmission of *L. (L.) chagasi* in metropolitan areas indicate the existence of factors that could contribute to the inefficiency of control programs, which have suffered questions, mainly on the adoption of measures such as the elimination of dogs serologically positive.

4. Rabies

Rabies is transmitted by an anthropozoonosis deposition of contaminated material and inoculation with the rabies virus by biting, scratching or licking the skin in healthy animals or humans. This infectious agent is a RNA virus of the *Rhabdoviridae* family, *Lyssavirus* genus present in saliva and secretions of infected animals.

This virus is composed of two units in its structure: ribonucleoprotein and viral envelope. There are also five proteins, including the viral envelope glycoprotein, of the most important due to stimulation of the immune system and production of neutralizing antibodies, which are able to confer protection against the disease. The virus affects the central nervous system (CNS) causing encephalitis, leading to around 100% of lethality and the high cost in preventing individuals at risk of illness and death. Despite being a disease studied since antiquity is still a public health problem. All mammals are considered sources of infection and therefore can transmit it to humans. The main animal species evolved in the transmission are: dogs, cats, bats, wild dog, marmosets, foxes, cattle, horses, pigs, goats, among others. Until a few years ago it was considered three transmission cycles (urban, rural, and wild) and is currently included another cycle observed among bats, denominated the air (Figure 5). Rabies is an urban problem in developing countries is characterized by the presence of disease in domestic animals such as pet dogs and cats. Rabies is mainly rural transmitter the hematophagous bat (*Desmodus rotundos*) that transmits the disease to herbivores, as these are the most common food source. Cycle in wild disease is transmitted to animals like fox, wolf, monkey, coon, skunk, among others. These animals can be a source of food for the hematophagous bat. It can capture bats and suffer injury or attacked by domestic animals. The air cycle is important for virus among species of bats, because these are the only mammals that fly. All species of bats, sucking are not susceptible to the virus. This disease has worldwide distribution. Only a few islands like Japan or Hawaii, there is no movement of the virus, even among the wild species considered natural reservoirs.

The incubation period is variable between different species of mammals. In humans this period can vary from two to ten weeks, on average 30 to 45 days. This variation is justified by the extent of the injury, viral inoculation and the virus strain. The infected animal usually begins transmission before presenting signs and symptoms of this disease. This period is well characterized in dogs and cats beginning two to four days prior to clinical manifestations and death occurring after five days of observation of clinical manifestations of disease.

The rabies virus multiplies in the initial period, at the site of inoculation and then reaches nerve endings. Dissemination occurs by retrograde axonal flow in centripetal movement to reach the CNS. That path remains protected by the sheath of nerves, not by stimulating an immune response. On reaching the CNS can replicate at various locations in the dog and cat, the target region is the hippocampus (Ammon's horn) and dentate gyrus (pyramidal neurons), spinal cord horses and cattle in the cerebellum (Purkinje cells). Only when a large amount of virus is produced stimulates the immune system and spreads to several sites, particularly the salivary glands, can also be found in the eyes, hair follicles and sweat glands.

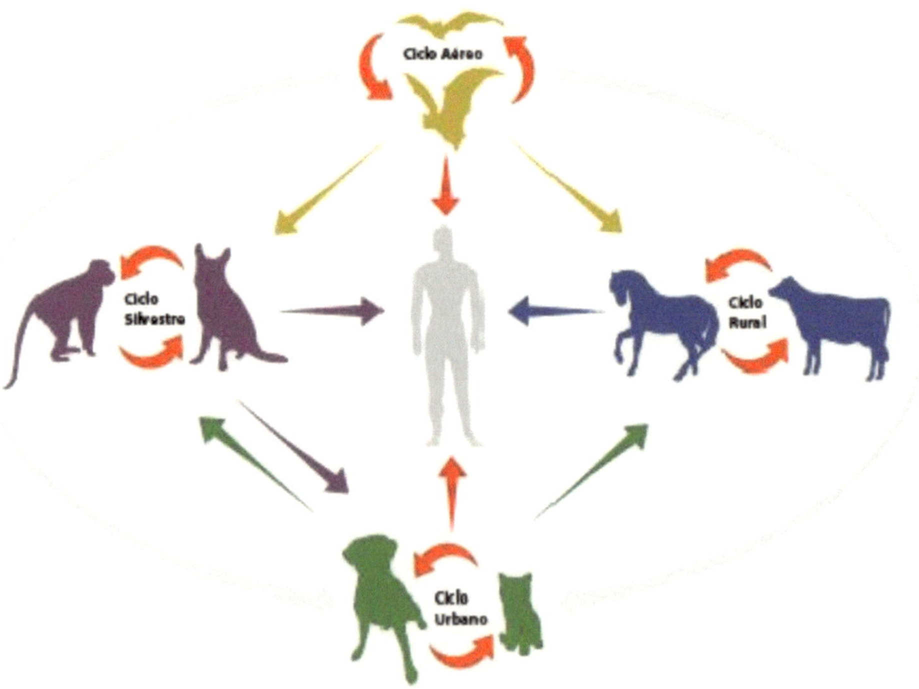

Source: Pasteur Institute -SES/SP

Fig. 5. Epidemiological cycles of rabies transmission in Brazil

4.1 Signs and symptoms in animals

The clinical condition of the animal is divided in podromic phase, furious rabies, paralytic and atypical. The podromic phase is characterized by a period of one to two days, the animals are uneasy with mild or apparent changes in behavior, dogs and cats, do not answer the call of the owners, have attention deficit, do not feed and can be isolated, seek hideouts. Large animals can move away from the group, not eating and isolate themselves. Passing this stage enter into a framework known as furious anger, where they show aggression, attack other animals that commonly live together and even the owner that are used to entertain. Other changes such as hunting boats and giving imaginary flies bite in the air, wander aimlessly, howling incessantly, unable to drink water by the pharyngeal nerve palsy recurrent, drooling, biting and attacking the cages, make changes as ophthalmic strabismus can also be observed. This phase is marked by aggressiveness and hyperexcitability due to encephalitis. The stage called paralytic rabies is characterized by the development of paralysis, especially in the hind limbs, followed by the jaw and forelimbs. When atypical rabies, characterized by slight changes in the behavior, is observed, there are difficulties to diagnose.

4.2 Signs and symptoms in humans

In humans the clinical picture may be divided into the following phases: neurology podromic, coma and death. The symptoms are nonspecific in early stages such as fever, headache, malaise, anorexia and sore throat. Sensitivity can occur at the site of biting, burning, numbness and itching. Then there are the manifestation in the CNS such as anxiety, restlessness, disorientation, hallucinations and seizures. It is commonly characterized by hydrophobia and spasms of swallowing difficulty, in which the person is thirsty, but cannot drink water. Struggling to swallow the saliva occurs which enhances dehydration. The disease progresses to severe psychomotor agitation, altered by seizures. The patient goes into coma, failure occurs breathe and death within five to eight days after onset of symptoms. Rabies is a notifiable shown.

4.3 Control rabies

The control of rabies in pets (dogs and cats) requires a series of measures such as: periodic vaccination against rabies; keep post vaccination against rabies fixed for the second dose in primed; vaccination of cats, among others; seize animals, keep them with quality of life and vaccinate them against rabies right away or when the redemption will be donated; performing euthanasia ethical method, the dogs that do not fit the above mentioned items; send material for laboratory diagnosis Rabies in quantity and frequency appropriate for observing the behavior of this virus; making epidemiological research in positive cases headed for prophylaxis of exposed persons; performing with focus lock vaccination actions and seizure of stray animals, within 72 hours; promote observation of aggressive dogs and cats for ten days from the date of the accident; stimulate the development of education initiatives and health promotion, using the held responsible.

Rabies is a fatal disease and only the development of the disease will take the animal to death, but euthanasia, conducted in an ethical manner, will alleviate the suffering of this animal is affected because this disease has no treatment in veterinary medicine.

The measure of control with greater relevance to rabies control is population control. This control should be accomplished through the castration of domestic animals, especially those who are wandering the street and placed collected for donation and mainly awareness of people to understand the true meaning of responsible ownership. The criteria of responsible ownership should be widely disseminated mainly in schools, because children will disseminate information to family practice and charge what they learned. The possession charge means: giving attention and affection for the animal; the animal out on the street should be conducted with collar and leash with individual controls and the strength to stop him; offering food and good quality water; bathe regularly; from three months to take the animal to receive the rabies vaccine and implement a booster dose after 30 days; routinely take the animal to the vet; take the animal with two months to vaccine other diseases; keeping the animal in space and where appropriate cannot attack other people or animals; if the animal impairs a person performs his observation for ten days; occur when mating these animals get homes for all puppies and not abandon them.

So we can decrease the use of the method of euthanasia to control and combat rabies

Some reports in Brazil, the USA and other countries approach a satisfactory response to treatment in human patients who had the disease. The research evaluating of the treatment effectiveness associated with awareness, the vast majority of people collaborate to minimize the euthanasia of pets.

5. Conclusions

From what has been discussed in this chapter with regard to leishmaniasis, we can conclude that euthanasia of dogs as one of the main measures used in the control of human disease has not proven very effective. Even with sacrifice of a high number of animals, the number of human cases has not decreased and the disease has spread even to urban areas. This is because other reservoirs may be involved in the biological cycle of the parasite and also because the very fast replacement of the dogs. It shows the need to establish other policies for control of the disease, associated or not to the euthanasia of dogs, such as vector control. In addition, efforts should be made towards prevention of the dog disease, such as the use of repellents to prevent the sand fly bite, and the development of effective vaccines candidates. Regarding to the rabies, the main control measure, animals vaccination has been shown effective in controlling the zoonosis, and the euthanasia is conducted only for sick animals since the treatment is not recommended.

6. References

Badaró, R.; Jones, TC.; Lorenço, R.; Cerf, BJ., Sampaio, D., Carvalho, EM., Rocha, H., Teixeira, R., Johnson, WD. (1986). The prospective study of visceral also reported in an endemic area of Brazil. Journal of Infectious Diseases, Vol.154, No.4, (October 1986), pp. 639-649,ISSN 1537-6613.

Barata, RA.; França-Silva, JC.; Mayrink, W.; Silva, JC.; Prata, A.; Lorosa, ES,Fiúza, JÁ.; Gonçalves, CM.; Paula, KM.; Dias, ES. (2005). Aspects of the ecology and behaviour of phlebotomines in endemic area for visceral leishmaniasis in State of Minas Gerais. Revista da Sociedade Brasileira de Medicina Tropical, Vol.38. No.5, (September/October 2005), pp. 421-425, ISSN 1678-9849.

Braga, MD.; Coêlho, IC.; Pompeu, MM.; Evans, TG.; MacAullife, IT.; Teixeira, MJ.; Lima, JW. (1998). Control of canine visceral leishmaniasis: comparison of results from a rapid elimination program of serum-reactive dogs using an immunoenzyme assay and slower elimination of serum-reactive dogs using filter paper elution indirect immunofluorescence. Revista da Sociedade Brasileira de Medicina Tropical, Vol.31, No.5, (September/October 1998), pp. 419-424, ISSN 1678-9849.

Brazilian Health Ministry. (2006). Manual de vigilância e controle da leishmaniose visceral. Brasília - DF.

Costa, CH.; Vieira, JB. (2001). Changes in the control of visceral leishmaniasis in Brazil. Revista da Sociedade Brasileira de Medicina Tropical, Vol.34, No.2, (March/April 2001), pp. 223-228, ISSN 1678-9849.

Dietze ,R.; Barros, GB.; Teixeira, L.; Harris, J.; Michelson, K.; Falqueto, A.; Corey, R. (1997). Effect of eliminating seropositive canines on the transmission of visceral leishmaniasis in Brazil. Clinical Infectious Diseases, Vol.25, No.5, (November 1997), pp. 1240-1242, ISSN 1537-6591.

Feitosa, MM.; Ikeda, FA.; Luvizotto, MCR.; Perri, SHV. (2000). Aspectos clínicos de cães com leishmaniose visceral no município de Araçatuba - São Paulo (Brasil). Clínica Veterinária. No.28, (September/October 2000), pp.36-44.

Figueiredo, FB.; Madeira, MF.; Menezes, RC.; Pacheco, RS.; Pires, MQ.; Furtado, MC.; Pinto, AG.; Schubach, TM. (2010). Efficacy of indirect immunofluorescence test in the diagnosis of canine leishmaniosis. Veterinary Journal, Vol.186, No.1, (August 2010), pp. 123-124 ISSN 1090-0233.

Genaro, O. (2002). Leishmaniose Tegumentar America / Leishmaniose Visceral America. In: Parasitologia Humana, eds: Neves, DP.; Melo, AL.; Genaro, O.; Linardi, PMP., 10th ed., pp. 36-72, Editora Atheneu, ISBN 857379243-4, São Paulo.

Lainson, R.; Shaw, JJ. (1998). New World leishmaniasis - The neotropical Leishmania species. In: Topley & Wilson's Microbiology and Microbial Infections: Parasitology, eds: Cox, FEG.; Kreier; Wakelin, D.; Topley & Wilson., 9th ed., Vol. 5, pp. 242–266, Hodder Arnold, ISBN 0340663200, London.

Lainson, R.; Shaw, JJ. (2005). Leishmaniasis in the New World. In: Topley & Wilson's Microbiology and Microbial Infections: Parasitology , eds: Collier, L.; Balows, A.; Sussman, M., 10th ed., Vol. 5, pp. 313–349, Hodder Arnold, ISBN 0340663200, London.

Laurenti, MD.; Corbett, CEP.; Sotto, NM.; Sinhorini, IL.; Goto, H. (1996). The role of complement in the acute inflammatory process in the skin and in the host-parasite interaction in hamster inoculated with *L. (L.) chagasi*. International Journal of Experimental Pathology. Vol.77, No.1,(February 1996), pp. 15-24, ISSN 1365-2613.

Leng, YJ. (1982). A review of kala-azar in China from 1949-1959. Transactions of the Royal Society of Tropical Medicine and Hygiene. Vol.76, No.4, pp. 531-537, ISSN 0035-9203.

Madeira, MF.; Schubach, AO.; Schubach, TMP.; Leal, CA.; Marzochi, MCA. (2004). Identification of *Leishmania (Leishmania) chagasi* isolated from health skin of symptomatic and asymptomatic dogs seropositive for leishmaniasis in the municipality of Rio de Janeiro, Brazil. The Brazilian Journal of Infectious Diseases. Vol.8, No.6, (December 2004), pp. 440-444, ISSN 1413-8670.

Nunes, CM.; Lima, VM.; Paula, HB.; Perri, SH.; Andrade, AM.; Dias, FE.; Burattini, MN. (2008). Dog culling and replacement in an area endemic for visceral leishmaniasis in Brazil. Veterinary Parasitology. Vol.153, No.1-2, (May 2008), pp. 19-23, ISSN 0304-4017.

Nunes, CM.; Pires, MM.; da Silva, KM.; Assis, FD.; Gonçalves Filho, J.; Perri, SH. (2010). Relationship between dog culling and incidence of human visceral leishmaniasis in an endemic area. Veterinary Parasitololy. Vol. 170, No.1-2, (February 2010), pp. 131-133, ISSN 0304-4017.

Pinelli, E.; Killick-Kendrick, R.; Wagenaar, J.; Bernadina, W.; del Real, G.; Ruitenberg, J. (1994). Cellular and humoral immune responses in dogs experimentally and naturally infected with *Leishmania infantum*. Infection and Immunity. Vol. 62. No.1, (January 1994), pp. 229-235, ISSN 1098-5522.

Silva, DA.; Madeira, MF.; Teixeira, AC.; de Souza, CM.; Figueiredo, FB. (2011). Laboratory tests performed on Leishmania seroreactive dogs euthanized by the leishmaniasis control program. Veterinary Parasitoly. Vol.179, No.1-3, (February 2011), pp. 257-261, ISSN 0304-4017.

Silveira, FT.; Lainson, R.; Corbett, CEP. (2004). Clinical and immunopathological spectrum of American cutaneous leishmaniasis with special reference to the disease in Amazonian Brazil: a review. Memórias do Instituto Oswaldo Cruz. Vol.99, No.3, (May 2004), pp. 239–251, ISSN 1678-8060.

Silveira, FT.; Lainson, R.; Corbett, CEP. (2005). Further observations on clinical, histopathological and immunological features of borderline disseminated cutaneous leishmaniasis caused by *Leishmania (Leishmania) amazonensis*. Memórias do Instituto Oswaldo Cruz. Vol.100, No.5, (August 2005), pp. 525–534, ISSN 1678-8060.

Silveira, FT.; Lainson, R.; Gomes, CMC.; Laurenti, MD.; Corbett, CEP. (2009). Immunopathogenic competences of *Leishmania (V.) braziliensis* and *L. (L.) amazonensis* in American cutaneous leishmaniasis. Parasite Immunology. Vol.31, No.8, (August 2009), pp. 423-431, ISSN 1365-3024.

World Health Organization (WHO). (2001). The World Health Report. Geneva.

12

Debate For and Against Euthanasia in the Control of Dog Populations

Antonio Ortega-Pacheco and Matilde Jiménez-Coello
Universidad Autonoma de Yucatan, Mexico

1. Introduction

Dogs share the same environment of humans and play an important role in their ecological adjustment. Since its domestication 12,000 to 15,000 years ago, they have been part of human evolution with increases on its population as humans settle down. Dogs provide social and health benefits to humans but they may also be involved in social conflicts such as bites, zoonosis, destruction of ecosystems, etc. As consequence of its uncontrolled and logarithmic growth on its population, several strategies have been taken in both developed and developing countries. Under these two scenarios, euthanasia is employed as part of the strategy to overcome the surplus of this species. However, ethical issues arise when healthy dogs are killed or methods used for euthanasia are inhumane and against international standards. Besides, euthanasia as a method to control the dog overpopulation has shown to be expensive and ineffective on long term. In humans euthanasia is restricted to compassion or "mercy" killing to relief the patient of an terminal disease or when life become too painful and with poor life expectative. In veterinary medicine the term euthanasia is broader since it also includes healthy animals such as dogs, for elective euthanasia considering owner convenience, reasons of overpopulation, for behavior problems or research purposes.

Canine overpopulation arises when uncontrolled breeding of dogs and irresponsible ownership act together. Dogs are promiscuous species by nature and since not a well defined seasonality occurs in this species, are ready to mate all through the year. Owners frequently claim their rights to own a dog but may be reluctant to take care of their responsibilities. If no laws to regulate dog ownership exist or if they exists but are not reinforced, the imminent consequence will be a surplus of the species ending on the streets or shelters. Even in shelters, it is estimated that 2 out of 3 animals entering a shelter won't have a chance to be adopted and have to be euthanized.

Several methods for euthanasia in dogs have been used. Some are recommended by international associations and others are considered illegal in some countries. Barbiturates (pentobarbitone or pentobarbital sodium) are by most the more common used drug for euthanasia in dogs; barbiturates cause deep anesthesia and unconsciousness before leading to respiratory failure. However, in case of anesthetized animals other methods such as Magnesium sulfate, potassium salts, carbon monoxide gas and even captive bolt shots can be administrated. Some inacceptable methods, still used in some countries are the use of strychnine, electrocutation, cyanide, decapitation, drowning and curariform drugs (for example, succinylcholine).

This manuscript describes the situation of canine overpopulation and strategies to control it with special reference to the use of euthanasia. The use of mass euthanasia of stray dogs in developing countries and euthanasia performed in dog shelters will also be addressed. A fair description of methods used for euthanasia will be described. A general discussion about ethical and moral issues about the use of euthanasia methods to control the population of dog over plus and better strategies to address the problem will be generated.

2. Canine overpopulation and welfare

Dogs may be classified according to the level of supervision as restricted or supervised dogs (Fully dependent and fully restricted or supervised), family dogs (fully dependent; semi-restricted) which can have access to the streets, neighbourhood dog (semi-dependent, semi-restricted or unrestricted) and feral dog (independent, unrestricted, nobody takes responsibilities for it) (World Health Organization [WHO], 1990). Neighbourhood dogs are recognized as the most common kind of dog present in urban and rural areas from developing countries (Brooks, 1990; Orihuela & Solano, 1995; Fielding & Plumridge, 2005); those dogs are not necessary straying since may be allowed for freely roaming. In figure 1 an owned free roaming dog can be seen. Dog populations are very dynamics; after an initial exponential growth, the birth rate begins to decrease and the rate of death increases reaching equilibrium depending on the capacity of the environment to keep this balance (carrying capacity of the environment). The carrying capacity of the environment varies with habitat and it depends on the availability, distribution, and quality of the resources (shelter, food, water). In most cases if no control measures are taken, the density of a population of dogs is near the carrying capacity of the environment (WHO, 1990). The increasing in the number of dogs in a community may vary according to different habitats, cultures, and socio-economical structures of human rural and urban populations and to different epidemiological situations (Brooks, 1990; Margawani & Robertson 1995; Fielding & Plumridge 2005). Attitudes towards dogs have a great impact on its abundance and welfare. In developing countries dogs are relinquished and abandon to the streets by several reasons and become part of a stray population. India has one of the highest densities of stray dogs due to a large amount of edible litters on the streets, cultural tolerance of dogs and lack of consistently employed, sustained control programs (Butcher, 1999). As consequence, general health status of stray dogs is bad with thin to emaciate body condition, skin conditions and tick infestation (Totton et al., 2011). One of the critical factors leading to a fast growth of the canine population is the lack of control of birth rates as a result of failure to spay and castrate or to supervise pets. Free-roaming dogs, as a consequence, have indiscriminate promiscuity and a high birth rate achieving their maximal breeding efficiency. As result, most dogs are donated to other owners. These low or no cost pups can be responsible for a high number of the abandoned dogs (Hsu et al., 2003) or high number of unwanted dogs sent to the pounds. In developed countries few dogs become stray but are relinquished to dog shelters including pure breeds. Although it is assumed that paying a large amount of money for a pure breed dog will ensure good care an permanent home, this is untrue and frequently the most popular breed are relinquished in greatest numbers (Available at: www.isaronline.citymax.com). A population model based on dogs in the USA, used a birth and death rate of 12% and a turnover rate of 14%, which included stray dogs returning to the population of owned dogs. Of the dogs that died in this model (6.2 million), over a third (2.4 million) died in shelters (Patronek & Rowan, 1995).

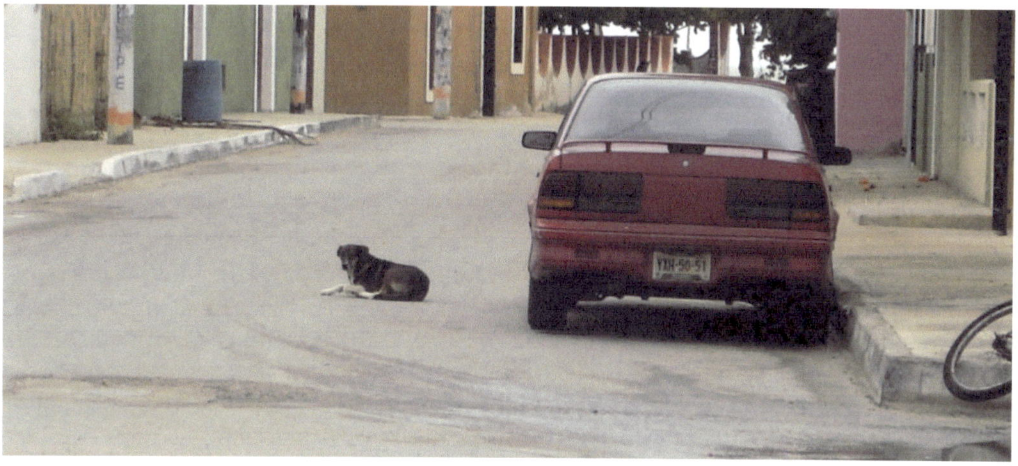

Fig. 1. An owned free roaming dog in a city

3. Methods of dog control population

There are many strategies to control dog populations but whatever the method used it should be based on ethical standpoints and/or practical experiences according to national/local situation avoiding animal suffering and when possible killing through effective, preventative programs. This ensures humane and sustainable solutions. Any program that only concentrates on the 'end result' such as euthanasia is provisional and do not solve the original problem. Strategies to control the overpopulation of free-roaming dogs include enforcement of law, education of owners and sterilization of pets. Dog-control programs are more widely used among the more-developed countries. In less-developed countries, dog control programs (when they existed at all) tended to employ killing methods (including poisoned baits), that are not recommended on animal-welfare grounds (Dalla Villa et al., 2010). Mass culling of stray dog population has historically been used to control rabies in India (Reece, 2007). Rabies has a high incidence in dogs in areas where dog populations reach high densities and where animals are poorly supervised (Wandeler & Bingham, 2000). Recommended control measures for dog rabies control include movement restriction, reproduction control, habitat control and removal of straying dogs. The removal of straying dogs by killing strategies cannot be effective in long term without the enforcement of laws and education of people. Free ranging domestic dogs are non-cooperative populations, i.e. they are not dependant on other animals of the same species to survive so any reduction in the population density through additional mortality is rapidly compensated by better reproduction and survival, and removal of the population to its maximum carrying capacity. In many developed countries stray dogs is a problem that has never risen because of different sanitary and ecological conditions but most important because of licensing programs, public education for responsible ownership and well-developed re-homing shelters.

Reducing birth rates may have a great influence in reducing dog relinquishment and consequently euthanasia. Surgical neutering is by far the most common method of birth control in dogs but it's too expensive to be performed at large scale so in many countries because of it costs it may be restricted or even prohibited. Neutering and release strategies for stray dogs have been recommended similarly as used in the TNR for cats known as Animal Birth control (ABC) program (Totton et al., 2011). The ABC program involve the capture, surgical sterilization and rabies vaccination of stray dogs with the whole idea to replace the sexually intact, unvaccinated stray dog population with a smaller population of infertile healthier dogs in order to reduce the population of dogs in a given area. To be effective in that, the work has to be intensive, 70% of the dogs should be neutered during one breeding cycle, which is approximately about the next six months (Butcher, 1999; Reece, 2007). Success of ABC program in controlling the stray dog population has been state in India (Reece and Chawla, 2006; Totton et al., 2010). However, dogs are always dependent on humans and releasing them back to the streets, although a progressively reduction in its numbers may occurs, that does not improve their health and still have the potential risk to bites and transmission of diseases. Under this panorama, euthanasia may be necessary considered. Besides, free-roaming cat populations have a high intrinsic growth rate, and euthanasia has proved to be more effective at reducing its populations than trap-neuter-return programs (Andersen et al., 2004). Overcrowd of dog shelters because of recruitment of many dogs and lack of adoptions is also a reason of mass dog euthanasia.

A special mention is the dog meat consumption in Asian countries such as South Korea, China, Vietnan and Phillipines. In these countries eating dog is a socially acceptable practice. In South Korea for instance dog meat is eaten nationwide all year round. Their industry involves about 1,000,000 dogs killed yearly to supply the approximately 6,000 restaurants serving this food. A typical Korean dog slaughterhouse could have dogs ranging from poodles to beagles to Korean Jindo dogs; dogs are also imported from Laos to cover the demand. In China the Saint Bernard breed is becoming popular for food consumption for the fast growth of the puppies and animals are slaughtered between 6 and 12 months of age for best size and tenderness. Under these circumstances, the population of dogs may be dramatically reduced. The controversy in this case is not because of the consumption of dog meat itself or the results of this practice on reduce the population, but factors like cruelty involved with the killing. No country in the world consuming dog meat has developed a humane method of dog slaughter under intensive farming practices. Currently, cruel methods are being used including beating, strangling, boiling and bleed to death (by cutting holes in their paws) and sometimes dogs are skinned while still alive.

4. Euthanasia in dogs

In veterinary medicine the alternative to euthanasia is in many cases considered as a "clinical act"; it doesn't mean a failure in veterinary practice, but rather a prudent withdraws in time to avoid further suffering, when we know that there is no alternative to ensure an adequate quality of life. In general, euthanasia of dogs is banned except in special justified cases such as seriously or incurably ill or proven to be dangerous dogs. However, in many countries due to the legal classification of animals as personal property, the owner has the right of ownership over his animal so that the pet can selling or killed (Passantino et al., 2006). In this view a request for euthanasia is licit, whatever the animal's state of health may be. Euthanasia must be carried out exclusively by an experienced veterinarian. When euthanasia of a healthy owned dog is requested by its owner, the veterinarian should reproach such a request based on their professional ethic code and look for more appropriate options. Veterinarians counsel pet owners on daily basis and have the knowledge and "authority" to heal human culture so they may have an important role in reducing dog euthanasia (Scarlett et al., 2002). Relinquishing of dogs is the beginning to the "euthanasia route" and in many cases behavioral problems such as inappropriate elimination (Voith & Borchel, 1982; Patronek et al., 1996), aggressive behavior (Patronek et al., 1996), and other behavioral problems are involve in the relinquishment. A study of dog euthanasia from Denmark in 1997-1998 showed that, of the 2,493 euthanized dogs surveyed, 23.6 % were euthanased in response to behavioural problems (Mikkelsen & Lund, 1999). A high proportion of adopted stray dogs from pounds are bringing back to the pounds for several reasons. In a dog pound from Italy, from 1,789 adopted dogs, 271 (15%) where brought back because of behavioral problems (Mondelli et al., 2002)

Several societies such as the World Society for the Protection of Animals does not condone mass destruction as a control population measure of dogs and cats when there are circumstances when euthanasia is the most humane option. Animals considered for euthanasia should include those sick or dangerous. However, euthanasia can also be acceptable in animals unsuitable for homing or returned to the streets or to alleviate shelter overcrowding which compromise the welfare of animals held there (World Society for the Protection of Animals [WSPA], 2000). In Italy since 1991, national legislation does not permit euthanasia of unwanted roaming dogs unless they have an incurable condition or are proven to be dangerous. Unattended dogs are placed in long-term shelters in questionable conditions where they often remain for most of their lives (Dalla Villa et al., 2008). Consequences of such decisions may alter the dynamic of dog populations if no other control measures are considered to reduce the number of dogs, especially those stray. For instance, in animal shelters from Barcelona Spain in 2003 routine euthanasia of unclaimed stray animals was discontinued, due to a political decision of the city council. However the suspension of routine euthanasia was associated with a marked increase in the number of stray dogs. Canine distemper became endemic in the shelter until late 2004, due to a certain unwillingness to use euthanasia to control infection transmission (García-Rodríguez et al., 2008).

When euthanasia is considered, several methods are available for dogs but not all are considered acceptable (Close et al., 1997). However, because of the safety for personnel, efficacy and costs, the preferred method is the intravenous injection of sodium pentabarbitone (Table 1). Different methods for euthanasia in dogs are well described elsewhere however some methods remain controversial (Andrews et al., 1993). A reliable method will produce rapid loss of consciousness until death occurs. Regardless of the method used, it is important to minimize distress, anxiety and pain. It is compulsory to confirm the death of dog when euthanasia is performed before the body is disposed or left unattended. If an animal is not dead, another method of euthanasia should be performed. Finally the carcass should be disposed according to the local ruling legislation avoiding the risk of residues. Incineration is considered the safest way of carcass disposal.

Agent	Remarks
Sodium Pentobarbitone	Best option for intravenous injection. Intracardiac or intrapulmonary routes of injection should not be used as they are extremely painful, unless under full anaesthesia.
T61	Very effective agent but only to be injected very slowly intravenously. Animals may require sedation prior to administration. It may cause convulsions in the unconscious animal, which may be aesthetically unpleasant.
Secobarbital/dibucaine	Secobarbital is a short-acting analogue of thiamylol sodium, whereas dibucaine is a highly toxic local anaesthetic causing rapid loss of consciousness, loss of respiration and cardiac arrest. The combination product produced a quiet and rapid death. Dibucaine alone is not desirable for use for euthanasia.
Halothane, isoflurane, enflurane	These are all acceptable methods of euthanasia for carnivores. Appropriate gas scavenging apparatus should be used to prevent operator exposure.
Captive bolt	Can be inhumane if shot is inaccurate and dog is only wounded. Animal should be restrained. Personnel must be trained in these techniques to ensure correct positioning of the pistol and immediate death. No risk to operator (see free bullet) unless risk of dog infected with rabies, due to potential contact with brain issue.
Electrocution	This method may produce severe pain due to cardiac fibrillation before onset of unconsciousness. Pain can also be caused by violent extension of the limbs, head and neck and may not be effective if insufficient current applied (a considered lethal shock is 1 kV passing from the ear to hindleg) so the equipment must be regularly checked and maintained to ensure correct voltage. Dogs should be unconscious before being electrocuted by electrical stunning (current through the brain to produce an instantaneous stun) or anaesthesia. Death would result from current passed through the heart of an unconscious. animal. Proper equipment and trained operator is essential. May be hazardous for operator, who should use protective equipment (boots and gloves). Low cost. Death must be confirmed.
Concussion	Only to be considered in small neonates
Shooting	Can be inhumane if shot is inaccurate and dog is only wounded; dog may also escape. Skilled operator essential. Risk of injury to operators and spectators. Not necessary to handle or capture dog. Brain tissue may be unavailable for rabies diagnosis. Shooting of carnivores using a free bullet is only acceptable under field conditions when no other methods can be used. Only specialized marksmen should be used.

Table 1. Must accepted methods for euthanasia in dogs

All the above mention agents or methods are in general fast and highly efficient. The following agents are unacceptable and are condemned for use as euthanasia agents in dogs: strychnine, nicotine, caffeine, magnesium sulfate, potassium chloride, cyclopropane, hydrogen cyanide gas, methoxyflurane, trichloroethylene, nitrous oxide cleaning agents, solvents, disinfectants and other toxins or salts, and all neuromuscular blocking agents. Other methods such as drowning, concussion (adults), decapitation, asphyxia, strangulation or air embolism are also not considered as euthanasic methods. When euthanasia is considered, besides the appropriate method used The World Organisation for Animal Health [OIE] (2010) suggests special attention to:

a. Restraint. When a dog needs to be restrained for euthanasia, this should always be done with full regard for operator security and animal welfare. Some euthanasia methods should be used in association with sedation or anaesthesia in order to be considered humane.
b. Special equipment. When special equipment is needed to perform euthanasia (e.g. gas chamber), the system should be designed for the purpose and regularly maintained in order to achieve operator security and animal welfare.

Because neonates and adults with impaired breathing or low blood pressure are resistant to hypoxia, methods that depend upon achieving a hypoxic state (e.g. CO2, CO, N2, Ar) should not be used. These methods should not be used in dogs aged less than 2 months, except to produce loss of consciousness and should be followed by another method to cause death. In general, neonates form carnivores should be treated as adults. Sodium pentobarbitone is the preferred method but concussion and cervical dislocation may be used in very small neonatal dogs and only in cases of emergency (OIE, 2010). However, operators must be well trained in the physical techniques to ensure that they are correctly and humanely carried out. When ovarian hysterectomies are performed, euthanasia of feti should be accomplished as soon as possible after removal from the dam.

5. Ethical concerns of euthanasia in stray dogs and animal shelters

Although in veterinary practice euthanasia in dogs is reasonably common, these "end of life decision" provoke an emotional period and in many instances ethical concerns occurs. For these reason, methods such as the undisclosed standardized client (USCs) and the measure of patient-centered consideration (MPCC) may reduce animal suffering and enhance the satisfaction and well-being of both clients and veterinarians (Nogueira et al., 2010).

However, when a healthy dog has to be euthanized a moral dilemma occurs in the profession. Dogs may be consider animals as sensitive beings, so they have the capacity to perceive pain and pleasure and are worthy of being under the protection of a law. Killing a healthy animal have legal consequences and may be considered a crime. In contrast euthanasia is legal in specific cases. For these reasons, people involved in dog pounds and dog shelters need to be aware of the use of euthanasia as part of the strategy dealing with dog overpopulation and be aware of the moral dilemma involved. Euthanasia only treats the symptoms but not the causes of the problems of overpopulation and should be considered as the last resource.

Three different scenarios of mass euthanasia of dogs to control its population may be found, dog pounds, animal shelters and municipal campaigns of dog population control.

5.1 Dog pounds

Also called "public shelters" or "animal control agencies" are common in many developing countries where laws regulate and justify the mass euthanasia. Dog pounds activities are generally limited to the custody and euthanasia of stray animals and are commonly finance by tax found from the municipalities. The pickup and reception of surplus and stray o relinquished animals have the objective to avoid damage to the community. The OIE (2010) considers euthanasia as a method to reduce the number of stray dogs to an acceptable level in order to reduce the risk of rabies and other zoonotic diseases and to prevent harm to the environment and other animals.

An example of dog pound facilities is shown in Figure 2. Dog are protected for 3-10 days to give them the opportunity to be re-homed to their original owners or being adopted. However in dog pound, very few dogs are claimed and the adoption rate is very low or practically non-existing. Under these situation an overflow of dogs rapidly occurs and the quickest way to obtain space is by eliminate them by "strategic euthanasia". Since practically all dogs are euthanized, no moral conflicts arise by selecting candidates.

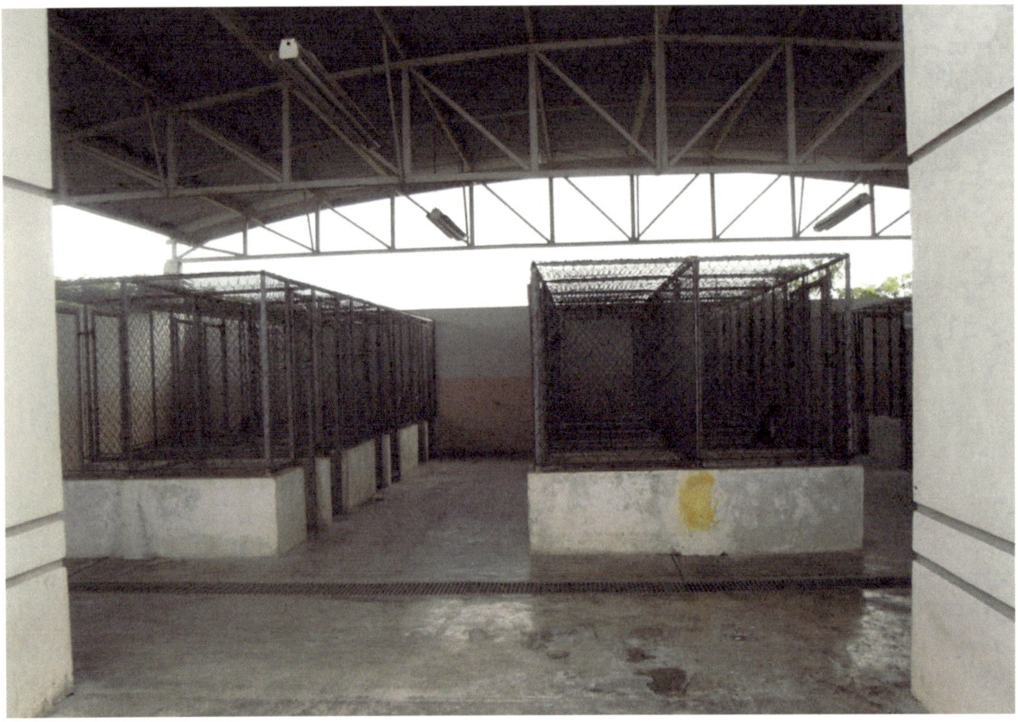

Fig. 2. A municipal dog pound building

Dogs that arrive in very bad conditions without few possibilities to be adopted should be immediately euthanized. In Figure 3 two typical case of dog going to immediate euthanasia are shown; in these cases there is no chance of treatment. It is estimated that 75% of the world's dog population are strays. Managing them presents a problem in many countries, and has serious implications for public health and animal welfare. Killing stray dogs often produces a short term effect, even when maximal catching rates (up to 24% of dog population/year) make no significant impact (WHO, 1988, 1990). Efforts of dog pounds should be focus on preventing these problems by public education including the supervision of breeding, management of behavioral problems and promoting the culture of adoption. In Barcelona Spain, with the formulation of a city Plan for Pet Animals, the activities were redirected, concentrating on services within the city limits and stimulating adoption. Participation of both professional and humane organizations was sought, premises were renovated, responsible ownership of animals was promoted, controlled urban colonies of cats were established, and adoptions become the cornerstone of policy, centering the activity of the pounds toward its clients. Changes in the dog pound's activity since 1998 reflects a clear decrease in the number of animals retained, as well as in the proportion subjected to euthanasia (from 83.4% of euthanasias of animals entered in 1993 to 47.2% in 2001). This decrease may reflect an improvement in the problem of stray animals. Besides, these developments have also resulted in a positive change in the relationship with the media and animal welfare organizations (Peracho et al., 2003).

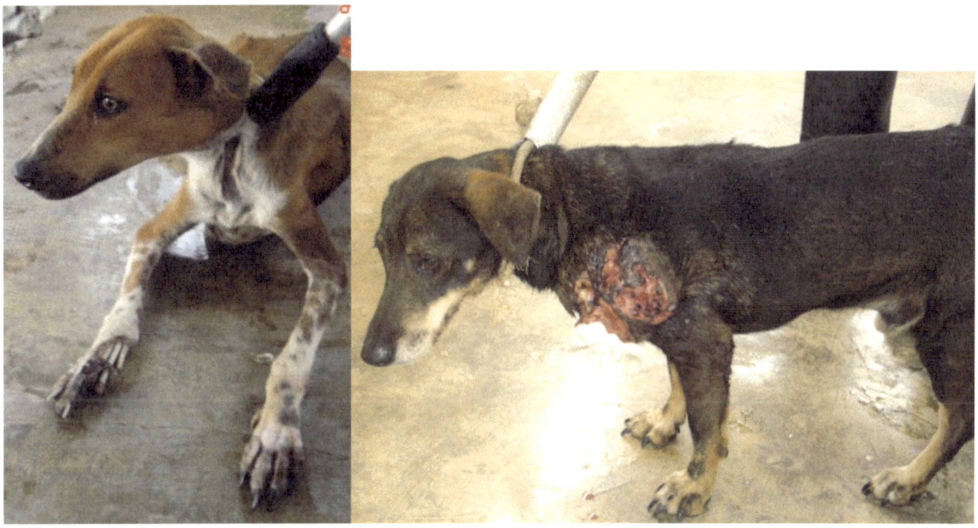

Fig. 3. Stray dogs from a dog pound apt for euthanasia

5.2 Dog shelters

Also called human agencies are usually non-profit agencies depending on charities and donations to fund their operations. In these agencies relinquished animals are accepted and educational programs on animal care and welfare to public are offer. Adoptions of dogs are also offered and this is fundamental for the flow of animals through the shelter. Ideally, no healthy, adoptable animal should be euthanized. However, euthanasia in dog shelters occurs frequently because of the flow of dogs is altered by the high income number of animals and limitations of space and funds, or when old age and terminal diseases requires to end a poor life quality. An estimation of euthanized rates in North American dog and cat shelters indicates figures of 10 to 20 million each year (Olson, 1990; Caras, 1993). In 2003, Michigan shelters discharged 140,653 dogs: Of these, 56,972 (40%) were euthanized and 40,005 (28%) were adopted (Bartlett et al., 2005). In Colorado shelters, after considerable efforts centered in increasing adoptions, increasing the number of dogs returned to owners by implementing licensing requirements and improving identification methods, education of public on animal welfare issues and subsidizing spay neuter programs, the number of unwanted dogs have decreased but after almost a decade, no changes in the euthanasia rate of dogs (3.7/1000 residents/year) have been observed indicating that the shelters dynamics of dogs appeared to reached an equilibrium with respect to euthanasia (Morris et al., 2011). A model suggests that the balance between supply and demand for dogs can be achieved such that euthanasia is never required (Frank, 2004).

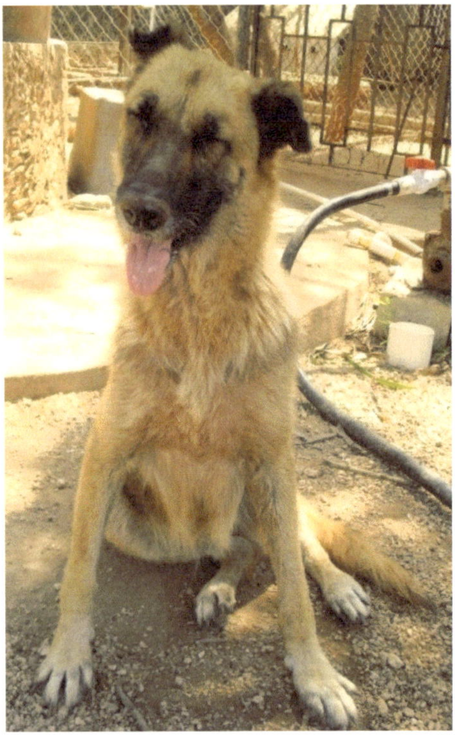

Fig. 4. A dog from a shelter considered for euthanasia

However, euthanasia is always required for the animals difficult to adopt (old, sick, unpopular breed, behavioral problem). As seen euthanasia in shelters is a used resource but it also generates moral issues. No kill shelter dog should be defined as one in where no adoptable dog is euthanize but where this resource may be used in old and dying dog in pain or suffering. In figure 4 an old dog in pain with bad life quality is shown. Although veterinarians have the professional knowledge and experience to euthanize dogs, other professionals, such as animal shelter workers, may also be trained to euthanize dogs. Killing shelters may bring a moral stress to their workers when dealing with euthanasia. Although workers realize that euthanasia of dog as a police to deal with over-population, this will not diminished the problem and they have to rationalize it even when they become enrolled to shelters with the idea of interacting and love caring of dogs. Euthanasia training for shelter workers also includes seminars on dealing with the irony that responsible animal care sometimes includes killing animals (Arluke, 1991).

The concept of canine health management is accord with the concept Shelter medicine or population medicine. Population medicine is based on setting production goal, identifying risk factors of disease, preventive disease and maximizing production. Production goals in companion animals would be an acceptable level of welfare and considerations of the incidence and prevalence of clinical and behavioral disease (Hurley, 2004). The implement of the shelter medicine in two Italian shelters (where laws do not currently allow euthanasia as a suitable method to control shelter population or used for scientific purposes) during three years and without admission of new dogs "closed system" resulted in improved dog health and welfare, as indicated by the significant reduction in both the prevalence and incidence of major pathologies during the next two years (Dalla Villa et al., 2008).

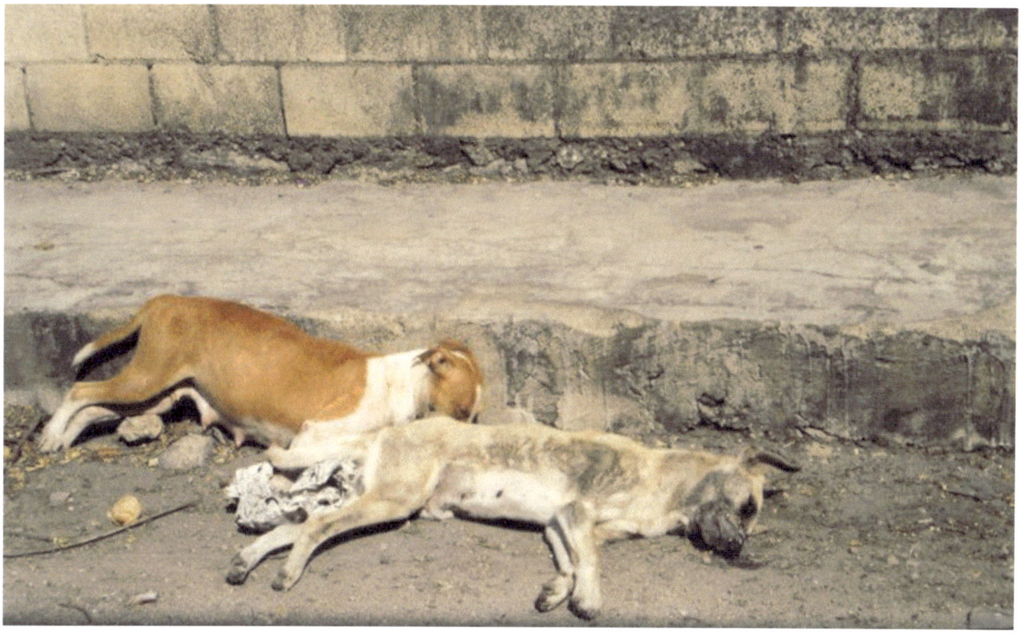

Fig. 5. Stray dogs poisoned during a municipal campaign

5.3 Municipal campaigns

Other scenario of mass destruction of dogs in order to control its population, specially stray dogs, is sometimes carried out in small rural municipalities using poisonous baits with strychnine or cyanide; strychnine causes violent convulsions and painful muscle contractions whereas cyanide pose extreme danger to personnel and the manner of death is aesthetically objectionable. Use of such method is totally unacceptable since are not considered euthanasic agents. In figure 5 an example of stray dogs poisoned during a campaign in Yucatán Mexico is shown; baits with strychnine were placed in the main streets were dogs were free roaming. Cats an opossums are also victims of the baits. Other variety of inhumane methods used in such campaigns include shooting, hanging and electrocution in a futile attempt to control the number of stray dogs. Such strategies are inhuman and potentially dangerous specially in kids and wild life consuming the baits and should be condemn. The prevention culture through education of the public should be considered by the local authorities to deal with this kind of problem.

In extreme situations for instance in provinces of Argentina, a recently promulgate law prohibit the function of dog pounds and euthanasia was banned in small animals, including animals with cases of terminal diseases or serious injuries (La Nación, 2011), these may result morally questioned because of the unnecessary suffering of the dog. In Mexico, despite the existence of laws regulating dog pounds and management of stray dogs (NOM-042-SSA2-2006), these are in most cases not conforming for several reasons. Many cases of mass killing of dogs and cats are reported throughout the country and condemned by the society. In some circumstances like in a small town in Mexico (Tlaxiaco, Oaxaca), with the increasing number of stray dogs (considered as pests), the Municipal Health Bureau announced that it expects the slaughter of over a thousand dogs in the streets because they are a source of pollution and the number of attacks to humans have been increasing for the large population of these pets. The sterilization campaigns which are made in order to prevent further proliferation of stray dogs in Tlaxiaco has been very erratic and no more than 55 animals had neutered, not even 10% of the estimated population. This is an example of municipal mismanagement and the consequent failure of campaign to sterilize dogs and cats, and most of all, a failure of public education about responsible pet ownership. In a different context in the Jaltenco municipality of Mexico city, were massacred with machetes and beaten to death around 30 dogs and cats that were under guard in a separate animal protection. Hooded men in black, with the approval of municipal police and some neighbors, the animals were attacked, leaving them very badly wounded amputees under cries of pain and fear. Only 12 of them managed to recover. This is an example of irresponsible brutality of ignorant authorities dealing with the problem of dog overpopulation.

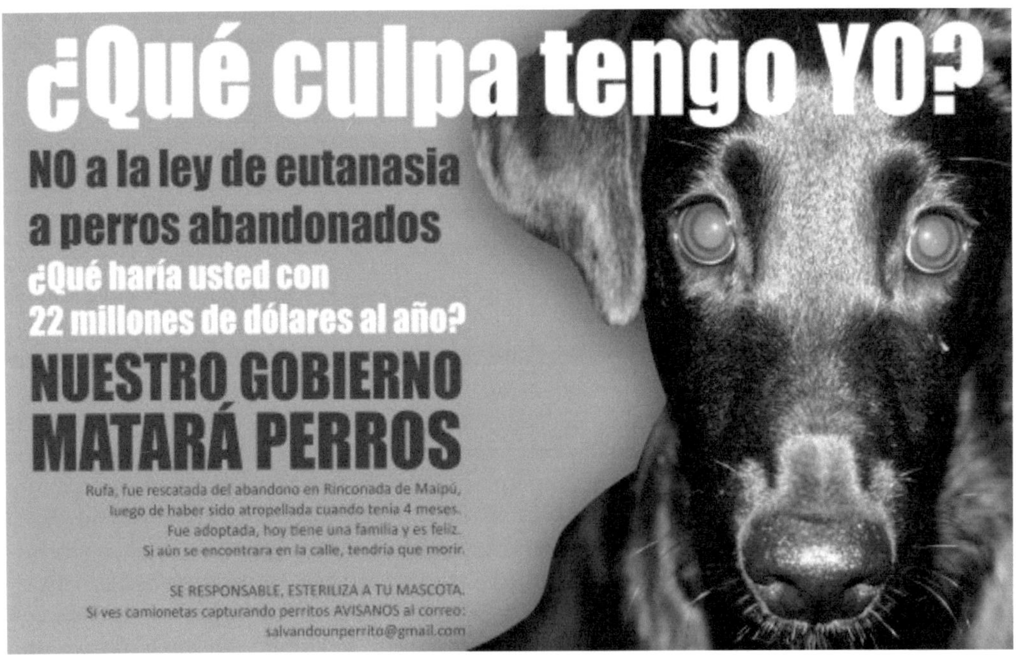

Fig. 6. Signal of protest against the decision of killing dogs in the city of Neuquen, Argentina. From the text "Why is my fault? No to the euthanasia law against stray dogs. What would you do with 22 millions of dollars a year? Our government will kill dogs" (available at: www.taringa.net/posts/solidaridad/6490679/Firma-el-petitorio-en-repudio-a-la-matanza-en-Neuquen_.html)

Fortunately, the society and animal protection associations are aware of these activities and accuse and expose the authorities responsible of such strategies to control stray dog populations. An example of society claims against massive dog killing is seen in the province of Neuquen in the Patagonia region of Argentina. After an outbreak of leptospirosis, a municipal resolution to sacrifice over 1100 dogs was announced. The resolution planned for the coming five days sacrificing 220 dogs, many of them delivered by their owners. These woke up the action from neighbors and animal welfare groups across the country. Authorities said that they will not kill animals, but called the neighbors to take charge of homeless pets. An example of protest and call to the society against this resolution is showed in figure 6.

6. Conclusion

The use of euthanasia in control programs of the canine population generally tends to generate controversy and misinterpretation of the criteria recommended by different agencies. In general society strongly opposes to euthanasia and condemns governments that employ this strategy as a means of dog population control. Euthanasia is only a temporal remedy to cure the symptoms rather than causes of the problem of overpopulation, and should be the last resource to use at the end of a long process of evaluation. Euthanasia may be required in specific scenarios to balance the flow of dog overcrowd, to reduce the risk of zoonotic transmission and damage to the environment and to avoid unnecessary suffering. However, ethical concerns come about when healthy animals have to be killed. Nothing is going to solve the dog overpopulation problem except the capacity of humans to understand the situation and take actions avoiding the born of unwanted puppies and become responsible owners avoiding the relinquishing of their pets.

7. Acknowledgments

Authors would like to thank the Dog pound (Canine & Feline Control Center) from the municipality of Merida Yucatan, Mexico, to the Arqta Silvia Cortés from the dog shelter "Evolución" and to Mrs Marcia Lara de Moreno from AMEDEA (Asociación Mexicana por los Derechos de los Animales, A.C. Yucatán) for their kindness collaboration and permission to take pictures included in this chapter.

8. References

Andersen, M.C.; Martin, B.J. & Roemer G.W (2004). Use of matrix population models to estimate the efficacy of euthanasia versus trap-neuter-return for management of free-roaming cats. *Journal of the American Veterinary Medical Association*, Vol.225, No.12, (December 2004), pp. 1871-1876, ISSN 0003-1488

Andrews, E.J.; Bennett, T.; Clark, J.D.; Houpt, K.A.; Pascoe, P.J.; Robinson, G.W. & Boyce, J.R. (1993). Report of the AVMA panel on euthanasia. *Journal of the American Veterinary Medical Association*, Vol.202, No.2, (January 1993), pp. 229-249, ISSN 0003-1488

Arluke, A. (1991). Coping with euthanasia: a case study of shelters culture. *Journal of the American Veterinary Medical Association* , Vol.198, No.7, (April, 1991), pp. 1176-1191, ISSN 0003-1488

Bartlett, P.C.; Bartlett, A.; Walshaw, S. & Halstead, S. (2005). Rates of Euthanasia and Adoption for Dogs and Cats in Michigan Animal Shelters *Journal of Applied Animal Welfare Science*, Vol.8, No.2, (January, 2005), pp. 97–104. ISSN 1088-8705

Brooks, R. (1990). Survey of the dog population in Zimbabwe and its levels of rabies vaccination. *Veterinary Record*, Vol.127, No.24, (December, 1990), pp. 592-596. ISSN 0042-4900

Butcher, R. (1999). Stray dogs- a worldwide problem. *Journal of Small Animal Practice*, Vol.40, No.9, (September, 1999), pp. 458-459. ISSN 0022-4510

Caras, R. (1993). One generation away from humanity. *Journal of the American Veterinary Medical Association*, Vol.202, No.6, (March, 1993), pp. 910-912. ISSN 0003-1488

Close, B.; Banister, K.; Baumans, V.; Bernoth, E.M.; Bromage, N.; Bunyan, J.; Erhardt, W.; Flecknell, P.; Gregory, N.; Hackbarth, H.; Morton, D. & Warwick, C. (1997). Recommendations for euthanasia of experimental animals: Part 2. *Laboratory Animals* Vol.31. No.1, (January, 1997), pp. 1-32. ISSN 0023-6772

Dalla Villa, P.; Kahn, S.; Stuardo, L.; Iannetti, L.; Di Nardo, A. & Serpell, J.A. (2010). Free-roaming dog control among OIE-member countries. *Preventive Veterinary Medicine*, Vol.97, No.1, (August, 2010), pp. 58-63. ISSN 0167-5877

Dalla Villa, P.; Iannetti, L.; Podaliri Vulpiani, M.; Maitino, A.; Trentini, R.; Del Papa, S.A. (2008). A management model applied in two 'no-kill' dog shelters in central Italy: use of population medicine for three consecutive years. *Veterinary Italy*, Vol.44, No.2, (April, 2008) pp. 347-359. ISSN 0505-401X

Fielding, W.J. & Plumridge, S.J. (2005). Characteristics of owned dogs on the island of New Providence, The Bahamas. *Journal of Applied Animal Welfare Science*, Vol.8, No.4, pp. 245–260. ISSN 1088-8705

Frank, J. (2004). An interactive model of human and companion animal dynamics: the ecology and economics of dog overpopulation and the human cost of addressing the problem. *Journal of Human Ecology*, Vol.32, No.1, (February, 2004) pp. 107-130. ISSN 0300-7839

García-Rodríguez, A.; Peracho, V.; Villalbí, J.R.; Bouis, S.; Duràn, J. & Guix J. (2008). Avances en la gestión de un centro de acogida de animales de compañía. *Gaceta Sanitaria* Vol.22, No.1, (July, 2007) pp. 76-78. ISSN 0213-9111

Hsu, Y.; Severinghaus, L.L. & Serpell, J.A. (2003). Dog keeping in Taiwan: its contribution to the problem of free-roaming dogs. *Journal of Applied Animal Welfare Science*, Vol.6, No.1, pp. 1-23. ISSN 1088-8705

Hurley, K.F. (2004). Implementing a population health plan in an animal shelter: goal setting, data collection and monitoring, and policy development. In: *Shelter Medicine for Veterinarians and Staff.* Miller L. & Zawistowski (Ed.), pp. 211-234, Blackwell Publishing Professional, ISBN 0-8138-24486, Oxord, UK.

La Nación.com, (December, 2016). Prohíben perreras y la eutanasia de mascotas. In: *La Nación*, 12.02.2011. Available from: http//www.lanacion.com.ar/866148-prohiben-perreras-y-la-eutanasia-de-mascotas.

Margawani, K.R. & Robertson, I.D. (1995). A survey of urban pet ownership in Bali. *Veterinary Record*, Vol.137, No.19, (November, 1995) pp. 486-488. ISSN 0042-4900

Mikkelsen, J. & Lund, J.D. (1999). Euthanasia of dogs because of behavioural problems. An epidemiological study on euthanasia of dogs in Denmark-with particular reference to aggression problems. *Dansk Veterinærtidsskrift* Vol.82, No.11, pp. 474-479. ISSN 0106-6854.

Mondelli, F.; Levi, D.; Magistrelli, S.; Prato Previde, E. & Valsecchi, P. (2002). Why people brings back to the pound? A questionnaire study in Milan Italy. *Proceedings of the British Society of Animal Science*. pp. 65. ISBN 0906562 392. Published by BSAS, York UK, April, 2002.

Morris, K.N.; Wolf, J.L. & Gies, D.L. (2011). Trends in intake and outcome data for animal shelters in Colorado, 2000 to 2007. *Journal of the American Veterinary Medical Association*, Vol.238, No.3, (February, 2009) pp. 329-336. ISSN 0003-1488

Nogueira, B.L.J.; Adams, C.L.; Bonnet, B.N.; Shaw, J.R. & Ribble, C.S. (2010). Use of the measure of patient-centered communication to analyze euthanasia discussion in companion animals practice. *Journal of the American Veterinary Medical Association*. Vol,237, No.11, (December, 2010) pp. 1275-1287. ISSN 0003-1488

OIE (July, 2010). Stray dog population control. In: *Terrestrial Animal Health Code* 6.03.2011. Available from:
http//www.oie.int/index.php?id=169&L=0&htmfile=chapitre_1.7.7.htm

Olson, P.N. (1990). Concerned about euthanasia of healthy homeless animals (Letter). *Journal of the American Veterinary Medical Association* Vol.196, No.1, (January, 1990) pp. 10. ISSN 0003-1488

Orihuela, T.A. & Solano, V.J. (1995). Demographics of the owned dog population in Miacatlan, Mor. Mexico. *Anthrozoös*, Vol.8, No.3, (January, 1995) pp. 171–175. ISSN 0892-7936

Passantino, A.; Fenga, C.; Morciano, C.; Morelli, C.; Russo, M.; Di Pietro, C. & Passantino, M. (2006) Euthanasia of companion animals: a legal and ethical analysis. *Annali dell Istituto Superiore di Sanita.* , Vol.42, No.4, (July, 2006) pp. 491-495. ISSN 0021-2571

Patronek, G.J. & Rowan, A.N. (1995) Determining dog and cat numbers and population dynamics. *Anthrozoös* Vol.8, No.4 (January, 1995) pp. 199-205. ISSN 0892-7936

Patronek, G.J.; Glickman, L.T.; Beck, A.M.; McCabe, G.P. & Ecker, C. (1996). Risk factors for relinquishment of dogs to an animal shelter. *Journal America Veterinary Medical Association*, Vol.209, No.3, (August, 1996) pp. 572-581. ISSN 0003-1488

Peracho, V.; Villalbí, J.R.; Llebaría, X.; Armengou, J.M. & Guix, J. (2003). De la perrera municipal al centro de acogida de animales de compañía de Barcelona. *Gaceta Sanitaria*, Vol.17, No.6 (September, 2003) pp. 515-519. ISSN 0213-9111

Reece, J.F. & Chawla, S.K. (2006). Control of rabies in Jaipur, India by the sterilisation and vaccination of neighbourhood dogs. *Veterinary Record*, Vol.159, No.16 (September, 2006) pp. 379-383. ISSN 0042-4900

Reece, J.F. (2007). Rabies in India: an ABC approach to combating the disease in street dogs. *Veterinary Record*, Vol.161, No.9 (September, 2007) pp. 292-293. ISSN 0042-4900

Scarlett, J.M.; Salman, M.D.; New, J.G. & Kass, P.H. (2002). The role of veterinary practitioners in reducing dog and cat relinquishments and euthanasias. *Journal of the American Veterinary Medical Association*, Vol.220, No.3 (February, 2002) pp. 306-311. ISSN 0003-1488

Totton, S.C.; Wandeler, A.I.; Ribble, C.S.; Rosatte, R.C. & McEwen, S.A. (2011). Stray dog population health in Jodhpur India in the wake of animal birth control (ABC) program. *Preventive Veterinary Medicine*, Vol.98, No. 2-3 (February, 2001) pp. 215-220. ISSN 0167-5877

Totton, S.C.; Wandeler, A.I.; Zinsstag, J.; Bauch, C.T.; Ribble, C.S.; Rosatte, R.C. & McEwen, S.A. (2010). Stray dog population demographics in Jodhpur, India following a population control/rabies vaccination program. *Preventive Veterinary Medicine*, Vol.97, No.1 (August, 2010) pp. 51-57. ISSN 0167-5877

Voith, V.L. & Borchelt, P.L. (1982) Diagnosis and treatment of elimination behavior problems in dogs. *Veterinary Clinics of North America Small Animal Practice*, Vol.World Health Organization (1990). Consultation of dog population management. *WHO.ZOON 90.166*, 6-37

World Health Organization (1988). Consultation on dog ecology studies related to rabies control. *WHO/Rab.Res 88.25*

WSPA (2000). Humane euthanasia for dogs and cats. Royal Society for the Prevention of Cruelty to Animals. pp. 1-4.

ISAR (1991). A prime source of canine overpopulation. In: *International Society of Animals Rights, law and education serving animals- Special report.* 11.02.2011, Available from: http//www. isaronline.org.citymax.com/f/a.pdf